MENOPAUSE:
PHYSIOLOGY AND PHARMACOLOGY

Menopause:
Physiology and Pharmacology

DANIEL R. MISHELL, JR., M.D.

Professor and Chairman
Department of Obstetrics and Gynecology
University of Southern California School of Medicine
Chief of Professional Services
Women's Hospital
Los Angeles County-USC Medical Center
Los Angeles, California

YEAR BOOK MEDICAL PUBLISHERS, INC.

CHICAGO • LONDON

2 3 4 5 6 7 8 9 KC 89, 88, 87

Library of Congress Cataloging-in-Publication Data

Menopause : physiology and pharmacology.

   Includes bibliographies and index.
   1. Menopause.   2. Estrogen--Therapeutic use.
I. Mishell, Daniel R.   [DNLM: 1. Estrogens--therapeutic
use. 2. Menopause.   3. Menopause--drug effects.
WP 580 M5485]
RG186.M483 1986   618.1'75'061   86-15652
ISBN 0-8151-5914-5

Sponsoring Editor: James D. Ryan, Jr.
Manager, Copyediting Services: Frances M. Perveiler
Production Project Manager: Robert Allen Reedtz
Proofroom Supervisor: Shirley E. Taylor

Contributors

RANDALL B. BARNES, M.D.

Assistant Professor, Department of Obstetrics and Gynecology, University of Chicago; Section of Reproductive Endocrinology, Chicago Lying-In Hospital, Chicago, Illinois

ARIEH BERGMAN, M.D.

Assistant Professor, Department of Obstetrics and Gynecology, University of Southern California School of Medicine, Los Angeles, California

RICHARD BORENSTEIN, M.D.

Clinical Associate Professor of Obstetrics and Gynecology, Hebrew University Medical School, Jerusalem, Israel; Deputy Chief, Department of Obstetrics and Gynecology, Chief, Infertility Unit, Kaplan Hospital, Rehovot, Israel

PAUL F. BRENNER, M.D.

Professor of Obstetrics and Gynecology and Pediatrics, University of Southern California School of Medicine, Los Angeles, California

MARK BRINCAT, Ph.D., M.R.C.O.G.

King's College Hospital School of Medicine and Dentistry, London; Registrar, Department of Obstetrics and Gynaecology, Dulwich Menopause Clinic, Dulwich, London

TRUDY L. BUSH, Ph.D., M.H.S.

Assistant Professor of Public Health, Columbia University, New York, New York

LORRAINE DENNERSTEIN, M.B., B.S., Ph.D., D.P.M., F.R.A.N.Z.C.P.

First Assistant, Department of Psychiatry, Austin Hospital, Heidelberg, Victoria, Australia

EGON DICZFALUSY, M.D.

Professor, Karolinska Institutet, Stockholm, Sweden

TAVIA GORDON

Research Professor of Statistics, George Washington University Medical Center, Washington, D.C.

BRIAN E. HENDERSON, M.D.

Professor and Chairman, Department of Preventive Medicine; Director, USC Comprehensive Cancer Center, University of Southern California School of Medicine, Los Angeles, California

HOWARD L. JUDD, M.D.

Professor and Chief, Division of Reproductive Endocrinology, UCLA School of Medicine, Los Angeles, California

WILLIAM B. KANNEL, M.D., M.P.H., F.A.C.C.; F.A.C.E.

Professor of Medicine, Chief, Section of Preventive Medicine and Epidemiology, Department of Medicine, Boston University Medical Center, Boston, Massachusetts

R. J. B. KING, B.Sc., M.Sc., Ph.D., D.Sc.

Head, Department of Hormone Biochemistry, Imperial Cancer Research Fund, London, England

OSCAR A. KLETZKY, M.D.

Professor of Obstetrics and Gynecology, University of Southern California School of Medicine, Los Angeles, California

GEOFFREY LANE, M.B., B.S., M.R.C.O.G.

Senior Registrar, Department of Obstetrics and Gynecology, King's College Hospital School of Medicine and Dentistry, London, England

NANCY C. LEE, M.D.

Medical Epidemiologist, Division of Reproductive Health, Center for Health Promotion and Education, Centers for Disease Control, Atlanta, Georgia

ROBERT LINDSAY, M.B., Ch.B., Ph.D., F.R.C.P.

Professor of Clinical Medicine, Department of Medicine, College of Physicians and Surgeons, Columbia University; Director of Internal Medicine, Director of Research, Helen Hayes Hospital, West Haverstraw, New York

ROGERIO A. LOBO, M.D.

Associate Professor of Obstetrics and Gynecology, Chief of Reproductive Endocrinology and Infertility, University of Southern California School of Medicine, Los Angeles, California

THOMAS M. MACK, M.D.

Professor of Epidemiology, Department of Preventive Medicine, Los Angeles County-USC Medical Center, Los Angeles, California

DAVID R. MELDRUM, M.D.

Associate Professor, Department of Obstetrics and Gynecology, Director and Chief, Division of Female Infertility, UCLA School of Medicine, Los Angeles, California

VALERY T. MILLER, M.D.

Assistant Research Professor in Medicine, George Washington University Medical Center, Washington, D.C.

MALCOLM PADWICK, M.B., B.S.

Research Fellow, Registrar, Department of Obstetrics and Gynaecology, King's College Hospital School of Medicine and Dentistry, London, England

ANNLIA PAGANINI-HILL, Ph.D.

Associate Professor, University of Southern California School of Medicine, Los Angeles, California

HERBERT B. PETERSON, M.D.

Deputy Chief, Epidemiology Studies Branch, Division of Reproductive Health, Center for Health Promotion and Education, Centers for Disease Control; Clinical Assistant Professor, Department of Gynecology and Obstetrics, Emory University School of Medicine, Atlanta, Georgia

MALCOLM C. PIKE, M.D.

Professor of Medicine, Oxford University; Director of Cancer Epidemiology and Clinical Trials of the Imperial Cancer Research Fund, Oxford, England

JOHN PRYSE-DAVIES, M.D., F.R.C. Path.

Senior Lecturer, Institute of Obstetrics and Gynaecology, University of London; Consultant Histopathologist, Chelsea Hospital for Women, London, England

RONALD K. ROSS, M.D.

Associate Professor, Department of Preventive
Medicine, University of Southern California
School of Medicine, Norris Cancer Hospital
and Research Institute, Los Angeles, California

GEORGE L. RUBIN, M.B., B.S.

Chief, Epidemiologic Studies Branch, Division
of Reproductive Health, Center for Health
Promotion and Education, Centers for Disease
Control, Atlanta, Georgia

TIMOTHY A. RYDER, M.Sc., Ph.D.

Senior Scientist, Queen Charlotte's Hospital for
Women, London, England

BARRY M. SHERMAN, M.D.

Director, Clinical Research, Genentech, Inc.;
Clinical Professor, Stanford University School
of Medicine, Stanford, California

DONNA SHOUPE, M.D.

Assistant Professor, Reproductive
Endocrinology Division, University of Southern
California School of Medicine, Los Angeles,
California

NICK SIDDLE, M.R.C.O.G.

Consultant Gynaecologist and Honorary Senior
Lecturer, University College and Middlesex
Hospital, London, England

WILLIAM N. SPELLACY, M.D.

Professor and Head, Department of Obstetrics
and Gynecology, University of Illinois College
of Medicine, Chicago, Illinois

JOHN STUDD, M.D., F.R.C.O.G.

King's College Hospital School of Medicine
and Dentistry; Consultant Gynaecologist and
Obstetrician, Dulwich Hospital, London,
England

JACK F. TOHMÉ, M.D.

Assistant Clinical Professor of Medicine,
College of Physicians and Surgeons, Columbia
University; Associate Clinical Director,
Regional Bone Center, Helen Hayes Hospital,
West Haverstraw, New York

RUTH B. WEG, Ph.D.

Professor of Gerontology, Research Associate,
Andrus Gerontology Center, Leonard Davis
School of Gerontology, Gerontology Research
Institute, Los Angeles, California

M. I. WHITEHEAD, M.R.C.O.G., M.B.B.S.

Senior Lecturer/Consultant Gynaecologist,
Academic Department of Obstetrics and
Gynaecology, King's College Hospital School
of Medicine and Dentistry, London, England

Preface

With improved health care, not only in the United States but in the less developed countries, the number of women living past the age of menopause is steadily increasing. In the 1980 U.S. census it was estimated that there were more than 30 million women older than 50 years of age. Postmenopausally, there is a marked increase in the number of various pathologic conditions in women. Some of these, such as hot flushes, atrophic vaginitis, atrophic urethritis, and osteoporosis, are definitely linked to a reduction in circulatory estrogen levels. Others, such as coronary heart disease, although increasing in incidence postmenopausally, have not been shown to have a definite causal relation to estrogen deficiency.

The use of postmenopausal exogenous hormonal replacement to alleviate or prevent these conditions is controversial. Although many authorities recommend the use of exogenous hormonal replacement by asymptomatic postmenopausal women, others, because of concern of the effect on the incidence of breast and endometrial cancer as well as hypertension, believe their use should be restricted to asymptomatic women.

Unfortunately, considering the magnitude of the problems of pathologic conditions associated with estrogen deficiency in postmenopausal women, there has been a relative paucity of research studies in this area. Also, very few large, well controlled studies concerning the benefits and risks of estrogen replacement exist and as a result, health care providers are confused about this issue. Because of this confusion, and because of the difficulty in correlating data about the pathology and treatment of menopausal women, it was decided to publish a book that summarizes the current information on this subject.

A group of investigators from several countries who have been performing research upon this subject for several years has graciously provided the time and effort to contribute chapters to this volume. This book is divided into four sections: physiology of the menopausal period; beneficial effects of pharmacologic agents; adverse effects of hormone replacement therapy; and formulations and pharmacology of treatment. An introduction concerning the effect of the increasing number of postmenopausal women in less developed countries has been provided by Egon Diczfalusy. There may be some duplication of certain areas in some of the chapters. There may also be apparent conflicts among the statements of different authors. These apparent discrepancies reflect the lack of scientific data and are not meant to confuse the reader. In many instances, conclusions have to be derived from incomplete data.

The editor wishes to thank all the contributors for taking the time and effort to provide the reader with the current state of knowledge in this area, and to thank Ms. Laurel Oden for her untiring efforts in coordinating and reviewing the manuscript.

DANIEL R. MISHELL, JR., M. D.

Contents

CHAPTER 1

Introduction: Menopause, Developing Countries, and the 21st Century*

EGON DICZFALUSY, M.D.

"There is nothing either good or bad, but thinking makes it so."

Hamlet II, ii.

THE CLASSICAL QUOTATION "tempora mutantur et nos mutamur in illis"[4]—times change and we change with them—has never been more valid than in our time. What represents the essentially new element of our epoch is the rate of change and its complexity. Times seem to change more rapidly than we do, and the changes around us are so rapid that our perception of the world in which we are living is lagging behind. Hence, it becomes difficult to assess in its entirety the state of art in a seemingly well-defined area, such as the "future of the menopause," without considering it in a global context, taking in account the complex relationships between population growth, resources, environment, and development.

I hope, therefore, that the reader will have an understanding for the strange format of this review, in which the introduction is much longer than the description of the subject proper and in which the presentation of the background almost assumes the appearance of a kind of "State of the World Message." I think, however, that even a sketchy and incomplete presentation of the global perspective may be helpful for an analysis of the problem of menopause in the 21st century and its likely impact on the developing world.

BACKGROUND

Various types of evidence indicate that human settlements existed in Africa at least a million years ago. Hence, a decade in the history of mankind is analogous to a split second in the lifespan of a human being. However, as stated in the United Nations Report of the International Conference on Population,[14] during the past decade the world population has increased by 770 million, or almost by 20%, and most of this increase (90%) has occurred in developing countries. This acceleration in population growth can best be illustrated by recalling that around year 1 A.D. the world had about 300 million people and that at the time of Napoleon's death on Sainte-Hélène (May 5, 1821) the global population was still below one billion. It was approximately in 1850 that the first billion was reached. Then the next century and a half witnessed an unprecedented population growth, as shown in Table 1–1.

---

*Based on a keynote address delivered at a symposium of the Swedish Society of Obstetrics and Gynecology in Stockholm on Sept. 14, 1985, to be published in *Acta Obstet Gynecol Scand* (1986).

TABLE 1–1.

The Growth of the Global Population Since 1850

YEAR	BILLIONS
1850	1
1930	2
1961	3
1976	4
1987	5

Hence, between 1950 and today, our generation has seen the birth of another world, equal in numbers, demands, hopes, and aspirations. How long can this rapid growth continue? Another hundred years, or so. According to the medium variant projection of the United Nations, the world population is expected to stabilize at 10.5 billion by the end of the 21st century. Ninety-five percent of this future growth of the world population will occur in the developing countries.[10] The above projection of the United Nations Population Division[16] can be compared with that prepared simultaneously, but independently, by the World Bank. According to the projections of the Bank, world population is expected to stabilize at a level over 11 billion in about year 2150.[20]

It is of course erroneous to consider population projections as predictions in the classical sense; rather, they are illustrations of what can happen given reasonable assumptions. Hence, if the assumptions underlying the medium variant projection of the U.N. Population Division (UNPD) and if the ''standard'' projections of the World Bank are correct, then by the year 2050 the population of today's developed countries would grow from 1.2 billion to approximately 1.4 billion, while that of those countries now classified as developing would grow from 3.6 billion to approximately 8.4 billion. By the time world population stabilized at 11 billion or so, sometime between year 2100 and 2150, India would be the most populous nation on Earth (1.7 billion), and the four most populous African countries, Nigeria, Ethiopia, Kenya, and Zaire, would have a total population of between 1.1 and 1.2 billion.[20] As a group, the poorest countries of today, those of sub-Saharan Africa and South Asia—which for the time being exhibit the fastest population growth—would account for about 50 percent of the global population, compared with approximately 30% today.

Based on the most recent projections of the World Bank[21] the hypothetical size of the predicted stationary populations of the ten most populous countries (with a projected minimum population of 200 million each) is expected to reach the figures indicated in Table 1–2.

It may be added that, whereas in 1950 approximately 67% of mankind was living in developing countries, by 1980 this figure was 75%; now it is expected that by the end of the next century 87% of the global population will live in countries now classified as developing. It was rightly emphasized in the 1984 World Developing Report by A. W. Clausen, the president of the World Bank, who said, ''Population growth does not provide the drama of financial crisis or political upheaval, but as this report shows, its significance for shaping the world of our children and grandchildren is at least as great.''[20] And whereas population should be viewed in its entirety—''as a resource, as a constraint, as a consequence, as a determinant, and as an integral element in life''— population growth should be viewed as ''the critical factor—to be considered in relation to an equally critical factor, the life-support system of this planet.''[10] Hence, granted that a complex and multifaceted relationship exists between population, environment,

TABLE 1–2.

Hypothetical Size of the Stationary Populations
of the Ten Most Populous Countries*†

COUNTRY	HYPOTHETICAL STATIONARY POPULATION (MILLIONS)	POPULATION SIZE IN 1983 (MILLIONS)
India	1,700	733
China	1,570	1,019
Nigeria	530	94
USSR	380	273
Indonesia	370	156
Pakistan	330	90
Bangladesh	310	96
Brazil	300	130
USA	290	235
Mexico	200	75

*Adapted from the World Bank: *World Development Report 1985*. London, Oxford University Press, 1985. Used by permission.
†Figures rounded to the nearest 10 million.

resources, and development, it can be predicted with a more than reasonable accuracy that "population growth will result in major strains on the already limited availability of food, clean water, shelter, energy, education, health services, and job opportunities. It will also speed up desertification, deforestation, and soil erosion."[1]

With regard to these factors, the present situation has been assessed in detail by the various specialized agencies of the United Nations.

As far as the global food situation is concerned, it shows a marked improvement for the time being. Nevertheless, cereal imports by many countries have considerably increased during the past decade. An example is presented in Table 1–3, which indicates

TABLE 1–3.

Cereal Imports of the 12 Most Populous Countries
of the World*

COUNTRY	POPULATION (MILLIONS) 1983	CEREAL IMPORTS (METRIC TONS × 1000) 1974	1983
China	1,019	9,176	19,167
India	733	5,261	4,280
USSR	273	7,755	32,132
USA	235	0,460	0,594
Indonesia	156	1,919	2,992
Brazil	130	2,485	4,925
Japan	119	19,557	25,296
Bangladesh	96	1,719	1,844
Nigeria	94	0,389	2,336
Pakistan	90	1,274	0,396
Mexico	75	2,881	4,483
Germany, Fed. Rep.	61	7,164	4,209
Total	3,081	60,040	106,654

*Adapted from the World Bank: *World Development Report 1985*. London, Oxford University Press, 1985. Used by permission.

the development of cereal imports by the 12 most populous countries of the world during the past decade.

It is apparent from the data of Table 1–3 that cereal imports further increased both by developed (USSR, Japan) and by developing (China, Mexico, Nigeria) countries. Furthermore, in other parts of the world (e.g., Africa) we have witnessed a major famine of alarming proportions as late as in 1985. What is perhaps more serious is that, according to the United Nations Environmental Programme (UNEP), in 1981–82 some 1.7 billion human beings lacked safe drinking water and 1.2 billion lacked any form of sanitation.[15]

The desperate debt situation of some developing countries is extensively covered by the news media and so is the energy situation of those that do not belong to the "club" of oil-producing countries. A summation of these two factors may create a major squeeze, even on the economy of a developed country, but in the case of a developing country the combined effect may seriously interfere with development. A few examples are presented in Table 1–4.

It can be seen that in 1983, debt service plus energy imports accounted for 95%, 85%, and 77%, respectively, of exports, in the case of Turkey, Brazil, and Pakistan. Furthermore, only energy imports accounted for 101%, 82%, 68%, 58%, and 57%, respectively, of the merchandise exports of Jordan, Panama, Guatemala, Senegal, and Sudan.[21]

Another change around us: the past 15 years witnessed an unprecedented worldwide increase in demand for education in general, and higher education in particular. A few examples are given in Table 1–5.

The data indicate that the number of students enrolled in higher education dramatically increased in both developing and developed countries. The situation in several developing countries certainly does not correspond to previous perceptions based on

TABLE 1–4.

Debt Service and Energy Imports in Selected Countries*

COUNTRY	POPULATION (MILLIONS)	DEBT SERVICE† YEAR		ENERGY IMPORTS‡ YEAR	
		1970	1983	1965	1983
Argentina	30	21	24	8	9
Bangladesh	96	—	15	—	20
Brazil	130	12	29	14	56
Burma	36	16	34	4	—
Egypt	45	36	28	11	12
Ethiopia	41	11	11	8	—
India	733	22	10	8	—
Indonesia	156	7	13	3	20
Mexico	75	24	36	4	—
Nigeria	94	4	19	7	—
Pakistan	90	24	28	7	49
Philippines	52	7	15	12	44
Thailand	49	3	11	11	39
Turkey	47	22	29	12	66

*Adapted from the World Bank: *World Development Report 1985*. London, Oxford University Press, 1985. Used by permission.
†As a percentage of exports of goods and services.
‡As a percentage of merchandise exports.

TABLE 1–5.

Number of Individuals Enrolled in Higher Education
as Percentage of the Population
Aged 20–24*

	YEAR	
COUNTRY	1965	1982
Argentina	14	25
Brazil	2	12
Bolivia	5	16
Costa Rica	6	27
Cuba	3	19
Honduras	1	10
India	5	9
Japan	13	30
Jordan	2	32
Korea, Rep. of	6	24
Peru	8	21
Sweden	13	38
Thailand	2	22
USA	40	58
USSR	30	21
Venezuela	7	22

*Adapted from the World Bank: *World Development Report
1985*. London, Oxford University Press, 1985. Used by permission.

information collected in the late sixties. Whereas a cadre of young people with higher education is not only an enormous asset, but also a prerequisite for developing countries on their road towards self-reliance and intellectual independence, a rapid increase of this "pool" may also create major problems in terms of massive unemployment among academically qualified individuals. An example is the major shortage of physicians in the countryside coupled with unemployment among medically qualified persons in countries such as Pakistan and India.[6]

This brings up the problem of the availability of health services in general and of well-trained physicians in particular, an aspect of considerable importance for our forthcoming discussion of the "aging society" and the menopause. In Table 1–6 the population per physician in the 12 most populous countries is related to their total fertility rate in 1965, and 15 years later, in 1980.

In 1980 among these 12 countries (not quite unexpectedly) the lowest "density" of physicians was in Nigeria and Indonesia and the highest in the USSR and in the Federal Republic of Germany.

Whereas the data of Table 1–6 are representative of 12 countries with a total of more than 3 billion inhabitants, they must be complemented with similar data from developing countries with very high fertility rates; such data are presented in Table 1–7.

It can be seen from the data that, during the 15 year period between 1965 and 1980, the previous critical situation did not improve at all in Ethiopia and even worsened in Mozambique and Uganda.

Unemployment is perhaps the greatest global plague of the 1980s in the developed world; however, it is even more serious in developing countries, which are lacking any supportive mechanisms for the jobless. In global terms, the International Labour Office (ILO) estimates that "between 1980 and 2000 employment must be found for 700 mil-

6 / Chapter 1

TABLE 1–6.

Total Fertility Rate and Population per Physician in the 12 Most Populous Countries of the World*

COUNTRY	POPULATION (MILLIONS) 1983	TOTAL FERTILITY RATE 1983	POPULATION PER PHYSICIAN	
			1965	1980
China	1,019	2.3	—	1,740
India	733	4.8	4,860	3,690
USSR	273	2.4	480	270
USA	235	1.8	670	520
Indonesia	156	4.3	31,800	11,500
Brazil	130	3.8	2,180	—
Japan	119	1.7	930	780
Bangladesh	96	6.0	—	7,800
Nigeria	94	6.9	45,000	12,000
Pakistan	90	5.8	3,160	3,480
Mexico	75	4.6	2,100	—
Germany, Fed. Rep.	61	1.4	630	450

*Adapted from the World Bank: *World Development Report 1985*. London, Oxford University Press, 1985. Used by permission.

lion new entrants into the labour force, approximately twice the number of the 1960–1980 period. Moreover, a back-up of unemployed or seriously underemployed workers need jobs. This group constitutes one third of the existing labour force of 1,200 million."[5]

Last but not least in these series of problems are recent environmental changes. The Stockholm Conference devoted to the Year of the Forest (1983) summarized succinctly and rather dramatically the daily changes taking place in our environment: "*This day* world population has increased by 175,000 persons. *This day* an additional 160 square kilometers have been converted into deserts. *This day* fully 300 square kilometers of

TABLE 1–7.

Total Fertility Rate and Population per Physician in 12 Developing Countries with High Fertility Rate*

COUNTRY	POPULATION (MILLIONS) 1983	TOTAL FERTILITY RATE 1983	POPULATION PER PHYSICIAN	
			1965	1980
Afghanistan	17	8.0	15,800	16,700
Algeria	21	7.0	8,400	2,600
Burma	36	5.3	11,700	4,700
Ethiopia	41	5.5	70,200	69,400
Ghana	13	7.0	12,000	7,200
Kenya	19	8.0	12,800	7,900
Morocco	21	5.8	12,100	10,800
Mozambique	13	6.5	18,700	39,100
Nepal	16	6.3	46,200	30,100
Sudan	21	6.6	23,500	8,900
Uganda	14	7.0	11,100	13,900
Zaire	30	6.3	39,000	13,900

*Adapted from the World Bank: *World Development Report 1985*. London, Oxford University Press, 1985. Used by permission.

tropical forests have been cut down.''[18] In fact, the UNEP considers at least one third of earth's land area at risk from desertification.[15]

The so-called population problem is not only a problem of growth but also that of a changing distribution and age structure. During the 21st century the former will be characterized by an increasing urbanization, the latter by an increasing aging. The urban population as a percentage of total population in selected countries is indicated in Table 1–8.

The data of Table 1–8 indicate major differences in the extent of urbanization, varying from 17% to 86%. It can also be seen that the population of many developing countries (e.g., Argentina, Chile, Mexico, Peru) is predominantly urban. However, irrespective of the relative extent of urbanization, the percentage of urban population uniformly increased between 1965 and 1983. Although the data of Table 1–8 do not include any projections, it should be noted that the UNPD calculates that, whereas in 1974 the number of cities with 4 million or more inhabitants was only 28 and only 15 of those were situated in developing countries, by the year 2000 there will be 66 such cities, of which 50 will be in the developing world. The UNPD projections also indicate that by the year 2025 there will be 135 such cities, 114 of them in developing countries.[16] Expressed in percentages, this would mean that by the year 2025 almost two thirds of the global population will live in a large metropolis.

The other important population change, that in age structure, relates to a rapid increase in life expectancy at birth. The increase in life expectancy at birth that occurred between 1965 and 1983 is illustrated by the data of Table 1–9.

The data indicate that major differences existed among the various countries even in 1983; the life expectancy at birth for Angolan women was still only 44 years, compared to 80 years for Swedish women. It also appears that, with the exception of the USSR,

TABLE 1–8.

Urban Population as Percentage of Total Population in Selected Countries*

| | YEAR | |
COUNTRY	1965	1983
Argentina	76	84
Bangladesh	6	17
Brazil	51	71
Chile	72	82
China	18	21
Germany, F.R.	79	86
India	18	24
Indonesia	16	24
Japan	67	76
Mexico	55	69
Nigeria	15	22
Pakistan	24	29
Peru	52	67
Thailand	13	18
USA	72	74
USSR	52	65

*Adapted from the World Bank: *World Development Report 1985*. London, Oxford University Press, 1985. Used by permission.

TABLE 1–9.

Life Expectancy at Birth (Years) in Selected Countries in 1965 and in 1983*

| | LIFE EXPECTANCY AT BIRTH | | | |
| | MEN | | WOMEN | |
COUNTRY	1965	1983	1965	1983
Angola	34	42	37	44
Argentina	63	66	69	73
Bangladesh	45	49	44	50
Brazil	55	61	59	66
China	55	65	59	69
Cuba	65	73	69	77
India	46	56	44	54
Indonesia	43	52	45	55
Japan	68	74	73	79
Jordan	49	63	51	65
Korea, Rep. of	55	64	58	71
Mexico	58	64	61	68
Nigeria	40	47	43	50
Pakistan	46	51	44	49
Sudan	39	47	41	49
Sweden	72	75	76	80
USA	67	72	74	79
USSR	65	65	74	74

*Adapted from the World Bank: *World Development Report 1985*. London, Oxford University Press, 1985. Used by permission.

the life expectancy at birth significantly increased for both men and women during the 18-year period between 1965 and 1983. Indeed, in China, India, and Indonesia, the increase was as much as a full decade.

It is expected that the increase in life expectancy will continue also into the 21st century and will eventually lead to the disappearance of the current geographic differences. As indicated by the projections of the United Nations (Table 1–10), it is expected that by year 2025 the global life expectancy at birth will be 70 years.[16]

It is easy to see that the combination of continued population growth and rapidly

TABLE 1–10.

Life Expectancy at Birth (Years) According to the Estimates and Medium Variant Projections of the United Nations Population Division*

YEAR	WORLD	DEVELOPING COUNTRIES
1974	55.4	52.7
1984	58.9	56.6
2000	63.5	61.8
2025	70.0	68.9

*Adapted from the United Nations Population Division: *World Population Prospects: Estimates and Projections as Assessed in 1982*. Report of the Secretary General, United Nations International Conference on Population, Mexico City, August 1984, pp. 29–30. Used by permission.

increasing life expectancy at birth will significantly alter not only the age structure, but also the dependency ratio.

Table 1–11 presents the age composition of the global population in 1980 as estimated by the World Health Organization.[23]

The data indicate that in 1980 some 35% of the global population was aged 14 or less and 21% aged 45 or more. The differences between developed and developing countries are considerable. However, these differences become even more conspicuous when assessed in the light of the data of Table 1–12, which shows the corresponding age composition of deaths.

The striking differences between developed and developing countries hardly necessitate any comments. According to the projections of the United Nations World Assembly on Aging (Vienna, 1982), which are based on a somewhat different grouping (Table 1–13), it is expected that by the year 2025 as much as 23% of the total population of the developed countries will consist of persons aged 60 and older and the number of such persons in developing countries will double between 1975 and 2025.[17]

The absolute figures hidden behind these percentages are even more impressive; as indicated by the data of Table 1–14; even in 1950 the global number of persons aged 60 and older did not exceed 200 million, and only 40% of those lived in developing countries.

According to the projections of the Vienna International Plan of Action on Aging (1982), within the next 40 years the number of persons aged 60 and older will increase to 1.1 billion, and by the year 2025 more than 70% of those will live in countries now classified as developing.[17]

TABLE 1–11.

Estimated Age Composition of Population
(in Percentages) in 1980*

AGE GROUP (YEARS)	DEVELOPED COUNTRIES	DEVELOPING COUNTRIES	WORLD TOTAL
0–14	23	39	35
15–44	45	44	44
45–64	21	13	15
>64	11	4	6

*Adapted from the World Health Organization: *World Health Statistics Annual*. Geneva, 1983. ISBN 92-4-067831X. Used by permission.

TABLE 1–12.

Estimated Age Composition of Deaths
(in Percentages) Around 1980*

AGE GROUP (YEARS)	DEVELOPED COUNTRIES	DEVELOPING COUNTRIES	WORLD TOTAL
0–14	4	40	32
15–44	7	12	11
45–64	21	18	19
>64	68	30	38

*Adapted from the World Health Organization: *World Health Statistics Annual*. Geneva, 1983. ISBN 92-4-067831X. Used by permission.

TABLE 1–13.

Projected Age Structure as Percentage
of Population*

	DEVELOPED COUNTRIES AGE GROUP		DEVELOPING COUNTRIES AGE GROUP	
YEAR	<15	>60	<15	>60
1975	25	15	41	6
2000	21	18	33	7
2025	20	23	26	12

*From the United Nations World Assembly on Aging, Vienna, 1982: The Vienna International Plan of Action on Aging, 1982. Used by permission.

TABLE 1–14.

Projected Size of the Global Population
of Persons Aged 60 and Over*

YEAR	WORLD (MILLIONS)	DEVELOPING COUNTRIES (MILLIONS)
1950	200	80
1975	350	178
2000	590	355
2025	1100	792

*From the United Nations World Assembly on Aging, Vienna, 1982: The Vienna International Plan of Action on Aging, 1982. Used by permission.

With this introduction and with the background information presented in Tables 1–1 through 1–14, we can now address the subject proper: menopause, developing countries, and the 21st century.

MENOPAUSE AND THE 21ST CENTURY

According to the estimates of the Vienna International Plan of Action on Aging, the present sex ratio, i.e., the number of men per 100 women in industrialized countries, is around 75 for the age group 60–69 and approximately 50 for those aged 80 and over.[17] Hence, it is reasonable to assume on the basis of the data of Table 1–14 that the total number of women aged 60 and older will approach 350 million by the year 2000 and that it will be in the neighborhood of 650 million 25 years later, in 2025. It is also plausible to assume that by the year 2025 as many as 475 million such women, or 73%, will live in developing countries. Furthermore, similar considerations based on the figures of Table 1–11 suggest that in 1980 21% of the global population (estimated by the World Bank at 4,435 million[20, 21]), or 930 million individuals, were aged 45 or older. Assuming a sex ratio of 85, it may be calculated that in 1980 the global population of women aged 45 or over was approximately half a billion. This figure is in close agreement with that calculated in a previous review[13] on the basis of the country-by-country data reported in the latest edition of the World Health Statistics.[23] These figures are reproduced in Table 1–15.

The data indicate that, whereas between 1980 and 2000 the population of women approaching or reaching menopause in the developed countries will increase by less than

TABLE 1–15.

The World Population of Women Aged 45
and Over (in Millions)*

	YEAR		
REGION	1960	1980	2000
Developed countries	155	204	251
Developing countries	175	274	468
Total	330	478	719

*Adapted from Diczfalusy[3] and the World Health Organi-
zation.[23]

50 million, during the same period the corresponding number of women in developing countries will increase by almost 200 million. In less than 15 years from now, in the year 2000, some 12% of the world population will consist of women aged 45 or older and almost half a billion of them will live in developing countries. From there on, their number and relative proportion will rapidly increase pari passu with the increasing life expectancy at birth in the developing countries. Hence, it is rather naive to think—and this is what I frequently hear from health administrators of developing countries—that the menopause as a problem mainly concerns the well-to-do Western societies. Within 15 years it could be a problem of considerable dimensions also in the developing world, and by the middle of the 21st century it may, or may not, develop into a problem of overwhelming proportions in certain developing countries which lack a suitable medical infrastructure.

Why "may, or may not"? Because there is virtually no information on the menopause in developing countries, be it the age distribution, sociocultural significance, or the prevalence of osteoporosis, cardiovascular disease, and musculoskeletal disorders.[22]

In the discussion below, the WHO definitions will be used: *Menopause* is the permanent cessation of menstruation resulting from loss of ovarian activity. *Perimenopause* (climacteric) is the period immediately prior to the menopause and at least the first years after it. *Postmenopause* is the period dating from the menopause, which can only be assessed in retrospect.[22] The only addendum to these definitions is that by now a considerable body of evidence indicates that the perimenopause is a much more protracted period than previously believed.

It is known that several factors influence the *age at menopause,* for instance, ethnic differences, secular trends, age at menarche, marital status, parity, occupation, smoking habits, altitude, socioeconomic conditions, and, possibly, contraceptive use.[22] However, the available information is mainly based on observations made in developed countries. Hence, there is little, if any, information available on the age distribution, sociocultural significance, and prevalence of various symptoms and major disorders in various developing countries. The absence of such data makes it very difficult to adequately assess the relevant health and social service requirements in developing countries today and especially tomorrow.

In fact, very little is known in various developing countries of the perception of women concerning the lack of menstruation and childlessness, the attitude of husbands, the social status and extent of economic deprivation of postmenopausal women, or the alternative roles they may play and the medical and social services available to them.[22] Similarly, information is extremely limited on the prevalence and sociocultural impact of the various vasomotor and psychologic symptoms, sexual decline, vaginal dryness, dyspareunia, insomnia, urinary problems, skin changes, and bleeding disturbances, or on the optimal hormonal therapy needed—a subject which is also controversial in the developed world.

Last but not least, it should be borne in mind that there is no such thing as a homogeneous group of developing countries. If you have seen one, you have certainly not seen the others. Developing countries markedly differ from each other, and to extrapolate from the prevailing conditions in one country to those of another may be at least as hazardous as extrapolating from developed to developing countries. Therefore, it will be essential to establish the age distribution, sociocultural impact, and the prevalence of symptoms and major disorders in as many developing countries as possible.

Osteoporosis

From the arguments advanced above, it follows that it will be extremely important to find out the prevalence of osteoporosis in various developing countries, in view of the rapid change in lifestyle and the equally rapid increase in life expectancy at birth. Osteoporosis is a major disorder of the greatest possible concern; it is a monumental problem in the developed world, since it is established that, by the age of 80, some 25% of Western women have sustained one or more fractures of the proximal femur, vertebrae, or distal radius.[22] In the United States osteoporosis is affecting as many as 15–20 million individuals, and about 1.3 million fractures attributable to osteoporosis occur annually in people aged 45 and older.[9] In fact, the cost of osteoporosis in the United States has been estimated at $3.8 billion annually. Among those who live to be 90, 32% of women and 17% of men will suffer a hip fracture, mostly due to osteoporosis. Most patients fail to recover normal activity, and mortality within one year approaches 20%.[9] It is easy to see that a rapidly increasing life expectancy at birth will further exaggerate the magnitude of the problem.

What are the risk factors? Epidemiologic studies point to a number of risk factors—but again, only in Western populations. The *established* risk factors include age, sex, race, body weight-for-height, menopause, estrogen and calcium deficiency, lack of exercise, immobilization, and prolonged bed rest. The risk increases with age and is higher in women than in men, and in whites than in blacks.[9] These estimates are based on data obtained in the United States; no information is available as far as developing countries are concerned.

Among *possible* risk factors, hereditary, smoking, and various dietary factors, such as alcohol, vitamins A and C, magnesium, and protein are under consideration. Again, no data are available from developing countries.

There has been a significant improvement in our diagnostic ability to ascertain accelerated bone loss, with methods ranging from simple spine radiography, radiogrammetry, photodensitometry, estimation of Singh index, photon absorptiometry, neutron activation techniques, Compton scattering, improved tomography, to classical histomorphometry.[9, 22] However, there still are many unsolved problems with regard to suitable methodology to assess bone loss during relatively short periods of time, especially in epidemiologic studies to be conducted in developing countries. It goes without saying that such studies will be of paramount importance in assessing the magnitude of risk in developing country populations. Computerized axial tomography will not be suitable for this purpose, not only because of the cost, but also because it requires a very high dose of radiation, some 15–30 times more than dual photon absorptiometry, which only necessitates 5–15 mrem. The disadvantage of the latter, in comparison with single-photon absorptiometry, is that the instrument is not mobile, a consideration of major importance in field studies conducted in developing countries. The accuracy and precision of both photon absorptiometric techniques (3%–6%) would seem to be satisfactory. Furthermore, certain biochemical parameters, such as urinary calcium/creatinine and proline/creatinine ratios, might have a certain value in relatively short-term comparative studies, with the important reservation that a lack of effect would have little, if any, predictive value.

With regard to preventive measures, it is established that in Western women, four factors are of cardinal importance for the reduction of the rate of bone loss: estrogen, calcium, vitamin D, and exercise.[9, 22] It is also agreed that adequate nutrition should include a daily dose of 1,500 mg elemental calcium in the absence, and 1,000 mg in the presence, of estrogen substitution therapy;[9] however, opinions greatly differ as to what dose, and particularly what type, of estrogen will provide an optimal substitution. A number of other agents are also under study.[9] They include sodium fluoride, calcitriol, calcitonin, anabolic steroids, large doses of progesterone, thiazides, bisphosphonates, and certain parathyroid preparations. The relative merits of these therapies remain to be evaluated.

However, an overwhelming problem is that we do not have an effective agent that could accelerate bone formation and replace bone that is lost. All that currently available therapeutic regimens can do is to reduce the rate of bone loss.

Why is it so important to establish whether or not osteoporosis is a major risk factor in Oriental or in Indian women? Is it not possible to simply extrapolate the data obtained in Western women? It is certainly possible, but very risky and of questionable scientific validity. It is known that genetic heterogeneity is frequently associated with metabolic heterogeneity, as indicated in the examples shown in Tables 1–16 and 1–17, which have been adapted from the classical paper of Kalow[7] and which indicate major population differences in the distribution of slow and fast acetylators and of "usual" and "atypical" variants of alcohol dehydrogenase. Furthermore, developing countries may markedly differ from developed ones with respect to environmental, nutritional, and other risk factors for disease, not to mention risk-benefit ratios. Also, as indicated above, developing countries may dramatically differ from each other with respect to several risk factors for osteoporosis.

Hence, an overall assessment of the research priorities with regard to osteoporosis strongly suggests that it will be important to study possible demographic differences,

TABLE 1–16.

Percentage Distribution of Slow Acetylators of Isoniazid in Various Populations*

POPULATION	SLOW ACETYLATOR	FAST ACETYLATOR	
		HETEROZYGOTES	HOMOZYGOTES
South Indians	59	36	5
Caucasians	59	36	5
Negroes	55	38	7
Chinese	22	50	28
Japanese	12	45	43
Eskimos	10	44	46

*Adapted from Kalow W.[7]

TABLE 1–17.

Percentage Distribution of Alcohol Dehydrogenase Variants in Liver Specimens from Various Populations*

COUNTRY OF ORIGIN	"USUAL"	"ATYPICAL"	
		HETEROZYGOTES	HOMOZYGOTES
Switzerland	82	18	0
Germany	93	7	0
England	93	7	0
Japan	13	44	43
China	11	44	45
India	100	0	0

*Adapted from Kalow W.[7]

the influence of nutritional factors, and the effect of socioeconomic conditions. It will also be of crucial importance to develop safe, simple, reliable, and inexpensive diagnostic procedures and preventive measures. A major effort is required to find a drug that will not only diminish the rate of bone loss, but which will accelerate bone formation.

Cardiovascular Disease

The second disorder of major importance is atherosclerotic cardiovascular disease. It is established that cessation of ovarian function is associated with a significantly increased risk of morbidity and mortality from such diseases,[22] as indicated in Table 1–18. This table was compiled on the basis of the data of the latest edition of the World Health Statistics.[23] The point is that the data indicate major differences not only between developing and developed countries, but also among various Western countries. The fact that senility without psychosis was indicated as the predominant cause of death in Thailand most probably indicates flaws in the diagnosis and data collection and reflects the fact that the diagnosis was not based on autopsy findings.

However, whereas it is relatively easy to dismiss the relevance of the Thai data shown in Table 1–18, it is more difficult to overlook the significance of the differences shown in Table 1–19. Indeed, the data strongly suggest that significant differences exist in the frequency of myocardial infarction and of other ischemic heart diseases as causes of death for women in the United States, compared to the figures reported not only from

TABLE 1–18.

Selected Causes of Death for Women Aged 65 and Over in Various Countries*

CAUSE OF DEATH	WHO CLASSIFICATION	PERCENTAGE OF WOMEN				
		USA	UK	FRANCE	JAPAN	THAILAND
Diseases of circulatory system	(25–30)	63	55	47	53	7.1
Malignant neoplasms	(08–14)	17	17	16	16	1.1
Senility without psychosis	(465)	0.1	0.4	3.4	7.6	67
Atherosclerosis	(300)	2.6	2.0	0.7	1.1	0.0
Number >65 who died		641,163	240,188	220,551	252,158	40,149

*Adapted from Diczfalusy[3] and the World Health Organization.[23]

TABLE 1–19.
Selected Causes of Death for Women Aged 65 and Over in Various Countries*

CAUSE OF DEATH	WHO CLASSIFICATION	PERCENTAGE OF WOMEN AGED 65 OR OLDER WHO DIED				
		USA	UK	FRANCE	JAPAN	THAILAND
Breast cancer	(113)	2.6	2.9	2.2	0.5	0.1
Uterine and cervical cc	(120 + 122)	1.0	0.8	1.1	1.1	0.2
Myocardial infarction	(270)	16	16	7.2	4.0	0.2
Other ischemic heart disease	(279)	18	8.4	2.2	3.8	0.1
Cerebrovascular disease	(29)	14	16	17	27	1.6
Number >65 who died		641,163	240,188	220,551	252,158	40,149

*Adapted from Diczfalusy[3] and the World Health Organization.[23]

Japan, but also from France. Therefore, a detailed study of the various risk factors involved appears to represent a very high priority. Also, as rightly emphasized by the WHO Scientific Group,[22] because of the overwhelming size of the underlying risk, in-depth epidemiologic studies on the effect of possible preventive agents, such as estrogens with or without added progestins, should be undertaken in various populations with the highest possible priority.

Musculoskeletal disorders

The third group of major disorders related to the menopause is represented by the various forms of rheumatic and degenerative musculoskeletal disorders. Here again, the same considerations apply as in the case of osteoporosis and cardiovascular disease; we have to find out the prevalence in different populations, including a large variety of developing countries; we have to ascertain whether or not estrogen administration is protective, and if so, what type of estrogen should be given and in what dose. The relative risks and benefits of such therapy must be carefully evaluated. What are those risks? The risks under discussion include endometrial and breast cancer, hypertension, cardiovascular complications, gall-bladder disease, and urinary tract stones (the last-mentioned in connection with high-calcium doses).

Risks of Estrogen Therapy

The benefits of estrogen substitution are well established and are rarely, if ever, debated. The debate is focused on the risks. This "estrogen risk" can be brought into focus by relating the established and/or probable risk factors for endometrial and breast cancer, as shown in Table 1–20. As indicated by the data in this table, there is indeed a strong association between exogenous estrogens and risk of endometrial cancer.[13] This poses an "estrogen dilemma," which is simply a reflection on the classical question: how much is too much? Excessive estrogen therapy, while decreasing the risk of osteoporosis may increase the frequency of endometrial hyperplasia and thus that of endometrial cancer. On the other hand, inadequate estrogen therapy will have little, if any, effect on osteoporosis. Two considerations may be helpful in this context. The first is that endometrial cancer is an infrequent condition and osteoporosis is a frequent one. The other consideration may sound rather philosophical although it has a very practical implication: Are all estrogens equal? What kind (weak, strong, inactive, active) of an

TABLE 1–20.

Risk Factors for Endometrial Cancer and Their Relation to Breast Cancer*

	RELATIVE STRENGTH OF ASSOCIATION†	
RISK FACTOR	ENDOMETRIAL CANCER	BREAST CANCER
Late menopause	+	+
Estrogen-secreting hormones	+ +	×
Polycystic ovary/anovulatory cycles	+ +	+
Obesity	+	±
Nulliparity	+	+
Low parity	+	±
Menstrual irregularity	+	−
Exogenous estrogens	+ +	+

*Adapted from Thomas DB: Do hormones cause breast cancer? *Cancer* 1984; 53:595.
† + +, strong; +, moderate; ±, probable; −, not a risk factor; ×, insufficient data

estrogen is, for instance, estrone sulphate, compared to estriol or to estradiol? Which compound, dose regimen, formulation, and route of administration provides an optimal substitution therapy in menopausal women? After 40 years of clinical research on estrogens, there still is a great hiatus and a definite need to learn more about the pharmacodynamic properties of natural estrogens to meet an increasing global need for an adequate, safe, and inexpensive estrogen substitution therapy.

CONCLUSION

The United Nations Vienna International Plan of Action on Aging[17] summarizes the ten basic principles to be observed in care of the elderly: equality, individuality, independence, choice, mobility, productivity, home care, access to services, cohesion among generations, promotion of self-care, and family care. The Plan of Action then states with emphasis that "diseases do not need to be essential components of aging" and predicts that "as men and women live to increasingly greater ages, major disabilities will largely be compressed into a narrow range just prior to death."[17] This sounds reassuring and inspires hope and confidence. However, with all due respect, how realistic is this prediction? How are we going to "compress into a narrow range just prior to death" the major disorders of the menopause—osteoporosis, atherosclerotic cardiovascular disease, musculoskeletal disorders, and senility?

It is clear that if we really wish to achieve the ambitious objectives set out by the Vienna International Plan of Action on Aging,[17] a number of urgent research tasks will confront the international scientific community, research tasks that can only be addressed by committed scientists, since in medical-technical terms only scientists can change the world.[2] Hence, in a rapidly changing world we have to establish on a country-by-country basis the age distribution and sociocultural significance of the menopause and the prevalence of the various disorders which to a large extent will determine the health and social service needs of individual developing countries. Furthermore, rapid progress must be made in the areas of diagnosis, prevention, and treatment of osteoporosis, atherosclerotic cardiovascular disease, musculoskeletal disorders, and senility. The risks associated with preventive hormone therapy must be significantly reduced or eliminated.

As far as the United Nations and its Specialized Agencies are concerned, there is a need to establish an international code of ethics for the protection of the elderly and to impress the member states to ratify it rapidly. What is even more urgently needed is to establish within the World Health Organization a Special Programme (in analogy with the Special Programme of Research, Development and Research Training in Human Reproduction or that on Tropical Diseases) to act as the main instrument of the United Nations system for conducting, promoting, coordinating, and evaluating international research related to the problems of aging, with special emphasis on the needs of developing countries.

It goes without saying, that the various national and international measures required to foot the bill will be very expensive. Hence, there must be a significant change in the international attitude that is so deep that . . . it reaches the purse. As the famous Austrian general Raimund von Montecuccoli said: three things are necessary to conduct a successful war: money, money, and money.[8] The tabulations given in Tables 1–21 to 1–23 might provide some ideas as to where to find the money required.

The data of Table 1–21 were published by the United Nations Environmental Programme[15] on the relationship between global expenditures on arms and health.

In this eight-year-old table, the ratio of military and health-related expenditures is more important than the figures, especially since the expenditures on arms appear to be underestimates when compared to the detailed country-by-country estimates published by the Stockholm International Peace Research Institute (SIPRI) in its latest Yearbook;[12] some of these data are shown in Table 1–22.

The figures of Table 1–22 relate to 1980 prices and exchange rates; therefore, in terms of the situation of 1986 the last figure ($649 billion in U.S. dollars) comes pretty close to $1 trillion.[12] A rather interesting mathematical exercise would be to divide this figure by 5 billion, the expected global population next year. This exercise gives U.S.

TABLE 1–21.

Expenditures on Arms and Health*

EXPENDITURE	DEVELOPED COUNTRIES		DEVELOPING COUNTRIES	
	1970	1978	1970	1978
Military	312	345	70	102
Health	126	213	13	22

*Figures rounded to nearest billion in U.S. dollars.

TABLE 1–22.

World Military Expenditure At 1980 Prices and Exchange Rates*

YEAR	EXPENDITURES U.S. BILLION $ 1976
1976	514.0
1978	537.7
1980	564.4
1982	609.9
1984	649.1

*Adapted from SIPRI Yearbook 1985, London, Taylor and Francis, 1985.

TABLE 1–23.

Official Development Assistance From Some
OECD† Members as Percentage of Donor Gross
National Product (GNP)*

COUNTRY	YEAR		
	1975	1980	1984
Denmark	.58	.74	.85
Canada	.54	.43	.47
France	.62	.64	.77
Germany, Fed. Rep.	.40	.44	.45
Italy	.11	.17	.32
Japan	.23	.32	.35
The Netherlands	.75	1.03	1.02
Norway	.66	.85	.99
Sweden	.82	.79	.80
Switzerland	.19	.24	.30
United Kingdom	.39	.35	.33
United States	.27	.27	.23

*Adapted from the World Bank: *World Development Report 1985*. London, Oxford University Press, 1985.
†The Organization for Economic Cooperation and Development; member states are, in addition to those indicated in the table, Australia, Austria, Belgium, Finland, Greece, Iceland, Ireland, Luxembourg, New Zealand, Portugal, Spain and Turkey.

$200, a yearly sum, which in another world could have been spent to improve the quality of life of every human being living on this planet today.

Obviously, neither the entire world as such, nor the developed nations, spend so much money on assistance to developing countries. How much do they spend on it then? The development assistance of some of the "great spender" countries is shown in Table 1–23.

It can be seen that, in terms of gross national product (GNP), development assistance in 1984 varied between 0.23% (United States) and 1.02% (The Netherlands). These percentages correspond to approximately 8.7 and 1.3 billion U.S. dollars, respectively. For a comparison which may not be entirely fair, the two great champions of another "club," the OPEC (the Organization of Petroleum Exporting Countries), namely Saudi Arabia and Kuwait, provided development assistance in 1983 amounting to approximately 3.9 and 1.0 billion US dollars, corresponding to 3.5% and 4.5% of their GNP, respectively.

As Ludwig Wittgenstein states it, "logic is not a body of doctrine but a mirror-image of the world."[19] In logical terms the next question is almost inevitable: how much should, or could the countries spend on international assistance *under the present circumstances?* Answers to this question might be variable and not always logical, since they will depend on the value systems of each individual. However, two reflections appear to be appropriate in this context: The first is that, during the past decade, certain responsible governments considered it both justified and possible to spend five times more of their countries' GNP on development assistance than other responsible governments. Secondly, based on past performance, it is most impressive to see what WHO Special Programmes could achieve in a global perspective with modest yearly budgets of the order of 10–20 million U.S. dollars. A similarly organized Special Programme systematically addressing the problems of aging with special emphasis on the developing countries would not cost more and could achieve a great deal. How did Shakespeare say it? "Delays have dangerous ends."[11]

REFERENCES

1. Delegation of Sweden to the United Nations International Conference on Population, Mexico City, August, 1984. Statement by Ms. Gertrud Sigurdsen, Minister of Health.
2. Diczfalusy E: Contraceptive futurology, or 1984 in 1984. *Contraception* 1985; 31:1.
3. Diczfalusy E: Keynote address: Menopause and the developing world. Chapter 1, in Notelovitz M (ed): *The Climacteric In Perspective*. Lancaster, MTP Press, 1986.
4. Harrison: Description of Britain Pt. III, ch. iii, p. 99 (1577) cf. also J. Owen: Epigrams. Both quoted by the *Oxford Dictionary of Quotations*, ed. 2. London, 1953.
5. International Labour Office (ILO), Geneva: Population, Development, Family Welfare. The ILO's contribution, p 55 (ISBN 92-2-103874-2).
6. Mr. Muhammad Khan Junejo, Prime Minister of Pakistan: Speech delivered at the Centenary Silver Jubilee of the King Edward Medical College, Lahore, Dec 15, 1985, *The Pakistan Times,* Dec 15, 16, 1985.
7. Kalow W: Ethnic differences in drug metabolism. *Clin Pharmacokinet* 1982; 7:373. (AIDS Press Australasia Pty Ltd).
8. Montecuccoli R von: *Memorie della guerra.* 1703.
9. National Institutes of Health: *Osteoporosis*. Consensus Development Conferences Statement vol 5, no 3, 1984. (US Government Printing Office: 1984-421-132:4652).
10. Salas RM: *Population: The Mexico Conference and the Future.* Opening Address for the International Conference on Population, Mexico City, August 6, 1984. UNFPA/ICP/84/E/2500.
11. Shakespeare W: *King Henry VI*. Part I, III, ii, 33.
12. Stockholm International Peace Research Institute (SIPRI): *Armaments and Disarmament. SIPRI Yearbook*. London, Taylor and Francis, 1985.
13. Thomas DB: Do hormones cause breast cancer? *Cancer* 1984; 53:595.
14. United Nations: Report of the International Conference on Population, 1984. Mexico City, 6–14 August 1984. E/CONF. 76/19. United Nations Publication Sales No E.84.XIII.8.
15. United Nations Environment Programme (UNEP): The state of the Environment 1984: The Environment and the Dialogue between and among developed and developing countries, UNEP, Nairobi, Kenya.
16. United Nations Population Division: *World Population Prospects: Estimates and Projections as Assessed in 1982,* to be issued as a United Nations Publication; data reproduced in the Review and Appraisal of the World Population Plan of Action; Report of the Secretary General, United Nations International Conference on Population, Mexico City, August 1984; E/Conf. 76/4 Corr. 1.26, July 1984, pp 29–30.
17. United Nations World Assembly on Aging, Vienna, 1982: The Vienna International Plan of Action on Aging, 1982, paras 9 and 11. Cf. Swedish Ministry for Foreign Affairs: Förenta Nationernas åldrandekonferens i Wien 26 juli-6 augusti 1982. Norstedt Tryckeri, Stockholm, 1983.
18. Declaration of the United Nations Conference on the Human Environment and the Action Plan for the Human Environment, Stockholm, 1972.
19. Wittgenstein L: *Tractatus Logico-philosophicus*. London, Routledge & Kegan Paul Ltd, 1961, ISBN 0710079230.
20. *World Development Report 1984*. Published for the World Bank by Oxford University Press, London. ISBN 0-19-520459-X.
21. *World Development Report 1985*. Published for the World Bank by Oxford University Press, London. ISBN 0-19-520481-6.
22. World Health Organization: Research on the menopause. *Techn Rep Ser* 1981; 670. Geneva.
23. World Health Organization: *World Health Statistics Annual,* Geneva, 1983. ISBN 92-4-067831X.

PART I

Physiology of the Menopausal Period

CHAPTER 2

Demography

RUTH B. WEG, Ph.D.

THE MYSTERIES OF MENSTRUATION and its cessation, menopause, are the bases for much mythology concerning the reproductive cycle of women. Many cultures had taboos relating to the menstruating and menopausal woman, and some have added taboos concerning pregnant and child-bearing women.[85, 92]

Historically and currently, the human family is characterized among its primate relatives, and the million and more other animal species on earth, by one of the lowest reproductive rates. Human parents generally bestow resources, affection, and time on their young for life, which is not typical of the majority of mammalian species. Another human primate attribute held in common with few other animals (e.g., elephants, some carnivores, and possibly whales and dolphins) is the strong intergenerational, familial bond that remains past the sexual maturity of the offspring.

More than 200 years ago, Linnaeus identified the human species *(Homo sapiens)* accurately as a member of the primates. As early as 1963, T. H. Huxley regarded great apes as the closest relatives of human beings. But the discovery of which of the apes was the closest relative of all awaited the work of King and Wilson,[52] who found that the polygamous chimpanzee rather than the monogamous gibbon (who took a ''wife'' for life) was genetically and therefore biochemically more like people.

A significant departure of the female human being from most of her nonhuman primate relatives is the presence of a menstrual cycle rather than an estrous cycle. The gibbon female is also not subject to an estrous cycle and is sexually receptive at any time. In contrast to the obvious vulvar swelling of the female chimpanzees and gorillas that occurs immediately prior to ovulation as a sign of invitation to males, ovulation in the human female is masked to others, although marked by a variety of changes in body odors, sensory modalities, body temperature, and at times, mood and attitudes.[22, 23, 79, 98]

This ''loss of estrous'' led to the lack of easily recognizable external signs at mid-cycle and the accompanying potential for human sexual activity throughout the menstrual cycle. We are still attempting to answer the questions of why and when this shift in hominid evolution took place. There have been some who view the opportunity for continuous sexual activity (the menstrual cycle) as useful in monogamous pair bonding.[71] More recent studies indicate there is no support for the belief that monogamous mammals are more sexually active than other species with different mating habits.[55] Geneticists and sociobiologists have a different opinion for the development of monogamy: Under the harsh conditions of paleolithic times, both parents were needed to ensure the survival of the young, and the monogamously bonded pair were more likely to pass on their genes. Under more favorable conditions, when the mother's care of the young was sufficient, the males would be more promiscuous, again for the sake of propagation and survival of their genes.[99] The "when" in human history and evolution of the human menstrual cycle remains unanswered.

A variety of theories and suggestions have addressed the "why," but none yet is sufficiently well-documented to be acceptable as definitive "truth." It is logical to assume that in the human, the estrous cycle was gradually replaced by the menstrual cycle. This change greatly affected human female sexuality and the interaction between men and women.[93] There have been much interest and study regarding the mystical significance to many cultures of blood and, particularly, menstrual blood. Blood is central to birth and, often, to death. Early hominids saw blood as a vital force, developed magic rituals with blood, and made bloody sacrifices to their gods and spirits, as did specific cults of the dead.[85] Menstrual taboos developed because the biologic role of menstruation had been a frightening mystery until recent times. It is no surprise that menstrual blood became basic to the practice of alchemy, magic, and witchcraft through the 17th century and, in some parts of the world (e.g., Tibet), into more recent times.[5] Menstrual blood can be produced only by women, and it flows for days without causing weakness or death, which makes it a mysterious, impressive difference between men and women. Since it is generally agreed that women in prehistory and early human recorded history were pregnant most of the time, even the irregular and infrequent appearance of female menstruation was sufficient to uphold its power.

It became apparent that menarche was a sign of sexual maturity and a necessary prelude to bearing children. Moreover, menstrual bleeding was absent during pregnancy and therefore was perceived as a necessary contribution to the creation of new life. Puberty rites practiced by men of tribes in 20th-century central Australia and New Guinea involve bloodletting by "slitting the underside of the penis from the point nearest the scrotum, sometimes for as little as an inch, sometimes for almost its whole length."[85, 44] This attempt to capture the magic, vitalizing energy of female bleeding is often referred to as "men's menstruation." Those undergoing these puberty rites, like menstruating women, were ritually isolated from the remainder of the community during the bleeding.[94]

With age, a woman gradually, naturally surrenders her maternal productivity, and menstruation along with it. Although both men and women experience a climacteric, only the woman knows menopause—a definite point in the climacteric, marking the diminution of ovarian function, the permanent cessation of menstruation (for a minimum of 12 months), and a more drastic fall in the levels of the female sex hormones, estrogens and progesterone.[97] The human male may never lose his capacity for paternity, whatever his age, although the male sex hormones gradually diminish with the years, as does spermatogenesis.[56]

WHY MENOPAUSE?

Although it has generally been assumed that nonhuman animals maintain their reproductive capacity till death, there is now some evidence to counter this belief. The way of animal life in the wild, characterized by survival of the fittest, would likely result in death of the aging animal before menopause. Laboratory research data involving aging animals within the last 10–15 years has indicated reproductive aging symptoms similar to human reproductive aging. A colony of monkeys observed from 1935 to 1975 provided the basis for reports on the menstrual and reproductive histories of three monkeys, including accurate dates of birth.[89] Most frequently noted signs of reproductive aging in animals are reduced litter size and cessation of fetal production well before death.

The consensus appears to be that the mechanism in most species for lowered fertility is outside the ovary, since instances are cited in which cyclic ovarian behavior remains until death or close to death.[27, 48] For example, Finn[27] conjectures that the diminished litter size may be a function of inability of the blastocyst to implant, which in turn could result from age-related, heightened autoimmune response or changes in hormonal interactions and/or DNA. In most captive, aging animals, although fertility decreases or ceases, the reproductive cycling continues, since follicles appear to be present in most species examined. The cycling is species-specific, suggesting genetic determination.[48] It would appear that human menopause, as now known and described, is unique to the human female, despite some demonstrated similarities in the CBA mouse and rhesus monkey.[42, 48, 88, 89]

But why does human menopause happen? On Melville Island in Northern Australia, the Tiwi women believe that infrequency or cessation of sexual intercourse is the cause of menopause.[33] In contrast, Victorian sex manuals indicated that excessive expression of women's passion accounted for menopausal problems.[31] A teleologic explanation holds that the forces of evolution sought to protect the older human female from the hazards to "conceive and bear and raise children."[70(234)] Evolution, however, is rarely concerned with the individual but rather with the progeny of a species. The assumption is more likely that the tribe/species was benefited by the mandatory retirement of the female from reproduction and her continued presence to a healthy old age. The human female, among all other primates, had developed a way to further species survival independent of the womb—the evolution of menopause. These elder women became sources of experience and wisdom for handling the small and large crises of the tribe, especially in the care of the young. At best, "why menopause," is poorly answered scientifically at this time, but conjecture stimulates thinking and will continue to do so until new data accumulate to support theories.

ETIOLOGY OF MENOPAUSE

The most widespread statement on the etiology of menopause is simply ovarian failure. Menopause is that stage of loss of viable oocytes, numbering between 400,000–500,000 at birth, finally unresponsive to stimulation by pituitary gonadotropins (GnH). There is agreement that, during the reproductive years, the maturing female experiences a continuous diminution in the number of follicles, yet data on the exact number of oocytes at different ages are scanty.[88] Early studies have suggested that after the menopause, the ovary still contains some oocytes.[9, 10, 49, 68] Ultrastructure investigation of such follicles and oocytes reveal relatively normal appearance,[17] although they may be functionally abnormal.[41] Ovarian structural changes with age appear to coincide with endocrine changes: theca interna and granulosa cells, the sites of estrogen and progesterone synthesis, diminish, while stromal or interstitial cells, considered the source of androgens, increase in number and activity.[7, 78, 83]

There is continuing discussion that no one event, but a disruption of the complex of interacting biologic events, is involved in menopause. The negative feedback loop which organizes and maintains the cyclic menses includes the interaction of hypothalamus, anterior pituitary, and ovaries. Changes in function in any one of these could conceivably play a major role in the initiation of menopause. Yen[102] considers the primary alteration to be in the ovary, which demonstrates decreasing responsivity to stimulation by pituitary gonadotropins, leading to a further drop in estrogen levels. He notes that ovarian synthesis of estrogen has dropped to 40% of premenopausal rate in women 50–60 years old and to 20% in most women older than 65. Further, he suggests that, due to this decrease in estrogen negative feedback effect on the anterior pituitary, follicle stimulating hormone (FSH) levels increase to roughly ten times greater, and luteinizing hormone (LH) levels about four times greater, than those in younger women. This rise in production of LH and FSH is, in part, also a function of the hypothalamic response to diminished ovarian estrogen and progesterone as evidenced by the increased output of gonadotropin releasing hormones (GnRH). Since the ovaries appear unable to respond to this intense stimulus with a larger output of estrogens and/or progesterone, the result is a high level of circulating gonadotropins and a level of female sex hormones that is typically lower than it was during earlier reproductive years.[37]

Finch,[25] Weiner and Ganong[95] also emphasize the interrelationship between the brain and the endocrine system in the determination of the cause of menopause. The recurrent menstrual cycles are seen as evidence of the inhibitory and stimulatory effect of hypothalamic neurotransmitters, gonadotropins, and ovarian steroids. With the beginning of reproductive aging, cycles become irregular, unpredictable, and finally cease, reflecting a break in the earlier balanced hypothalamic pituitary-ovarian feedback system. As suggested, alterations in any part of that system could have consequences for further disorder and the end to productive cycling, e.g., loss of secretory cells, decrease in hormonal output of existing cells, reduced sensitivity to feedback control, and decline in neurotransmitter activity.[40] Some ovarian function is observable after menopause; there may be a small number of follicles, even occasional corpora lutea, and hyperplasia of interstitial and stromal cells.[72] The plasma estrone in older women is a result of the peripheral conversion of adrenal androstenedione and, to a lesser degree, of the postmenopausal ovaries.[74, 82, 90]

Although, as stated earlier, the involutionary changes in the ovary could easily be considered the cause of cessation of cycling, the alteration in responsivity of the ovary to the gonadotropin is a logical alternative explanation that is in keeping with research on aging that identifies reduced efficiency and number of hormone receptors in many target organs.[80] One study[73] did report an increase in urinary estrogens after stimulation with gonadotropin. More recent studies confirm the steady decrease in responsiveness of the perimenopausal ovary and the absence of ovarian response to gonadotropin in the postmenopausal period.[82, 90]

In contrast to this ovarian decline, the aging human anterior pituitary response to hypothalamic GnRH appears to be fairly intact. Although the postmenopausal pituitary response is not augmented, as reported by several investigators,[7, 58] there is an increased response to GnRH infusion, similar to that measurable during the midfollicular phase, which is characterized by relatively low circulating levels of gonadotropin and estrogens.[96]

There are studies that suggest the aging hypothalamus and pituitary do show changes in sensitivity to estrogen feedback. Some evidence can be interpreted to show that there is increased sensitivity; for example, doses of ethinyl estradiol that are too small to lower gonadotropin concentration in young women can lower the GnH level in postmenopausal women.[66] Other data indicate a decrease in this feedback sensitivity; for example, suppression of gonadotropin levels and ovulatory surges of LH can take place in postmenopausal women only after doses of estrogens that are higher than those used in oral contraceptives.[100]

In addition to the most common explanation for increased levels of·gonadotropin in older women as the absence of negative feedback resulting from lowered levels of ovarian sex hormones, some investigators have suggested that an "inhibin" substance for FSH is present in the ovary, since FSH level is markedly different from that of LH. The ovaries of younger women would normally secrete both estrogens and "inhibin" to control FSH concentration. However, in the postmenopausal woman, the very low levels or absence of both "inhibin" and estrogens permit a marked rise in FSH levels in excess of LH.[82]

There are ambiguous data regarding the positive feedback system in aging women. An increase in anovulatory cycles imply an impairment. Other studies demonstrate a delayed rebound effect or ovulatory-like surge of LH after large doses of estrogen or estrogen-progesten and indicate that, under particular circumstances, the postmenopausal positive feedback system is functioning adequately.[100]

A general characteristic of the aging human brain is some neuronal loss in several areas. There is no investigated evidence of such changes in the human estrogen-sensitive supraoptic and paraventricular nuclei.[12] Reports do indicate an increase with age in concentration of estrogen receptors in cases of mammary cancer, but whether alterations in the estrogen binding capacity of the human brain and pituitary occur with age is not known.[51] Despite reports of deficiencies in neurotransmitter activity with age, it is not certain that human reproductive aging is mediated by this decline.[25] In a recent study on the neuroendocrine/aging processes in female rodents, there is information that (1) there is an ovary-dependent neuroendocrine syndrome of aging, and (2) ovariectomy attentuates the complex steroid dependent neuroendocrine aging, but not steroid-independent neuroendocrine aging. Nevertheless, Finch et al[26] conclude for now that estradiol-induced neuroendocrine damage in human adults is less likely than in rodents. These data do suggest that this possibility may exist, and neuroendocrine study of human females who have different hormone treatment patterns after natural menopause or hysterectomy should be pursued.

As the details of the hypothalamic-pituitary ovarian (HPO) reproductive interdependencies are examined, many questions remain as to cause and effect in the etiology of menopause. The decreased sensitivity of the aging ovary, in combination with lowered concentrations of ovarian steroids, can mask other deficiencies of the HPO system, e.g., alterations in the negative and positive feedback action by gonadal steroid hormones.[40] Although inhibition (negative feedback) of pituitary gonadotropin release can be achieved in postmenopausal women, the threshold of response to estrogens generally seems to be increased. Combined with the declining levels of estrogen, the increased threshold could contribute to incomplete inhibition of gonadotropin secretion; the consequent high concentration of gonadotropin could conceivably overstimulate the ovary and possibly lead to a final exhaustion of its steroid synthesis and secretion capacity.[24] Whatever the initial cause, the ultimate question still remains: Is ovarian failure physiologic or pathologic?[88]

It appears reasonable that future studies must examine the transitional stages from full reproduction to menopause more carefully. In this way, it would be possible to investigate those periods when the neuroendocrine system is still optimally or fully functional. Moreover, the comparisons of the preclimacteric, climacteric, and postmenopausal HPO systems should be concerned with the neuroendocrine profile of women rather than their chronology.[40] Information is needed regarding the sensitivity of gonad-otropin and GnRH stimulation, the responsiveness of the negative as well as the positive feedback systems, and the changes in receptor activity during that time period. Emphasis on the declining rather than the nonfunctional reproductive/sexual system permits a picture of continuous aging changes in the reciprocal interactions between the brain and the endocrine glands. In understanding the consequences of a slight change in one aspect of the system on the altered function of another, which in turn further alters the first part, the mechanism involved may be elucidated.

WHEN MENOPAUSE?

The perimenopausal, menopausal, and postmenopausal women make up a relatively large number of the total population of the Western world. About a third of the entire female population is postmenopausal, and 25% are aged 44–55 years, potentially perimenopausal and postmenopausal.[61] Approximately 50 years is the current median age at menopause, though about 8% experience premature menopause before age 40. Preliminary estimates of these women in the American resident population by the Bureau of the Census (1984) indicate they are indeed present in significant numbers (Table 2–1).

Many past studies that purported to estimate the mean or median age at menopause,

TABLE 2–1.

Estimates of the U.S. Resident Population by Sex and Age (July 1, 1984, Bureau of Census)*†

AGE	TOTAL	FEMALE	MALE
all ages	236,158	121,393	114,765
under 5	17,816	8,702	9,115
5–9	16,351	7,984	8,367
10–14	17,567	8,573	8,994
15–19	18,768	9,216	9,551
20–24	21,311	10,626	10,684
25–29	21,309	10,694	10,615
30–34	19,602	9,887	9,715
35–39	16,812	8,535	8,278
40–44	13,836	7,052	6,784
45–49	11,417	5,847	5,570
50–54	11,013	5,694	5,319
55–59	11,449	6,037	5,412
60–64	10,867	5,805	5,062
65–69	9,300	5,133	4,168
70–74	7,446	4,296	3,150
75–79	5,369	3,288	2,081
80–84	3,251	2,123	1,128
85 +	2,674	1,902	772

*Adapted from *Current Population Reports*, Series P 25 #965, p 17, Estimates of the Population of the United States by Age, Sex, and Race: 1980–1984, U.S. Department of Commerce, Bureau of Census.
†Numbers in thousands; computations based on rounded numbers.

and the variables which may modify this age, have had methodologic differences and problems.[36, 2, 4, 47] Interpretations and generalizations drawn from these data are difficult to compare, since they are marked by "biases and memory errors resulting from retrospective interviews, the method of selection and size of sample under study, variations in the definitions of menopause and use of inappropriate statistical procedures."[36(25)] Women who are more than five years past menopause "consistently understate their age at menopause."[63, 66, 36(25)] This underestimation of age at menopause can be explained by the tendency for women to recall their age at last birthday, rather than exact menopausal age. The habit of numerous interviewees to round off their age to the nearest 0 or 5 has resulted in a higher reported incidence of menopause at 40, 45, and 50 years.

Recent data are more reliable, having overcome some of the aforementioned major difficulties by combining two methods. First, in a cross-sectional study approach, a determination of the menopausal status and the current age is made at the interview. Secondly, a longitudinal cohort design is used to follow a group of women over time until natural menopause occurs. Nevertheless, it is still possible with this paradigm to include more women who experience an early climacterium, so a risk remains of underestimating age at menopause.[36] Most of the more recent studies have used the median age rather than the arithmetic mean age at menopause; the former is that age which finds one half of the study sample already postmenopausal. It has been demonstrated that the use of the mean or average gives more weight to "wider scatter of observations at younger ages."[36(27)]

Since the mid 20th century, those who have studied the history of the age at menopause compare it frequently to menarche, which has demonstrated a natural history of secular change. Over the centuries, the age at menarche has shown a secular change, from 17 years in northern Europe around 1800 to the present age of 13. In the United States, menarche now occurs at an average age of 12.8, with a range of 9–18 years.[50] This gradual worldwide decline has become fairly stable for the past few decades. Despite the fact that the frequency of age of menopause since early Greek days has remained at approximately 50 years, the possibility of a secular change in age of menopause resulting in a gradually later age at menopause over time persists.[2, 4, 28, 31, 60] Thus far, the data are heavily on the side of no such secular change for menopause. Investigations also have pursued the potential effects of a series of environmental, situational variables, few of which appear to be significantly correlated with age at menopause.

Classical Period

Amundsen and Diers,[2] who summarized the classical sources concerned with age at menopause, found an age range between 40 and 50 and a maximum of 60 years, similar to current information (Table 2–2). They also cite Backman[5] and Frommer,[30] who concluded that age at menopause did undergo a secular change. Backman believed that menopause was reached at about 40 years in ancient times, approximately 45 years during 1500–1800, and finally increasing to 48 years. Frommer found an increase of four years in 19th-century Great Britain, reaching a median age of about 50 years. However, a number of other authors did not concur, pointing out that there were minimal data to defend this claim.[15, 14, 60]

The works of Aristotle (384–332 B.C.) and Hippocrates (460?–?377 B.C.) carry the

TABLE 2–2.

Summary of the Age of Menopause According to Classical Sources*

AUTHOR	CENTURY	AGE CITED		
		MINIMUM	AVERAGE	MAXIMUM
Aristotle	4th B.C.		40	50
Diocles	4th B.C.			60
Hippocratic Corpus	4th B.C.		42	
Pliny	1st A.D.		40	50
Soranus	1st/and A.D.		40–50	60
Oribasius	4th A.D.	35	50	60
Aëtius	6th A.D.	35	50	60
Paulus Aegineta	7th A.D.	35	50	60

*From Amundsen DW, Diers CJ: Age of menopause in classical Greece and Rome. *Human Biol* 1970; 42:79–86. Used by permission.

earliest references to age at menopause (as they did of menarche). Aristotle wrote in *Historia Animalium* (VII5, 585a):

"The menses cease in most women around the 40th year, and in those in whom it goes on longer the menses continue until the 50th year, and at this time some women of that age have borne children, but none beyond that age."

Pliny the Elder (1st century A.D.) mentioned menopause in *Historia Naturalis* (VII, XIV, 61): "A woman does not bear children after age of 50, and with the majority menstruation ceases at 40."

Oriabasius (4th century A.D.) reported a wider range in the age of menopause and a later average age (*Eclogae Medicamentorum,* 142): "The menses cease around the 50th year, very few menstruate until 60, and in some, especially those who are very fat, the menses begins to abate from the 35th year." He commented on the relationship of obesity to menarche and menopause. Enlarging on an earlier treatise by Rufus Medicus (2nd century A.D.) regarding puberty, Oriabasius concluded that girls of moderate weight attained puberty earlier than those who were either lean or fat. Fat women also generally stopped menstruation as early as 35. For the obese, there appeared to be a correlation between a later menarche and early menopause.

Aetius, a 6th century physician, generally supported Oriabasius. Aegineta, a 7th century medical compiler, used Oriabasius or a common source as bases for his discussion of age at menopause. Backman in his works used only Pliny and Aristotle as quotable resources and selectively concluded: "This little survey makes it therefore not entirely improbable that in classical antiquity menopause began about the 40th year."[5(459)] He went further in his interpretation of the works of the ancients and stated they believed that an early menarche was inevitably a prelude to an early menopause. These men of antiquity perceived rapid development as a predictor of a short life, contrary to Backman's earlier comment regarding obese women (late menarche, early menopause).

Medieval Period

In their investigation into the age at menopause in medieval Europe (from the 6th through the 15th centuries), Amundsen and Diers[4] again found that the most cited age was 50 years. As with the classical literature, menopausal studies were not as well documented as were those of menarche (Table 2–3). It is not surprising that such a

TABLE 2–3.

Summary of the Age at Menopause According to Medieval Sources*

		AGE CITED		
AUTHOR	CENTURY	MINIMUM	AVERAGE	MAXIMUM
Aëtius	6th	35	50	60
Paulus Aegineta	7th	35	50	60
"Trotula"	11th/12th	35	50	75
John Platearius the Younger	11th/12th		60†	
Copho I	11th/12th		60†	
Copho II	11th/12th		50†	
Hildegard	12th		50	60–80
Thomas of Cantimpre	13th		50	
Gilbertus Anglicus	13th		50	
Bartholomaeus Anglicus	13th		50†	
John of Gaddesden	14th	35	50	
Ortloff the Bavarian	15th		40–50	

*From Amundsen DW, Diers CJ: The age of menopause in medieval Europe. *Human Biol* 1973; 45:610.
†Reported in a context suggesting the lower limit warranting medical concern.

difference in data exists when the nature and significance of the two events during medieval times are noted. A number of factors contribute to this dearth of reliable data concerning menopausal age in medieval Europe (and even in early America): the high death rate, the differential significance of the two events, the heightened difficulty in remembering an event which no longer exists, and biased, inadequate statistical analyses.[4]

For a long period, age of menopause appeared to be of little concern to authors of medical subjects in Western Europe. Attention to this important event awaited the arrival of the medical school of Salerno.[53, 76] After reviewing several unpublished manuscripts of Tortula, a physician, probably a Salernitan, whose works have been dated from the late 11th or early 12th century, possibly the 13th century, Post[76] found the most noted age at menopause was 50 years. He also mentioned the range was from 35 to 75 years, and a greater frequency of ages over 50 were indicated in these manuscripts.

During the first half of the 12th century Hildegard of Bingen also cited the 50th year as that time for the lack of menses, with the exception of some women who were so healthy and strong that menses could continue to the 70th year. Another three authors from the 13th century are thought to have used classical commentary as major authorities: Thomas of Cantimpre said, "A woman conceives clear up to the 50th year." Gilbert Angelicus said, "The menses are naturally retained below the 12th year and above the fiftieth." To Bartholomaeus Anglicus, the menses were "generally from the 14th up to the 50th year."[4(609)]

In the 14th century John of Gaddesden wrote that the menses "are withheld naturally until 12 or 14 years and after 50, although in some cases they cease earlier, at 35, 40, or 45, according to the various natures of women."[76(87)] By the 15th century, the age at menopause had not varied, and Ortloff of Bavaria described the span of menses as that which "comes to women who are over 12 years and continues to the fortieth year or to the fiftieth."[4(609)] Laslett[57(223)] has argued that Tortula's comments deserve little credence, since he used the humoral theory (now considered unscientific and ancient ignorance) to describe menstruation "until the 50th year if the woman is thin; until 60 or 65 or 55 if she is moist; until 35 if moderately fat." Post[76] did note these apparent "tales" may have been due to the few number of cases considered.

Amundsen and Diers[4] conclude that, despite such questionable approaches, the various observations of age at menopause among medieval authors "ought not be labeled as absurdities."[4(610)] It is worthwhile noting that the ages in Table 2–3 indicate the range in age at menopause (no one age was chosen), and the possible correlation between body build and menopausal age is still of interest to some investigators.[4, 45]

Twentieth Century Age at Menopause: Factors of Potential Influence

Selected studies are referred to repeatedly in various sources, and these appear to be minimally distorted by the biases and primitive statistical analyses mentioned earlier. What is most noteworthy is the consistency of age estimates at menopause for Caucasian women: from the median age of 50.78 in Britain[63] to 49.8 years in the United States[87, 36] (Table 2–4).

TABLE 2–4.

Estimates of the Age at Menopause from Selected Studies*

COUNTRY AND YEAR OF STUDY	RACE	MEAN OR MEDIAN AGE AT MENOPAUSE IN YEARS		TYPE OF STUDY	SOURCE
Scotland 1970	White	50.1	median	Cross sectional	Thompson et al. (1973)
England 1965	White	50.78	median	Cross sectional	McKinlay et al. (1972)
		47.49	mean		
England 1951–61	White	49.82	median	Cross sectional	Frommer (1964)
U.S.A. 1934–74	White	†49.8	median	Cohort	Treloar (1974)
		49.5	mean		
U.S.A. 1966	White	50.02	median	Cross sectional	MacMahon (1966)
	Negro	49.31	median		
	Both races	49.8	median		
Germany 1972	White	49.06	mean	Retrospective	Hofmann et al. (1972)
Finland 1961	White	49.8	mean	Retrospective	Hauser et al. (1961)
Switzerland 1961	White	49.8	mean	Retrospective	Hauser et al. (1961)
Israel 1963	White	49.5	mean	Retrospective	Hauser et al. (1963)
Netherlands 1969	White	51.4	median	Cross sectional	Jaszmann et al. (1969)
New Zealand 1967	White	50.7	median	Cross sectional	Burch et al. (1967)
South Africa 1971	White	50.4	median	Cross sectional	Frere (1971)
	Negro	49.7	median		
South Africa 1960	Negro	48.1	median	Retrospective	Abramson et al. (1960)
		47.7	mean		
South Africa 1960	White	48.7	mean	Retrospective	Benjamin (1960)
Punjab 1966	Asian	44.0	median	Cohort and cross sectional	Wyon (1966)
New Guinea 1973	Melanesian (nonmalnourished)	‡47.3	median	Cross sectional	Scragg (1973)
	(malnourished)	43.6	median		

*From Gray RH: The menopause—Epidemiological and demographic considerations, in Beard RJ (ed): *The Menopause*. Baltimore, University Park Press, 1976, p 28.
†Median estimates calculated by Gray RH.
‡Median estimates calculated by Dr. J. C. Barrett.

There is a difference between median and mean estimates of age at menopause. Median estimates are higher than mean estimates in cross-sectional or cohort investigations; this is not the case in earlier retrospective studies. For example, the mean ages at menopause range from 49.8 years in Switzerland and Finland[38] to 48.7 years among white South Africans.[8] The median age at menopause in industrialized societies is approximately 50 years—not unlike that described in the classical and medieval ages, with little change throughout recorded history.[88, 36, 31] This appears to imply the possibility of some internal clock, a message in the genes of the human family, similar to what has been found in captive animals who maintain a species-specific reproductive cycle (though fertility ceases) until near death.[48]

However, for the non-European women, the median age at menopause tends to be lower. A median age range has been reported from 49.7 years among the Bantu women in South Africa[29] to 43.6 years among women in New Guinea who have low nutritional status. A probit analysis of South African black women produced a median age of 50.70 years.[29] The probit method calculates the proportion of menopausal women at any particular age without knowing the age of menopause of any of the women under study. Frommer[30] also used the probit transformation and found modal and median age to be 50.1 years. Scragg[81] gives mean estimates of these same groups of approximately 47.7 years.

It is noteworthy that investigations of variables that may influence the age of menarche have been more carefully and intensively studied than those that may influence when menopause arrives. It is probable that any factor that has affected the reproductive history of the woman is a potential modifier of age at menopause. Most studies related to menopause have been retrospective, with all the difficulties inherent in that approach.

Some researchers suggest a possible relationship between heredity and age at menopause, e.g., the consistency of age estimates at menopause for white women.[63, 87] But the lack of twin, sister, or mother-daughter studies leave little control study proof for support.[28] Authors have noted familial patterns in menopausal age that are suggestive of genetic predetermination.[19, 35, 62, 75, 91] However, until longitudinal studies are undertaken with different generations and cultures, results to date cannot be considered unquestionably genetically based.

Ethnic differences cannot be compared with any validity, since the majority of the surveys used varied methods. However, two surveys that suggest the importance of an environmental variable did include different ethnic peoples in the same sample. One South African study found the median age at menopause was significantly lower among Bantu women as compared to the white women.[29] An American investigation supported this finding, although the results were not statistically significant: black women had a lower median age at menopause than white women.[29] Very low median ages, noted in the New Guinea and Punjabi work, point to poor nutrition as a probable cause of premature menopause.[81, 101] One group of New Guinea women with a median age of 43.6 years, mean height of 144.5 cm, and mean weight of 40.22 kg were found to have experienced severe and prolonged malnutrition. Another New Guinea sample with a higher median age at menopause of 47.3 years were better nourished, with a mean height of 153.8 cm and mean weight of 51.14 kg.

Both modern American studies and medieval records also make note of earlier menopause for thinner females.[60, 4] In well nourished samples of women in a number of studies, there was no correlation between age of menarche and age of menopause.[8, 38, 45, 63, 87] It is not unexpected that a significant decrease in the reproductive life span is positively correlated with serious malnutrition, since there are continuing reports of a negative correlation between age of menarche and menopause with poor nutrition.[36, 67, 81] Ethnicity has importance to the degree that poverty, lack of education, and malnutrition are more common among some ethnic groups than others.

The effect of parity on age of menopause remains ambiguous. Their interaction is complex and muddied with other intervening variables. Two studies have shown no correlation between menopausal age and childbearing.[45, 69] But British and Mexican surveys have presented data that are difficult to interpret: they found a positive correlation between later menopause and higher parity in women of upper socioeconomic status, but not so with women of lower socioeconomic status.[63, 84] Only one study in Israel looked at the relationship between the number of abortions and menopausal age.[77] There was a direct correlation—an earlier menopause as the number of abortions increased. More research is necessary in view of the present escalation of legal abortions cross culturally.

Marital status has been reported to have relatively inconsistent effects on age of menopause. Some evidence has been presented that age at menopause may be lower in nulliparous women.[8, 39] Some investigations have noted a younger age at menopause among unmarried women, although these data are frequently contradictory from one study to another.[45, 63]

Inconclusive evidence has been presented concerning the relation of disease and age at menopause. Generally noted is a delay of menopause in women with carcinoma of the uterus, breast, uterine fibroids, and diabetes.[39, 91]

The oral contraceptive pill has been in wide use for approximately 35 years, and this may not yet be enough time to determine the definitive, long-term influence on natural menopause. However, large numbers of women who were in their late 20s and 30s in the 1960s are approaching menopausal age, making this an appropriate time to implement study with adequate control groups to examine the effects of the pill on early and late menopause. There is no agreement that age at menopause is a function of the maturation and discharge of all eggs in the aging ovaries.[62, 17] The pill prevents ovulation and maintains monthly menses, so that its use may mask the initiation of menopause. No evidence exists yet that the pill will, in fact, delay the physiologic onset of menopause.

There is one environmental effect, cigarette smoking, that may play a critical role: "Smokers as a group have an earlier, natural menopause than nonsmokers."[47(1355),59] The Jick, Porter and Morrison data were a result of two large independent investigations designed and analyzed by the Boston Collaborative Drug Surveillance Program: the first included a 1972 survey of patients in 24 Boston area hospitals (1973); the second study used data from ongoing hospital monitoring of about 32,000 medical patients in seven countries.[46] The positive correlation found was very similar in the United States and other countries. For any given age, heavy smokers can expect to have a decreased age of menopause. Though the mechanism remains unelucidated, two theories have proposed that (1) liver enzymes induced by cigarette smoke may also affect steroid hormone metabolism and (2) the neuroendocrine system is affected directly by nicotine.[34]

Only one other factor has not been studied since the 1930s: climate. This was probably because the investigations to that time gave little evidence for any correlation.[21, 54] Of all the climatic variables, only altitude has been looked at more recently.[20, 28] Flint found a 1.5-year acceleration of menopausal age at 2,283 meters, 47.3 years as compared with 48.9 years for women living at 300 meters. Cruz-Coke found a similar result (a one-year acceleration) in a study of Chilean women living at 3,000 meters and over as compared to those living below 1,000 meters. These results may be a function of the lowered oxygen pressure at higher altitudes, and they are similar to the findings of Fusancha and Baker[32] of a later menarche among Quechua females living at high altitudes.

MacMahon and Worcester[60] have concluded that the multiple factors studied—socioeconomic conditions, race, marital status, income, geography, parity, height and skinfold thickness—appear to have little influence on age at menopause.

It is conceivable that a host of socioeconomic factors may be indirectly involved in the timing of menopause, since socioeconomic status has been demonstrated to influence education, nutrition, and health. A high standard of living could possibly moderate the incidence of disease and possibly the rate of aging, and so postpone the age at menopause.

SUMMARY

The reproductive and sexual behavior and histories of women have been topics of mystery, cultural rituals, taboos, and conjecture from ancient times forward. Recent scientific hypotheses and studies contribute to an increasingly realistic, but still incomplete, picture of the human female's menstrual and menopausal patterns.

In spite of the long-term concern and suppositions of ancient, medieval, contemporary philosophers, physicians, and scientists, many important questions remain essentially unanswered by contradictory, conflicting data. "When" the human female departed from other primate estrous cycles to the menstrual cycle is largely a guesstimate. Investigations into the "why" of menopause has thus far produced inadequate, unreliable data that do not identify the particular mechanisms involved in the hypothalamic-pituitary-ovarian interactions that are responsible for the human menopause. These include the reciprocal effects of the aging ovary, its steroids and neuroendocrine aging on the timing and course of menopause.

One prospective longitudinal study begun in the 1920s appears to have proven that age at menopause has no relationship to the age of menarche: women who reached menopause at 50 years included those with menarches at various ages.[87] A group of freshman coeds with documented menarches were followed for 40 years through menopause to the present, and no correlation was found. By considering a woman postmenopausal only after two calendar years had passed without menstruation, the errors of anomalous interruptions of menstruation were minimized.

Although some investigators believe that age of menopause is being achieved somewhat later, the secular trend typical of the menarche over the last 100 years has not yet been demonstrated for the age at menopause. The increase in the life expectancy of women (about 31 years since the turn of the century) makes it more feasible to explore a menopausal secular trend, if it exists, with longitudinal cross-cultural studies. Similar investigations to Treolar's[87] are necessary to confirm his conclusion.

What is striking about the comparison of age at menopause from the classical period through the present is the most frequent mention of the age of 50 years. In each period, classical (ancient), medieval, and modern, a range exists, but 50 years remains the mode. In spite of discussed methodologic problems and differences among all attempts to discover a specific age of menopause, current sophisticated, analytical studies also demonstrate a range, but a median (especially for white women) close to 50 years.

The primary difference between age at menopause in classical Greece and Rome and that of today's industrialized nations is that women in ancient times did not usually live beyond fertility to menopause. Contemporary women in America are living longer, and a much greater number are surviving to and beyond menopause (see Table 2–1). Budoff reported that in 1983 about 40 million women in the United States were postmenopausal, with an average age at menopause of approximately 51.4 years.[13] This similar median age at menopause from ancient times to the present is suggestive of a species program, a built-in genetic plan, and the range is a reflection of the multiple environmental factors that can modify the genetic potential.

Of other specific variables (race, familial patterns, parity, marital status, disease, altitude) studied for possible influence on age at menopause, relatively few have been demonstrated as statistically significant. Socioeconomic variables can reasonably be perceived to influence age of menopause indirectly through their effect on education, overall health status, and nutrition.

Some evidence, although not consistent, has been presented that marital status and parity could be factors in age at menopause, independent of one another. The same variables undoubtedly affect the total experience of menopause, regardless of age. Only two of the factors carefully investigated appear to play a significant part in the determination of age at menopause: altitude and cigarette smoking. Higher altitudes were found to accelerate menopausal age. More heavy smokers can expect to be postmenopausal at any given age as compared to nonsmokers.

A new 20th century biologic intervention, the oral contraceptive pill, has not been explored for its short- and long-term effects on age and/or experience of natural menopause. Now, all that can be said is that the pill masks the superficial recognition of menopause. The possible delay of menopause which has been suggested must be studied as part of a prospective longitudinal, biochemical investigation of the changes during the transitions between peri-, menopausal, and postmenopausal stages.

Because of the worldwide and historical repetition of the age of 50 years as the modal age of menopause, the importance of a genetic program is persuasive. The ranges found from the late 30s to the middle and later 50s or beyond address the environmental variables unique to various cultures, countries, eras, and individuals.

CONCLUSIONS

1. The median age at menopause throughout recorded history appears to have changed very little and hovers around 50 years of age (plus or minus 10–15 years). There is no reasonable way to escape the significance of genetic input.

2. Students of the reproductive history of the human female over the centuries have produced methodologically biased and inappropriately analyzed data. Current efforts have eliminated some of the barriers to valid, reproducible, statistically sound information.

3. There is considerable agreement that the use of the median age at menopause is a more reliable measure than the average or mean.

4. Many studies of potential influential factors for age at menopause have suffered from the lack of control groups, inadequate analysis, and retrospective approach. A few have provided reasonable and testable conclusions. One factor, the use of the contraceptive pill, has finally been present long enough to be seriously studied for its real effects, if any, on age at menopause.

5. Anthropologic support of the human female's shift from the estrous of other primates to menstrual cycles is of historical value, but not significant to the present issues of concern.

6. The etiology of menopause and the consequent course of this stage in the climacteric is under serious investigation in the continuing elucidation of the hypothalamic-pituitary-gonadal interaction throughout the human female's reproductive/sexual life.

7. A review of past and ongoing research can only leave us with the conclusion that what is urgently required are prospective, longitudinal, cross-cultural studies with adequate control groups. Further, the biases and ignorance of early history must be put in perspective, so that inquiries are undertaken without prior assumptions and conclusions that have resulted in false prophesies.

REFERENCES

1. Abramson JH, Gampel B, Slome C, et al: Age at menopause of urban Zulu women. *Science* 1960; 132:356.
2. Amundsen DW, Diers CJ: The age of menopause in classical Greece and Rome. *Human Biol* 1970; 42:79.
3. Amundsen DW, Diers CJ: The age of menarche in medieval Europe. *Human Biol* 1973a; 45:363.
4. Amundsen DW, Diers CJ: The age of menopause in medieval Europe. *Human Biol* 1973b; 45:605.
5. Backman von G: Die beschlanigte entwicklund der jugend. *Acta Anat* 1948; 4:421.
6. Beckett AH, Triggs EJ: Enzyme induction in man caused by smoking. *Nature* 1967; 216:587.
7. Ben-David M, van Look PFA: Hypothalamic-pituitary-ovarian relationships around the menopause, in van Keep PA, Serr DM, Greenblatt RB (eds): *Female and Male Climacteric: Current Opinion, 1978*. Proceedings of the 2nd International Congress on the Menopause, Jerusaleum, 1978. Baltimore, University Park Press, 1979.
8. Benjamin F: The age of the menarche and of the menopause in white Southern African women and certain factors influencing these times. *S Afr Med J* 1960; 34:316.
9. Bloch E: Quantitative morphological investigations of the follicular system in women. Variations at different ages. *Acta Anat (Basel)* 1952; 14:108.
10. Bloch E: A quantitative morphological investigation of the follicular system in newborn female infants. *Acta Anat (Basel)* 1953; 17:201.
11. Boston Collaborative Drug Surveillance Program: *Lancet* 1973; 1:1399.
12. Brody J, Vijayashankar N: Anatomical changes in the nervous system, in Finch CE, Hayflick L (eds): *The Handbook of the Biology of Aging*. New York, Van Nostrand Reinhold Co, 1977, pp 241–261.
13. Budoff PW: *No More Hot Flashes*. New York, Putnam & Sons, 1983.
14. Burch PRJ, Gunz FW: The distribution of the menopausal age in New Zealand. An exploratory study. *NZ Med J* 1967; 66:6.
15. Burch PRJ, Powell NR: Menarche and menopause. *Lancet* 1963; 2:784.
16. Conney AH, Jacobson M, Schneiderman K, et al: Induction of liver microsomal cortisol 68-hydroxylase by diphenylhydantoin, or phenobarbital: An explanation for the increased excretion of 6-hydroxycortisol in humans treated with these drugs. *Life Sci* 1965; 4:1091.
17. Costoff A: An ultrastructural study of ovarian changes in the menopause, in Greenblatt RB, Mahesh UB, McDonough PG (eds): *The Menopausal Syndrome*. New York, Medcom, 1974, p 12.
18. Costoff A, Mahesh V: Primordial follicles with normal oocytes in the ovaries of postmenopausal women. *J Am Geriatr Soc* 1975; 23:93.
19. Cruz-Coke R: Genetic characteristics of high altitude in Chile. Paper presented at the Meeting of Investigators on Population Biology of Altitude. Washington, D.C., November 13–17, 1967.
20. Curjel D: The reproductive life of Indian women. *Indian J Med Res* 1920; 8:366.
21. Currier A: *The Menopause* New York, D. Appleton & Co, 1897.

22. Diamond M, Diamond AL, Mast M: Visual sensitivity and sexual arousal levels during the menstrual cycle. *J Nerv Ment Disease* 1972; 155:170.

23. Doty RL: Olfactory communications in humans. *Chem Senses* 1981; 6:351.

24. Everitt AV: The hypothalamic pituitary control of aging and age-related pathology. *Exp Gerontol* 1973; 8:265–277.

25. Finch CE: Neuroendocrine mechanisms and aging. *Fed Proc* 1979; 38:178.

26. Finch CE, Felicio LS, Mobbs CV, et al: Ovarian and steroidal influences on neuroendocrine aging processes in female rodents. *Endocr Rev* 1984; 5:467.

27. Finn CA: Investigations into reproductive aging in experimental animals, in Beard RD (ed): *The Menopause*. Lancester, MTP Press, 1976, pp 1–23.

28. Flint M: Cross cultural factors that affect age of menopause, in VanKeep PA, Greenblatt RB, Albeaux-Fernet M (eds): *Consensus on Menopause Research*. Baltimore, University Park Press, 1976, pp 73–83.

29. Frere G: Mean age at menopause and menarche in South Africa. *S Afr J Med Sci* 1971; 36:21.

30. Frommer DJ: Changing age at the menopause. *Br Med J* 1964; 2:349.

31. Fuchs E: *The Second Season: Life, Love and Sex—Women in the Middle Years*. Garden City, NY, Anchor Press, Doubleday, 1977.

32. Fusancha A, Baker P: Attitude and growth: A study of pattern of growth of a high altitude Peruvian Quechua population. *Am J Phys Anthropol* 1970; 32:279.

33. Goodale JC: *Tiwi Wives*. Seattle, University of Washington Press, 1971.

34. Goodman LS, Gilman A: *The Pharmacological Basis of Therapeutics*. New York, Mac-Millan Publishing Co, 1975.

35. Gould H, Gould M: Age at first menstruation in mothers and daughters. *JAMA* 1932; 98:1349.

36. Gray RH: The menopause-epidemiological and demographic considerations, in Beard RJ (ed): *The Menopause*. Baltimore, University Park Press, 1976, pp 25–40.

37. Greenblatt RB, College ML, Mahesh VB: Ovarian and adrenal steroid production in the postmenopausal woman. *Obstet Gynecol* 1976; 47:383.

38. Hauser GA, Oribi JA, Valaer M, et al: Der einfluss des menarchealters auf des menopausealter. *Gynaecologia* 1961; 152:279.

39. Hauser GA, Remen U, Valaer M, et al: Menarche and menopause in Israel. *Gynaecologia* 1963; 155:39.

40. Henrik E: Neuroendocrine mechanisms of reproductive aging in women and female rats, in Voda AN, Dinnerstein M, O'Donnell SR (eds): *Changing Perspectives on Menopause*. Austin, University of Texas Press, 1982, pp 100–123.

41. Hertig AT: The aging ovary. *J Clin Endocrinol Metab* 1944; 4:581.

42. Hodgen GD, Goodman AL, O'Conner A, et al: Menopause in rhesus monkeys. Model for study of disorders in human climacteric. *Am J Obstet Gynecol* 1977; 127:581.

43. Hofmann D, Soergel T: Studies on age of the menarche and the age of menopause. Geburtshilfe Frauenheilkd 1972; 32:969.

44. Huxley TH: *Evidence as to Man's Place in Nature*. London, Williams & Norgate, 1863.

45. Jaszmann L, van Lith NO, Zaat JCA: The age at menopause in the Netherlands—the statistical analysis of a survey. *Int J Fertil* 1969; 14:106.

46. Jick H, Mietlinen OS, Shapiro S, et al: *JAMA* 1970; 213:1455.

47. Jick H, Porter J, Morrison AS: Relation between smoking and age of natural menopause. *Lancet* 1977; 1:1354.

48. Jones EC: The post reproductive phase in mammals, in *Estrogens in the Postmenopause Front. Horm Res* 1975; 3:1.

49. Jones EC, Krohn PL: The relationship between age, number of oocytes and fertility in virgin and nulliparous mice. *J Endocrinol* 1961; 21:469.

50. Katchadourian HA: *Fundamentals of Human Sexuality,* ed 4. New York, Holt, Rinehart & Winston, 1985.

51. Kaye AM: Oestrogen and Progesterone Receptors, in van Keep PA, Serr DM, Greenblatt RB (eds): *Female and Male Climacteric: Current Opinion 1978*. Proceedings of the 2nd International Congress on the Menopause, Jerusalem 1978. Baltimore, University Park Press, 1979.

52. King MC, Wilson AC: Evolution at two levels in humans and chimpanzees. *Science* 1975; 188:107.
53. Kirsteller PO: The school of Salerno. *Bulletin History of Med* 1945; 17:138.
54. Kirsch EH: *The Sexual Life of Women and the Physiological and Hygienic Aspects* (translated from German by N. Paul). New York, Allied Book Co, 1928.
55. Kleiman DG: Monogamy in mammals. *Q Rev Biol* 1977; 52:39.
56. Kolodny RC, Masters WH, Johnson VE: *Textbook of Sexual Medicine*. Boston, Little, Brown & Co, 1979.
57. Laslett P: Age at menarche in Europe since the eighteenth century. *J Interdisciplinary History* 1971; 2:221.
58. Lazarus L, Eastman CJ: Assessment of Hypothalamic Pituitary Function in Old Age, in Everitt AV, Burgess JA (eds): *Hypothalamus, Pituitary and Aging*. Springfield, Ill, Charles C Thomas, 1976.
59. Linquist O, Bengtsson C: The effect of smoking on menopausal age. *Maturitas* 1979; 1:171.
60. MacMahon B, Worcester J: Age at menopause U.S. 1960–62. *Vital Health Stat* 1966; 11:1.
61. McArthur JW: The contemporary menopause. *Primary Care* 1981; 8:141.
62. McCary J: *Sexual Myths and Fallacies*. New York, Van Nostrand Reinhold Co, 1973.
63. McKinlay S, Jeffreys M, Thompson B: An investigation of the age at menopause. *J Biosoc Sci* 1972; 4:161.
64. McKinlay S, Jeffreys M, Thompson B: An investigation of the age at menopause. *Br J Prev Soc Med* 1974; 28:16.
65. McKinlay S, McKinlay J: Selected studies on the menopause. *J Biosoc Sci* 1973; 5:533.
66. Mahesh VB: Gonadotrophins in the menopause, in van Keep PA, Greenblatt RB, Albeaux-Fernet M (eds): *Consensus on Menopause Research: A Summary of International Opinion*. Proceedings of 1st International Congress on the Menopause, La Grande Motte, France, 1976. Baltimore, University Park Press, 1976.
67. Malcolm LA: Growth and development in New Guinea—a study of the Bundi people of the Madang District. Institute of Human Biology, *Papua-New Guinea Monograph Series* 1970; 1:51.
68. Mandl AM, Shelton M: A quantitative study of oocytes in young and old nulliparous rats. *J Endocrinol* 1959; 18:444.
69. Masters WH, Johnson VE: *Human Sexual Response*. London, Churchill, 1966.
70. Morgan E: *The Descent of Woman*. New York, Stein & Day, 1972.
71. Morris D: *The Naked Ape: A Zoölogist's Study of the Human Animal*. New York, McGraw Hill, 1967.
72. Novak ER: Ovulation after fifty. *Obstet Gynecol* 1970; 36:903.
73. Paulson CA, Leach RB, Sandberg H, et al: Function of the postmenopausal ovary urinary estrogen excretion and the response to administered FSH. *J Clin Endocrinol* 1955; 15:846.
74. Peters H: The Aging Ovary, in van Keep PA, Serr DM, Greenblatt RB, et al (eds): *Female and Male Climacteric: Current Opinion 1978*. Proceedings of the 2nd International Congress on the Menopause, Jerusalem, 1978. Baltimore, University Park Press, 1979.
75. Popenhoe P: Inheritance of age of onset of menstruation. *Eugen News* 1928; 13:101.
76. Post JB: Ages at menarche and menopause: Some medieval authorities. *Popul Stud* 1971; 25:83.
77. Pumpianski R: Age at natural menopause. *Harefuah* 1967; 77:513.
78. Rice BV, Savard K: Steroid hormone formation in the ovary. *J Clin Endocrinol* 1966; 26:593.
79. Robinson JE, Short RV: Changes in breast sensitivity at puberty, during the menstrual cycle, and at parturition. *Br Med J* 1977; 1:1188.
80. Roth GS: Altered Biochemical Responsiveness and Hormone Receptor Changes During Aging, in Behnke JA, Finch CE, Moment GB (eds): *The Biology of Aging*. New York, Plenum Press, 1978, pp 291–300.
81. Scragg RFR: Menopause and reproductive span in rural Niugini. Presented at the Annual Symposium of the Papua New Guinea Medical Society, Port Moresby, 1973, p 126.
82. Sherman BM, West JH, Korenman SG: The menopausal transition: Analysis of LH, FSH, estradiol and progesterone concentrations during menstrual cycles of older women. *J Clin Endocrinol Metab* 1976; 42:629.

83. Smith OW, Ryan KJ: Estrogen in human ovary. *Am J Obstet Gynecol* 1962; 84:141.
84. Soberon J, Calderon JJ, Goldzieher JW: Relation of parity to age at menopause. *Am J Obstet Gynecol* 1966; 96:96.
85. Tannahill R: *Sex in History.* New York, Stein & Day, 1980.
86. Thompson B, Hart SA, Durno D: Menopausal age and symptomatology in a general practice. *J Biosoc Sci* 1973; 5:71.
87. Treolar AE: Menarche, menopause and intervening fecundability. *Human Biol* 1974; 46:89.
88. Utian WH: *Menopause in Modern Perspective.* New York, Appleton-Century Crofts, 1980.
89. van Wagen G: Vital statistics from a breeding colony. *J Med Primatol* 1972; 1:3.
90. Vermeulen A: The hormonal activity of the postmenopausal ovary. *J Clin Endocrinol Metabolism* 1976; 42:247,253.
91. Way S: The aetiology of carcinoma of the body of the uterus. *J Obstet Gynecol Br Emp* 1954; 61:46.
92. Weber C: Menopause: An older woman's view, in Little VC (ed): *The Older Woman.* (a collection of papers for a new course). Storrs, CT, University of Connecticut, 1980.
93. Weg RB: Introduction: Beyond intercourse and orgasm, in Weg RB (ed): *Sexuality in the Later Years: Roles and Behavior.* New York, Academic Press, 1983, pp 1–10.
94. Weideger P: *Menstruation and Menopause.* New York, Knopf, 1976.
95. Weiner RF, Ganong WF: Role of brain monoamines and histamine in regulation of anterior pituitary secretion. *Physiol Rev* 1978; 58:905.
96. Wentz AC, Jones GS, Rocco L: Gonadotropin responses following luteinizing hormone-releasing hormone administration in normal subjects. *Obstet Gynecol* 1975; 45:239.
97. WHO scientific group on research on the menopause: Research on the menopause. WHO Technical Report #670, 1981, pp 7–119.
98. Wilcoxon LA, Schrader SL, Sherif CW: Daily self reports on activities, life events, moods and somatic changes during the menstrual cycle. *Psychosomatic Med* 1976; 38:399.
99. Wilson EO: *Sociobiology: The New Synthesis.* Cambridge, Mass, Belknap Press of Harvard University Press, 1975.
100. Wise AJ, Gross MA, Schalch DS: Quantitative relationships of the pituitary-gonadal axis in postmenopausal women. *J Lab Clin Med* 1973; 81:28.
101. Wyon JB, Finner SL, Gordon JE: Differential age at menopause in the rural Punjab, India. *Popul Index* 1966; 32:328.
102. Yen SSC: The biology of menopause. *J Reprod Med* 1977; 18:287.

CHAPTER 3

Endocrinologic and Menstrual Alterations

BARRY M. SHERMAN, M.D.

THE MENOPAUSE is usually defined as that time when a woman ceases menstruation, an event that occurs around the age of 50 years in most women. The menopause is a dramatic expression of irreversible changes in both the reproductive and hormonal function of the ovary. The relatively abrupt onset of the menopause contrasts with the fact that it is the consequence of a gradual process that begins during the embryologic development of the ovary.

Follicular maturation that leads to ovulation and, on occasion, to fertilization and pregnancy is the dominant function of the ovary from the viewpoint of its importance to the maintenance of the species and the biologic development of the individual. Between menarche and menopause, the average woman undergoes about 400 ovulatory cycles. This represents a very small percentage of the several million oocytes present around the 20th week of fetal development or the 700,000 preantral follicles and oocytes present at birth.[1] The vast number of follicles degenerate, in a process referred to as atresia. Atresia is the exclusive outcome of the follicular development that goes on during fetal life and childhood, so that at puberty only about 400,000 oocytes remain. During the reproductive years, only one of a cohort of follicles that is recruited during each cycle progresses through the full process of maturation and goes on to ovulation. The rest undergo atresia. The morphologic features that accompany atresia have been well described, but its biochemical basis remains poorly understood. Regulation of atresia is probably related to the interaction of hormones and growth factors within the ovarian micro environment.[2, 3]

In a sense, atresia, not ovulation, is the dominant process in the ovary, and the menopause is due to atresia rather than to the loss of ovarian follicular elements due to ovulation. This is probably the reason that the age of menopause occurs over a rather narrow age span and is uninfluenced by prolonged periods of hypothalamic amenorrhea, suppression of ovulation by oral contraceptives, or number of pregnancies.

Morphologically, the menopausal ovary is somewhat smaller than that found during midreproductive life and may be irregular in shape. A few primordial follicles may be found for several years after cessation of menses. These residual follicles are often histologically abnormal. The stromal elements of the ovary predominate but cytologic studies indicate they have low steroidogenic activity.

The hormonal contribution of the ovary changes with both its functional state and with age. The measurement of hormone concentrations in blood and urine and the assessment of hormone production are the most direct means of assessing the biochemical function of the ovary. However, less precise indices, such as age itself, changes in secondary sex characteristics, fertility rates, patterns of menstrual cycle length, and basal body temperature have all been used to provide indirect information about ovarian function, and they provide useful background for the direct studies of hormones.

Ovarian hormonal activity increases during childhood, particularly from around age six until puberty. An increase in estrogen production is reflected in breast maturation, which precedes the onset of menses by one or two years. The increase in estrogen output during childhood is a response to greater pituitary gonadotropin release. Even in childhood, plasma LH and FSH demonstrate rudimentary cyclic patterns.

Recent studies of subhuman primates have convincingly shown that the onset of follicular maturation, ovulation, and menstruation is dependent on the appropriate amount and pattern of pituitary gonadotropin release.[4, 5] The process can be initiated in prepubertal monkeys when gonadotropin-releasing hormone (GRH) is administered in hourly pulses over several months. Simultaneous measurement of LH, FSH, estradiol, and progesterone reflect normal patterns of follicular development, ovulation, and corpus luteum function. Morphologic changes consistent with pubertal maturation were also observed. Dependence on pituitary stimulation was confirmed by the failure of menses to persist and the regression of pubertal development in the absence of gonadotropin stimulation. There is reason to believe that the prepubertal human ovary is also fully capable of responding to gonadotropin stimulation and that the onset of menses at puberty requires maturation of the hypothalamic mechanism for gonadotropin release. Further evidence for this is derived from patients with true precocious puberty.

After menarche, the two major clinical indices of the integrity of ovarian function are fertility, or the lack thereof, and the menstrual pattern. Stated in another way, women readily seek medical consultation for suspected infertility or because of irregular menstrual cycles or amenorrhea.

While most recent investigations have focused on directly measuring the changes in endocrine function of the ovary, human biologists have long been interested in the change in reproductive capacity of women with advancing years. It is virtually impossible to study this question today because of the widespread use of voluntary means of fertility control. Natural fertility is a term used to define reproduction in the absence of deliberate fertility control, and this has been studied from a historical perspective in European populations and in several developing countries during this century. Figure 3–1 shows some examples of fertility rates of married women in different populations. The rapid decline in fertility that occurs after age 30–35 is quite uniform in all groups.[6] Similar historical analyses show that the mean age at the birth of the last child is around age 40, 10 years before cessation of menses. Certainly, pregnancies after age 40 are not unusual, and individual women conceive up to, and occasionally even after, presumptive menopause. Nevertheless, these population data suggest that the biologic potential of the ovary declines a decade or more before menopause.

Other evidence that supports these suggestions have been derived from historical data. Treloar and his colleagues prospectively collected information on menstrual cycle length from over 3,000 women.[7] This study clearly established that within a population there are systematic, age-related changes in menstrual cycle length. The years following menarche are characterized by irregularity of cycle length, with the occurrence of both unusually long and short cycle intervals. Cycles during the mid years of reproductive life, ages 20–40, are in general regular, and there is a gradual decrease in mean cycle length of two to three days. Beginning around the age of 40, there is a resumption of cycle irregularity. This change in menstrual pattern is a characteristic of the menopausal

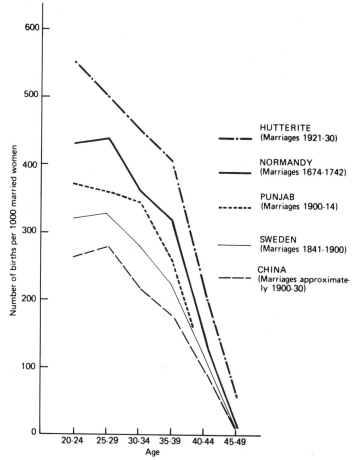

FIG 3–1.
Age-specific marital fertility for selected populations. (From Gray RH: Biological and social interactions in the determination of late fertility, in Parkes AS, et al (eds): *Fertility in Middle Age.* Cambridge, Galton Foundation, 1979, suppl 6, pp 97–115. Used by permission.)

transition and is often the first sign of approaching menopause. It is possible to relate these different cycle patterns to concomitant hormonal changes.[8]

Vollman added a dimension to the study of menstrual cycles by having participating women record daily basal body temperatures.[9] Based on the assumptions that a midcycle elevation in basal body temperature is evidence of ovulation and that the duration of the temperature rise is an index of corpus luteum function, Vollman was able to comment on the age-related changes in follicular and luteal phase length, rates of ovulation, and integrity of corpus luteum function. The decrease in cycle length with age is due to a shortening of the preovulatory or follicular phase of the cycle. The cycle irregularity that occurs with advancing years is associated with a greater proportion of anovulatory cycles when there is no increase in basal body temperature or short luteal phase cycles when the temperature rise is abbreviated. A similar study by Doring also showed that after age 40, 30%–50% of cycles were abnormal as judged from examination of basal body temperature records. These observations provide some biologic basis for the historical observations of diminishing ovarian function reflected by reduced fertility in women past the age of 35 (see Fig 3–1).

The normal menstrual cycle in women age 20–40 represents the integration of a complex series of hormonal and physiologic changes designed to optimize follicle development, fertilization, implantation, and sustenance of early pregnancy. A review of those findings provides the perspective from which to appreciate the changes that occur prior to and after the menopause.[10, 11]

As its name implies, follicle-stimulating hormone (FSH) is believed to initiate each cycle of follicular maturation. Plasma FSH increases from its nadir during the second half of the luteal phase. This increase is presumably critical to the recruitment of a new cohort of ovarian follicles from which one is ultimately selected for complete maturation and ovulation. The development of that follicle is reflected by a steady increase in plasma estradiol that begins during the midfollicular phase. Estradiol levels increase from 70–100 pg/ml during the early follicular phase to peak values of 300–400 pg/ml. Follicle-stimulating hormone falls reciprocally as estradiol rises. Plasma LH, which increases slowly and steadily during the follicular phase of the cycle, increases sharply at midcycle, coincident with or usually 12–18 hours after the estradiol peak. Both estradiol and LH decrease sharply after the midcycle, ovulatory event. Progesterone, which is in the 100 pg/ml range during the preovulatory phase of the cycle, begins to increase at the time of the midcycle LH surge as the graafian follicle is transformed into a functioning corpus luteum after ovulation. The normal luteal phase lasts 10–14 days, and progesterone levels are sustained at values of 10–15 ng/ml for at least 3–5 days during the midportion of the luteal phase. There is a secondary increase in estradiol during the luteal phase, with levels reaching 150–250 pg/ml.

Estradiol is the major circulating estrogen in premenopausal women. The pattern of plasma estrone parallels that of estradiol with concentrations that are 30%–50% those of estradiol. However, only about one third of the plasma estrone is derived directly from the ovary; the remainder is converted from androstendione. Both androstendione and testosterone levels increase during follicular maturation, reach maximum levels at midcycle, and often demonstrate a secondary increase during the luteal phase.

The systematic hormonal changes that reflect follicular maturation, ovulation, and corpus luteum function are observed during the menstrual cycles of women of all ages and can be presumed to occur in a reasonably normal fashion if a woman is menstruating at regular intervals. However, subtle changes in these parameters are observed in regularly menstruating women after the age of 40 (Fig 3–2):[12] (1) Cycles are somewhat shorter, and this is always due to a decrease in the length of the follicular phase; (2) plasma levels of FSH are increased, particularly in the early follicular phase; (3) plasma estradiol concentrations at midcycle and during the luteal phase may not be as great as in younger women; (4) plasma LH levels are not different from those measured in younger women, and (5) corpus luteum function remains robust. These hormonal changes provide further evidence that there is an alteration in the biologic potential of the ovary (i.e. estradiol response to FSH) that occurs before the onset of the irregular cycles, symptoms, or amenorrhea that herald the onset of menopause.

Most women experience some irregularity in cycle length before the onset of the menopause. The hormonal correlates of these irregular cycles are as unpredictable as their occurrence, although several generalizations can be made.[12–15] The irregular vaginal bleeding usually follows some increase in plasma estradiol, which may or may not be accompanied by an increase in plasma progesterone. This increase in estrogen and

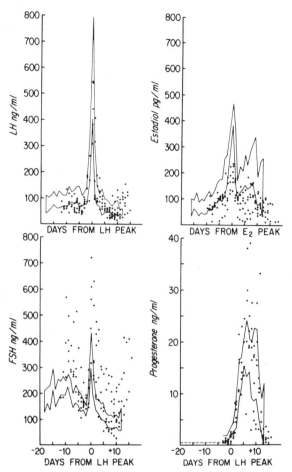

FIG 3–2.
Serum concentrations of LH, FSH, E$_2$, and P in eight cycles in women aged 46–56 years are compared with the mean $\pm$ 2 SEM in ten cycles in women aged 18–30 years (*enclosed area*). The LH, FSH, and P levels are synchronized around the day of the LH peak, and E$_2$ levels are synchronized around the day of the E$_2$ peak. (From Sherman BM, et al: *J Clin Endocrinol Metab* 1976; 42:629. Used by permission.)

progesterone reflects some degree of maturation of residual ovarian follicles. The spectrum of hormonal changes extends from cycles with hormonal fluctuations that resemble those of younger women to prolonged episodes of amenorrhea that are terminated by several days during which there is a rise and fall in plasma estradiol with or without some increase in plasma progesterone. During the intervals between the episodes of follicular activity the concentrations of one or both gonadotropins may reach menopausal levels. However, these may decrease to premenopausal levels as the ovarian output of estrogens increases.

Figure 3–3 illustrates the altered hormonal relationships observed during the menopausal transition of one woman studied at intervals for almost two years. This figure dramatically illustrates information gleaned from both cross-sectional and longitudinal studies that show early monotropic increases in FSH, gonadotropin levels fluctuating

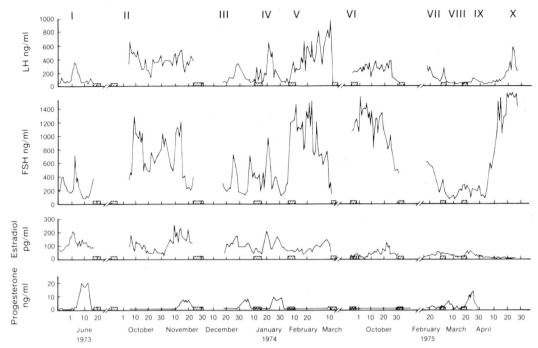

FIG 3–3.
Concentrations of LH, FSH, estradiol, and progesterone over several years in one woman who
was 50 years old at the start of sampling. Hormone levels are arrayed by calendar date;
hatched areas indicate menstruation.

between menopausal and premenopausal values despite basal estrogen values in the
range of premenopausal women, and variable evidence of corpus luteum function prior
to episodes of vaginal bleeding.

The first cycle (I) is typical of that seen in older women who menstruate regularly.
The plasma FSH concentration is increased with prominent peaks in the early follicular
phase as well as at midcycle. By contrast, the plasma LH is in the normal range although the midcycle peak is somewhat prolonged. The plasma estradiol concentration
at midcycle and during the luteal phase does not reach the levels seen in younger
women, while the luteal phase progesterone values duplicate those seen in normal
women both in magnitude and duration. Several months later, this woman experienced
her first long intermenstrual interval. At this time both LH and FSH were elevated into
the menopausal range and fell reciprocally as the plasma estradiol concentration increased prior to menses. It is of importance to note that the menopausal gonadotropin
levels persisted despite plasma estradiol concentrations that were always at least equal
to those observed during the follicular phase of menstrual cycles in younger women.
Cycle III shows similar changes, although the plasma LH concentration is not elevated
to the same degree. Cycle IV illustrates an extraordinarily short cycle with a minimum
interval from the menses of cycle III to the midcycle peaks of estradiol LH and FSH.
Cycle V is characterized by the lack of increase in progesterone prior to menses and by
very high levels of both LH and FSH. Cycle VI could be classified as anovulatory,
although the increase in plasma estradiol that preceded menses was presumably due to
limited development of one or more residual follicles. Cycles VII and VIII show lower

levels of gonadotropins and episodes of vaginal bleeding that were not clearly associated with systematic changes in ovarian steroids. Cycle IX shows yet a different phenomenon, in that an increase in both plasma estradiol and progesterone was not followed by vaginal bleeding.

Recall that in younger women a substantial number of follicles is recruited each cycle, from which one is selected for complete maturation. The chaotic hormonal patterns that accompany irregular cycles in older women probably reflect a limited number of follicles available for recruitment as well as their varied and usually diminished potential for development.

The study of hormonal changes during menstrual cycles of older women have raised several questions about pituitary ovarian regulation. The disparate patterns of plasma LH and FSH as illustrated in Cycle I suggest that these two hormones can be regulated independently. There is increasing evidence for the existence of an ovarian hormone, termed inhibin or folliculostatin, that may specifically influence pituitary FSH release. This material has been recovered from follicular fluid and has been demonstrated to suppress pituitary FSH.[16] It has been postulated that there is a decrease in inhibin in older women consequent to a diminished complement of ovarian follicles. This may explain the increase in plasma FSH that is observed with increasing age. Since FSH is presumed to initiate succeeding waves of follicular maturation, the increased plasma FSH concentrations in older women may also be responsible for the fact that follicular maturation occurs at a more rapid rate, with a consequent decrease in follicular phase and menstrual cycle length.

The increased concentrations of immunoassayable LH and FSH measured when plasma estradiol levels remain in the normal range, as vividly illustrated in cycle II, has been taken as additional evidence for a nonsteroidal regulation of pituitary gonadotropin secretion. Alternatively there may be a decrease in hypothalamic-pituitary sensitivity to estrogen feedback with age. Others have postulated a change in the ratio of immunologic-to-biologic potency of circulating gonadotropins in older women.

A woman's last episode of menstrual bleeding is difficult to identify, except in retrospect. The older the subject and the longer the duration of amenorrhea, the more unlikely it is that the subject will have another episode of vaginal bleeding (Fig 3–4).[17] Plasma estradiol levels decrease gradually over the first year or so of menopausal amenorrhea. Occasionally, increased plasma levels of estradiol can be measured for several days, presumably reflecting the activity of some remaining ovarian follicular elements. However, with eventual loss of all follicular activity, the ovary ceases to be an estrogen-secreting organ.

The hormonal status of postmenopausal women has been carefully studied. Table 3–1 summarizes and contrasts plasma hormone concentrations in pre- and postmenopausal women. The most important feature of the menopause is that estradiol ceases to be the major circulating estrogen and is present at levels of 20–25 pg/ml or less. Direct catheterization of the ovarian circulation has shown a small contribution of estradiol from the postmenopausal ovary, with the remainder derived from conversion from estrone, which in turn is derived from aromatization of androstendione.[18–20] Cessation of ovarian function also means the absence of cyclic increases in plasma progesterone, so that plasma levels remain at 0.5 ng/ml or less. Progesterone is derived entirely from the adrenal glands.

The menopause is an estrogen-progesterone deficient state compared with the premenopausal condition. However, cytologic examination of vaginal epithelium from post-

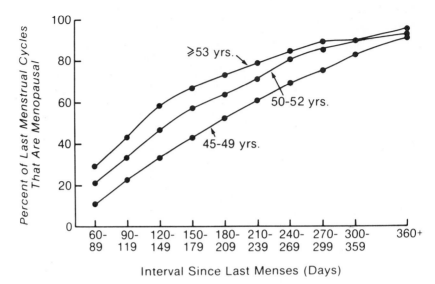

FIG 3–4.
The probability of the occurrence of menopause according to the interval of amenorrhea and age. (From Wallace RB, et al: *Am J Obstet Gynecol* 1979; 135:1021. Used by permission.)

menopausal women has demonstrated a wide range of biologic estrogen effect.[21] This raises questions concerning the source and regulation of estrogen production in postmenopausal women.

Estrone, a less potent estrogen than estradiol, is the major circulating estrogen in postmenopausal women. Circulating levels are in the range of 20–60 pg/ml, which may equal or exceed values during the follicular phase in premenopausal women, but there is no cyclic increase in estrone as there is in premenopausal women.[22] Plasma concentrations correlate well with the estrogenic effect reflected on vaginal cytology. Since the adrenal does not secrete estrogens and since the direct ovarian contribution is miniscule, there has been a great interest in the origin of circulating estrone in postmenopausal women and the reasons for its variability among individuals.

Based upon the observation that the placental estrogen production is totally dependent on conversion from C19 androgenic precursors, investigators postulated that in postmenopausal women estrogens might be derived largely from conversion of circulating androgens. It is now well established that androstendione is the major precursor of

TABLE 3–1.

Comparison of Plasma Sex Hormone Concentrations in Pre- and Postmenopausal Women

HORMONE CONCENTRATION	PREMENOPAUSAL		POSTMENOPAUSAL
	MIN	MAX	
Estradiol pg/ml	50–60	300–500	5–25
Estrone pg/ml	30–40	150–300	20–60
Progesterone ng/ml	0.5–1.0	10–20	0.5
Androstenedione ng/ml		1.0–2.0	0.3–1.0
Testosterone ng/ml		0.3–0.8	0.1–0.5

estrone and that the conversion is carried out by aromatase, an enzyme system responsible for the biosynthesis of estrogens from C19 precursors located in several tissues, including adipose, muscle, and bone marrow.[23, 24]

The regulation of extraglandular conversion of androstendione to estrone is of importance, because it is related to the differences in estrone concentration and estrogenic effects observed among women. Those differences could be determined by the production of androstendione and/or the extent of its conversion to estrone. Total androstendione production is actually less in postmenopausal compared with premenopausal women, but the extent of its conversion to estrone is increased from about 1.4% in premenopausal to 2.7% in postmenopausal women. The adrenal glands are the major site of sex hormone production in postmenopausal women, contributing about one half of the plasma testosterone and two thirds of the plasma androstendione concentration.[25] Evidence for the adrenal origin of these hormones includes observation of a diurnal rhythm, diminished levels after dexamethasone administration, increased levels after adrenocorticotropin (ACTH) administration, and significantly diminished concentrations in patients with Addison's disease.[22] The ovarian contribution has been documented by arterial venous differences for both androstendione and testosterone in the ovarian circulation. Furthermore, oophorectomized women have lower circulating levels of these hormones than women of comparable age with intact ovaries. These androgens arise from the stromal and hilar cells of the ovary in response to stimulation by high circulating concentrations of LH.[19, 20]

Among healthy women, the extent of aromatization of androstendione to estrone is determined by differences in rates of conversion rather than by differences in production of the androgen precursor. Adiposity and age are the major factors contributing to increased rates of hormone conversion. There is a strong relationship between body weight and the extent of aromatization of plasma androstendione that parallels the relationship between adipose tissue mass and the plasma estrone concentration.[26–29] Within the adipose tissue the major site of aromatization has been localized to stromal or vascular cells rather than to the adipose cell itself. This helps explain why substantial weight loss is not accompanied by a decrease in the conversion of androstendione to estrone.

There are several important clinical correlations of these biochemical observations. Estrone can be further metabolized to estradiol at the cellular level in estrogen-sensitive target tissues, so that the plasma estrone concentration may not accurately reflect the biologic estrogen effect. Nevertheless, the differing plasma estrone concentrations are reflected in the spectrum of estrogenic activity in vaginal cytologies. The association of endometrial carcinoma with obesity has been linked to higher plasma estrone concentrations. However, the greater rates of conversion of androstendione to estrone in patients with endometrial carcinoma cannot be explained totally on the basis of increased adipose tissue mass and these patients may have additional reasons for enhanced rates of aromatization. A contrasting situation concerns reported higher incidences of menopausal symptoms among women of lower body weight who have lower plasma estrone concentrations. Inhibition of the conversion of androstendione to estrone by the aromatase inhibitor aminoglutethamide has been used effectively to treat patients with estrogen receptor-positive metastatic breast cancer.

Plasma FSH concentrations remain elevated even into old age and are persistently higher than plasma LH concentrations, reversing the ratio measured in premenopausal women. There is evidence that plasma LH may decrease somewhat with advancing years. The pulsatile pattern of gonadotropin release persists in the menopause, and the pulse frequency has been associated with but is not causally related to episodes of menopausal flushing. The gonadotropin concentrations of older women appear sensitive to the subject's nutritional status, since illness and weight loss are associated with a decrease in plasma concentrations of both hormones.[30] This may be an analogous situation to the hypogonadotropic states observed in younger women with anorexia nervosa or other forms of nutritionally related amenorrhea.

REFERENCES

1. Nicosia SV: Morphological changes of the human ovary throughout life, in Serra GB (ed): *The Ovary*. New York, Raven Press, 1983, pp 57–81.
2. Harman SM, Louvet J-P, Ross GT: Interaction of estrogen and gonadotropins on follicular atresia. *Endocrinology* 1975; 96:1145.
3. Richards JS: Maturation of ovarian follicles: Action and interactions of pituitary and ovarian hormones in follicular cell differentiation. *Physiol Rev* 1980; 60:51.
4. Knobil E: The neuroendocrine control of the menstrual cycle. *Horm Res* 1980; 36:53.
5. Wildt L, Marshall G, Knobil E: Experimental induction of puberty in the infantile female rhesus monkey. *Science* 1980; 207:1373.
6. Gray RH: Biological and social interactions in the determination of late fertility, in Parkes AS, Herbertson MA, Cole J (eds): *Fertility in Middle Age*. Cambridge, England, Galton Foundation, 1979, pp 97–115.
7. Treloar AE, Boynton RE, Behn BG, et al: Variation of the human menstrual cycle through reproductive life. *Int J Fertil* 1967; 12:77.
8. Sherman BM, Korenman SG: Hormonal characteristics of the human menstrual cycle throughout reproductive life. *J Clin Invest* 1975; 55:699.
9. Vollman RF: *The Menstrual Cycle*. Philadelphia, WB Saunders Co, 1977.
10. Ross GT, Cargille CM, Lipsett MB, et al: Pituitary and gonadal hormones in women during spontaneous and induced ovulatory cycles. *Recent Prog Horm Res* 1970; 26:1.
11. Vande Wiele RL, Bogumil J, Dyrenfurth I, et al: Mechanisms regulating the menstrual cycle in women. *Recent Prog Horm Res* 1970; 26:63.
12. Sherman BM, West JH, Korenman SG: The menopausal transition: Analysis of LH, FSH, estradiol, and progesterone concentrations during menstrual cycles of older women. *J Clin Endocrinol Metab* 1976; 42:629.
13. Metcalf MG, Donald RA, Livesey JH: Pituitary-ovarian function before, during and after the menopause: A longitudinal study. *Clin Endocrinol* 1982; 17:489.
14. Reyes FI, Winter JSD, Faiman C: Pituitary-ovarian relationships preceding the menopause. I. A cross-sectional study of serum follicle-stimulating hormone, luteinizing hormone, prolactin, estradiol, and progesterone levels. *Am J Obstet Gynecol* 1977; 129:557.
15. Van Look PFA, Lothian H, Hunter WM, et al: Hypothalamic-pituitary-ovarian function in perimenopausal women. *Clin Endocrinol* 1977; 7:13.
16. Channing CP, Anderson LD, Hoover DJ, et al: The role of nonsteroidal regulators in control of oocyte and follicular maturation. *Recent Prog Horm Res* 1982; 38:331.
17. Wallace RB, Sherman BM, Bean JA, et al: Probability of menopause with increasing duration of amenorrhea in middle-aged women. *Am J Obstet Gynecol* 1979; 135:1021.
18. Judd HL, Judd GE, Lucas WE, et al: Endocrine function of the postmenopausal ovary: Concentration of androgens and estrogens in ovarian and peripheral vein blood. *J Clin Endocrinol Metab* 1974; 39:1020.
19. Longcope C, Hunter R, Franz C: Steroid secretion by the postmenopausal ovary. *Am J Obstet Gynecol* 1980; 138:564.
20. Judd HL, Shamonki IM, Frumar AM, et al: Origin of serum estradiol in postmenopausal women. *Obstet Gynecol* 1982; 59:680.
21. Efstratiades M, Tamvakopoulou E, Papatheodorou B, et al: Postmenopausal vaginal cytohormonal pattern in 597 healthy women and 301 patients with genital cancer. *Acta Cytol (Baltimore)* 1982; 26:126.
22. Vermeulen A: The hormonal activity of postmenopausal ovary. *J Clin Endocrinol Metab* 1976; 42:247.

23. Edman CD, MacDonald PC: The role of extraglandular estrogen in women in health and disease, in James VHT, Serio M, Giusti G (eds): *The Endocrine Function of the Human Ovary*. London, Academic Press Inc, 1976, pp 135–140.
24. Longcope C: The significance of steroid production by peripheral tissue, in Scholler R (ed): *Endocrinology of the Ovary*. Paris, Editions SEPE, 1978, pp 23–40.
25. Maroulis GB, Abraham GE: Ovarian and adrenal contributions to peripheral steroid levels in postmenopausal women. *Obstet Gynecol* 1976; 48:150.
26. Forney JP, Milewich L, Chen GT, et al: Aromatization of androstenedione to estrone by human adipose tissue in vitro. Correlation with adipose tissue mass, age, and endometrial neoplasia. *J Clin Endocrinol Metab* 1981; 53:192.
27. Ackerman GE, Smith ME, Mendelson CR, et al: Aromatization of androstenedione by human adipose tissue stromal cells in monolayer culture. *J Clin Endocrinol Metab* 1981; 53:412.
28. Vermeulen A, Verdonck L: Factors affecting sex hormone levels in postmenopausal women. *J Steroid Biochem* 1979; 11:899.
29. Meldrum DR, Davidson BJ, Tataryn IV, et al: Changes in circulating steroids with aging in postmenopausal women. *Obstet Gynecol* 1981; 57:624.
30. Warren MP, Siris ES, Petrovich C: The influence of severe illness on gonadotropin secretion in the postmenopausal female. *J Clin Endocrinol Metab* 1977; 45:99.

CHAPTER 4

Vasomotor Instability of the Menopause

OSCAR A. KLETZKY, M.D.
RICHARD BORENSTEIN, M.D.

HOT FLUSHES are the most common and troublesome symptom of the climacteric. They are a reflection of the vasomotor instability which may precede the menopause (cessation of ovarian function) by months or years before the last menses. Hot flushes are characterized by a sensation of intense heat of the upper part of the body, accompanied by an ascending flushing of the thorax, neck and face, which is usually followed by profuse sweating. Unlike some other symptoms or signs of the climacteric, such as bone demineralization, vaginal dryness, and dyspareunia, which gradually increase in intensity, the hot flush symptom lessens in frequency and intensity with advancing age. It has been reported that 50%–76% of women with physiologic or surgical (ovariectomy) menopause complain of hot flushes.[1–3] Of all the women having hot flushes, 85% will suffer from this disturbance for more than a year, and 25%–50% will experience it for more than five years.[1, 3, 4] Vasomotor flushes occur at irregular intervals during the day and night and may be severe enough to affect the patient's normal life pattern, resulting in severe insomnia or nervousness. Insomnia may be produced by the sudden occurrence of the hot flush or by a central nervous system disturbance, since the waking episode can occur before the flush.[5–8] A premonitory phase, consisting of palpitation and sensation of pressure in the head, has been described.[5] However, such prodromal symptoms are not felt by all menopausal women. Hot flushes can be triggered by some environmental changes. In the single patient extensively studied by Molnar, a finger prick or the sound of a door bell or telephone were sufficient to evoke a flush episode.[9] Similarly, the simple vision or smelling of a meal or hot weather can be conducive to flushing. On the other hand, the absence of obvious external or conscious stimuli during sleep is not sufficient to prevent the occurrence of hot flushes and, in fact, flushes usually occur more frequently during sleeping hours.[9] It is currently unclear whether the increased frequency of flushes during sleep is because of physiologic or subconscious stimuli. The duration of the subjective symptoms varies between 30 seconds to about five minutes with a mean duration of four minutes. The frequency of flushes varies from one every few minutes to one or two per week.[10] Other symptoms that occur with less frequency than the hot flushes but may accompany them are palpitations, vertigo, weakness, and faintness. It has been estimated that there are more than 25 million women in the United States with either natural or surgical menopause.[10] Although hot flushes are one of the most frequent of all gynecologic complaints, little is known about their pathogenesis.

PATHOPHYSIOLOGY OF HOT FLUSHES

Until recently, few attempts have been made to clearly define the physiologic changes associated with hot flushes. During the hot flush, an increase in oxygen consumption and cheek temperature as well as an increase in finger volume, which probably indicates peripheral dilatation, has been reported previously.[11, 12] In addition to peripheral vasodilatation, other cardiovascular changes, such as an increase of the heart rate by 15% and fluctuations in baseline electrocardiogram, have been observed.[9, 13] Electrocardiogram changes can also reflect skin perspiration with poor conductance and not be due to real dynamic heart changes. No alterations in blood pressure have yet been reported.

The very extensive study of peripheral temperature changes during several hot flushes of a single postmenopausal woman described by Molnar was followed by several reports confirming a close temporal relationship of the beginning of the hot flush and an increase in peripheral temperature (Fig 4–1).[9, 10, 14–16] Changes in skin conductance and peripheral and core temperature were described in association with the onset of the subjective feeling (Fig 4–2).[16–17]

Mashchak et al. demonstrated the temporal relationship between objective parameters

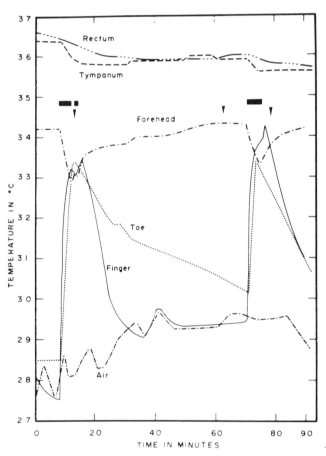

FIG 4–1.
Measurement of peripheral, tympanic and rectal temperature in two spontaneous flushes. (From Molnar GW: *J Appl Physiol* 1975; 38:499. Used by permission.)

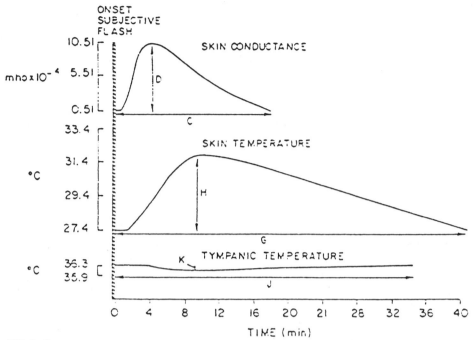

FIG 4–2.
Schematic representation of skin conductance, and skin and tympanic temperature based on measurements in menopausal hot flushes. (From Tataryn IV, *Maturitas* 1980; 2:101. Used by permission.)

such as augmented digital perfusion (ADP), peripheral temperature, serum luteinizing hormone (LH) concentration, and the vasomotor flush.[18] The onset of ADP consistently occurred before the initiation of the flush by 1.5 minutes and outlasted it (8.5 ± 1.0 vs. 4.2 ± 0.6 minutes) (Fig 4–3). Using the beginning of ADP as the starting point of the physiologic changes that occurred in a cyclic fashion, these authors showed a pattern in which ADP was followed by the increase in peripheral temperature, and finally by an increase of serum LH (Fig 4–4). It was also reported that a drop in core temperature, as determined by esophageal or tympanic membrane measurements, occurs almost four minutes after the beginning of the flush.[16–19] It is during this time that patients complain of chills. The decrease in core temperature is indicative of a central mechanism changing the thermoregulatory set point, and thus it could become the trigger stimuli for all physiologic changes associated with vasomotor flushes. Interestingly enough, asymptomatic menopausal women who were never treated with estrogen were found to have similar alterations of these objective parameters.[18] These women lacked only the flush-related increase in serum LH (Fig 4–5). Thus, the recording of the objective parameters is a more specific and reliable indicator of vasomotor instability than the recording of the subjective sensation of hot flushes.

The analysis of the time sequence has demonstrated that the subjective feeling of the vasomotor flush starts at the mean time of 1.5 ± 0.2 (SEM) minutes following the initiation of ADP. The maximal increase in digital temperature occurs six minutes after the beginning of ADP and lasts for 27.4 ± 12 minutes. The increase in plasma LH occurs after the increase in digital temperature and reaches a peak 12 minutes after the

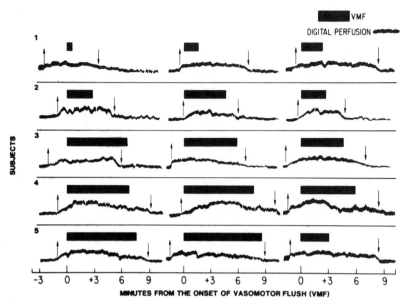

FIG 4–3.
Temporal relationship between the beginning and end of augmented digital perfusion and hot flushes. (From Mashchak CA, et al: *Maturitas* 1985; 6:301. Used by permission.)

onset of ADP. The beginning of ADP coincides with a serum LH nadir, probably reflecting the tail end of a previous episode. Furthermore, a significant increase in plasma epinephrine occurs three to six minutes after the beginning of ADP (see Fig 4–4). The plasma epinephrine increase is most likely of adrenal origin and represents either the homeostatic mechanism controlling the peripheral vasodilatation or a stress-related phenomenon. The above description of all objective parameters indicates that the increase in digital temperature is the result of the augmented digital perfusion.

The subjective feeling of the vasomotor flush probably is unrelated to either ADP or the increase in temperature, because these last two parameters were also observed in menopausal women who never complained of hot flushes and/or received estrogen treatment. Furthermore, symptomatic patients can have the same cyclic changes described above without the subjective feeling of the flushes as well as full symptomatic episodes. Thus, the physiologic changes are universal to all menopausal women, while the presence of the subjective feeling of the flush may be related to a given threshold of sensitivity. Since hot flushes are more frequently felt during the resting hours than when performing some activity, it is clear that the degree of mental awareness plays an important role. It can also be hypothesized that central adrenergic activation followed by a peripheral mechanism may be involved in the objective manifestations of these episodic menopausal changes.

The peripheral temperature increments during hot flushes are similar in different areas of the body (finger, toe, chest, or head) (see Fig 4–1). Because sweating is more prominent in the forehead and chest, the temperature in these areas returns to baseline faster than others. The degree of temperature increase is inversely related to its baseline; thus, when studying menopausal women, it has been recommended to maintain the room temperature at 23°C in order to record a larger peripheral temperature increase (mean of

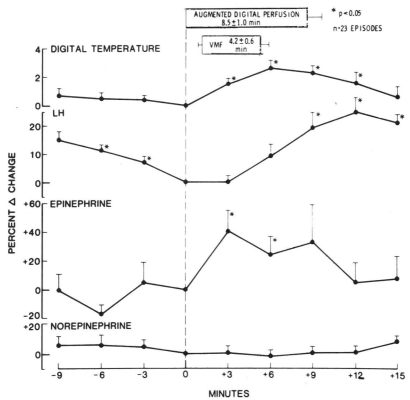

FIG 4–4
Composite graph of objective parameters obtained in 23 hot flushes from menopausal women. Data were normalized to the beginning of augmented digital perfusion. (From Mashchak CA, et al: *Maturitas* 1985; 6:301. Used by permission.)

4°C).[10] Digital temperature has been reported to be closely related to only 69% of subjective hot flushes.[10] In addition to the cardiovascular and temperature changes associated with vasomotor flushes (Fig 4–6) a decrease in skin resistance has also been reported.[16] Increments in skin resistance occur about one minute after the beginning of the hot flush and last for about 18 minutes. However, since skin resistance depends on the degree of perspiration, its measurement may give variable results, depending on the body areas of determination and the degree of perspiration.

HORMONAL STUDIES

Since hot flushes occur only in women who become hypoestrogenic following physiologic or surgical menopause or treatment with gonadotropin-releasing hormone (GnRH) agonists,[20, 21] it is logical to assume that the phenomenon may be associated or influenced by alterations in hormone levels. Therefore, several studies have attempted to correlate the blood concentration of several hormones with the occurrence of hot flushes. Earlier studies on gonadotropin levels during hot flushes demonstrated contradictory results.[22–24] Some authors reported a positive correlation,[22] while others demonstrated no correlation with hot flushes.[23, 24] However, in 1979, Tataryn et al. reported

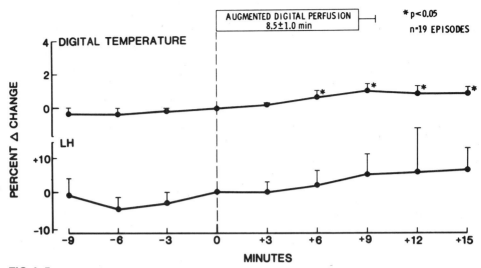

FIG 4–5.
Objective parameters obtained in asymptomatic menopausal women. Data are centered around the beginning of augmented digital perfusion. (From Mashchack CA, et al: *Maturitas* 1985; 6:301. Used by permission.)

a close temporal relationship between serum LH pulses, finger temperature, and hot flushes (Fig 4–7).[25] A nadir of serum LH preceded the temperature rise and the beginning of the hot flush, which was followed 14 minutes later by an LH peak. These observations were confirmed by other investigators who also found a lack of correlation with concentrations of serum FSH.[18, 19, 26] These results have suggested that the secretion of LH or the factor(s) responsible for the pulsatile LH release may be involved in the mechanism triggering these thermoregulatory events.[16] However, hot flushes were observed in patients after total hypophysectomy[27] or following a partial resection of the pituitary, cryotherapy, or irradiation of a chromophobe adenoma (Fig 4–8).[28]

Further evidence demonstrating that pulsatile serum LH does not cause the subjective feeling of the flush was recently reported.[20, 21] A potent GnRH analog was administered to menopausal women and was found to inhibit the pulsatile release of LH, while the vasomotor flushes persisted with similar incidence and intensity. The same analog given to menstruating women produced the same inhibition of LH pulsatility; however, these women also complained of hot flushes at the end of three weeks of treatment. Also, postmenopausal women treated with 5 µg of ethinyl estradiol for only two weeks showed the same objective changes of ADP and temperature without the corresponding serum LH increase (Fig 4–9).[18] These results are similar to those obtained in asymptomatic women, and therefore, it can be concluded that the presence of hot flushes and the temporally related increase in serum LH may not be related (see Fig 4–9). Because of the temporal relationship between flushes and pulsatile LH level, it is conceivable that a stimuli initiated in suprapituitary area(s) may initiate the hot flushes and also be related to the hypothalamic pathway controlling the pulsatile LH release.[29, 30]

The belief that estrogens play a role in the pathogenesis of vasomotor instability of the menopause is based on several lines of evidence. Vasomotor instability occurs only in women who have lost their ovarian function by either natural or surgical means, and thus it occurs with a sudden discontinuation of estrogen secretion.[31, 34] Furthermore,

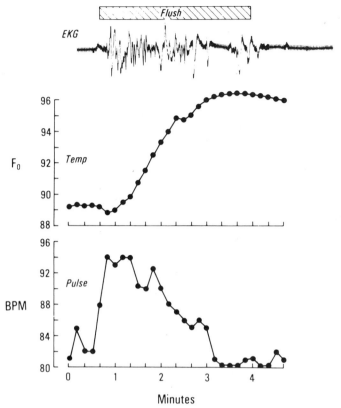

FIG 4–6.
Increases of fluctuations of baseline recording of ECG, skin temperature, and pulse rate during hot flush. (Courtesy of Yen SSC and Casper R.)

vasomotor flushes occur only in individuals who had previously been exposed to the influence of either exogenous or endogenous estrogens. Women with Turner's Syndrome have hot flushes only if first treated with estrogens.[36] Similarly, men treated with estrogens for prostatic carcinoma complain of hot flushes only after the medication is discontinued. However, initial reports on the association of estrone or estradiol and hot flushes have given conflicting results.[31–34] When factors such as age, body size, and bioavailability of estrogen were considered, a positive correlation between estrogens and hot flushes was demonstrated.[33] Younger (46 ± 2.1 years) and thinner (135 ± 5.3 lbs) menopausal women were found to have more flushes than older (55 ± 1.8 years) and fatter (159 ± 7.9 lbs) women (Fig 4–10). Furthermore, significantly lower levels of serum estrone (19.8 ± 1.7 vs. 31.7 ± 5.3 pg/ml), estradiol (8.8 ± 0.7 vs. 13.5 ± 1.3) and non-sex hormone-binding globulin (SHBG)-bound estradiol (3.6 ± 0.4 vs. 6.9 ± 1.1 pg/ml) were found in symptomatic than in asymptomatic postmenopausal women (Fig 4–11). Serum androstenedione and testosterone were not different in these two groups of women. These results will indicate the importance of endogenous estrogen metabolism in the genesis of hot flushes. The bioavailability of estrogens to the hypothalamic centers through the blood brain barrier may be the determining factor in the occurrence of hot flushes.[36, 37] The free estrogen and that loosely bound to albumin (non-SHBG-bound) are the only components that can cross the blood-brain barrier and

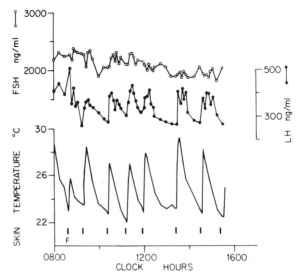

FIG 4–7.
Temporal relationship between hot flushes, peripheral temperature and serum LH concentration. No correlation is seen with serum FSH release. (From Tataryn IV, et al: *J Clin Endocrinol Metab* 1979; 49:152. Used by permission.)

induce a biologic effect. In vivo and in vitro studies have demonstrated that women with hot flushes have less estrogen available to the brain centers.[37, 38]

The participation of the adrenal medulla in the events surrounding the vasomotor instability of the menopause has recently been demonstrated.[18, 19] Significant increases of plasma epinephrine and decreases of norepinephrine have been found to accompany

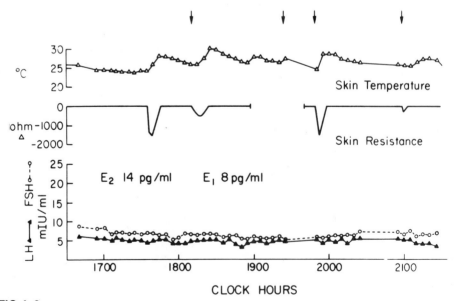

FIG 4–8.
Skin resistance, peripheral temperature and gonadotropin in a patient after resection of a pituitary adenoma. (Meldrum DR, et al: *J Clin Endocrinol Metab* 1981; 52:684. Used by permission.)

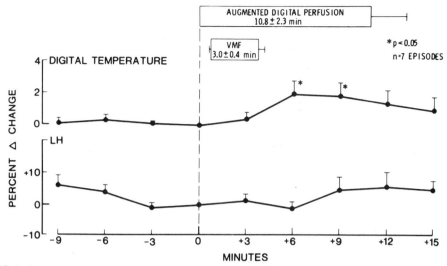

FIG 4–9.
Findings in seven menopausal hot flushes in women treated for two weeks with ethinyl estradiol. Data are centered around the beginning of augmented digital perfusion. (From Mashchak CA, et al: *Maturitas* 1985; 6:301. Used by permission.)

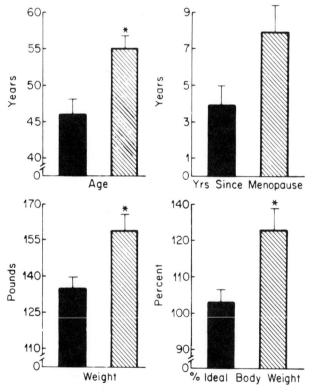

FIG 4–10.
Comparison of age and weight in symptomatic (*solid bars*) and asymptomatic (*striped bars*) menopausal women. *Asterisks* represent significance from asymptomatic women. (From Erlik Y, et al: *Obstet Gynecol* 1982; 59:403. Reprinted by permission from the American College of Obstetricians and Gynecologists.)

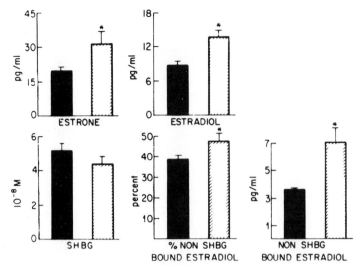

FIG 4–11.
Mean ± SEM levels of estrone, estradiol, SHBG-bound estradiol in symptomatic (*solid bars*) and asymptomatic (*striped bars*) menopausal women. *Asterisks* represent significance from symptomatic women. (From Erlik Y, et al: *Obstet Gynecol* 1982; 59:403. Reprinted by permission from the American College of Obstetricians and Gynecologists.)

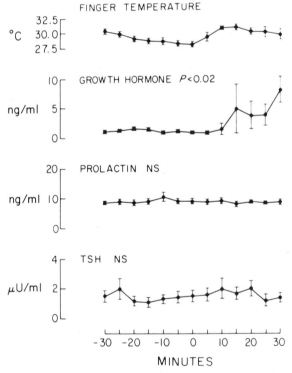

FIG 4–12.
Serum growth hormone, prolactin and thyroid-stimulating hormone concentrations before and after the increase in digital temperature. (From Meldrum DR, et al: *Obstet Gynecol* 1984; 64:752–756. Reprinted by permission from the American College of Obstetricians and Gynecologists.)

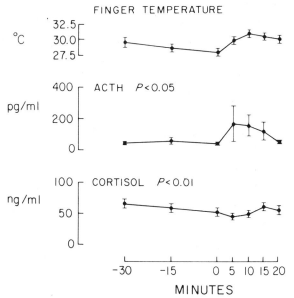

FIG 4–13.
Correlation between increase of peripheral temperature and increase in serum ACTH and cortisol concentrations. (From Meldrum DR, et al: *Obstet Gynecol* 1984; 64:752–756. Reprinted with permission from the American College of Obstetricians and Gynecologists.)

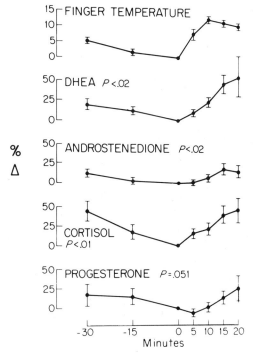

FIG 4–14.
Significant changes of serum DHEA, androstenedione and cortisol at the time of increase in peripheral temperature in menopausal women. (From Meldrum DR, et al: *J Clin Endocrinol Metab* 1980; 50:685. Used by permission.)

the hot flush when these catecholamines were measured every one to three minutes. These changes could not be confirmed in studies which obtained blood samples at intervals of five minutes or longer.[26] The action of catecholamines, histamine, serotonin, and prostaglandin on the central nervous systems of subjects complaining of hot flushes has not yet been completely elucidated.

Additional correlations between other pituitary hormones and hot flushes were further demonstrated by Meldrum et al.[34, 35] Significant increases in growth hormone (GH) and adrenocorticotropin (ACTH) occurred 30 and 5 minutes, respectively, following the rise of skin temperature (Figs 4–12 and 4–13). Illner et al. have suggested that ACTH release may be secondary to a hypothalamic reaction to the peripheral cooling that follows the hot flush.[39] In addition, mean serum cortisol concentrations increase 15 minutes after the hot flush, presumably as a consequence of the preceding elevation of ACTH. A significant increase in serum dehydroepiandrosterone and androstenedione in addition to cortisol at the time of flushes might indicate an adrenal response to the stress or the flush (Fig 4–14). It was recently reported that endogenous opioids do not play an important role in the genesis of hot flushes, since the administration of naloxon, an opioid antagonist, failed to alter the flushes, finger temperature, skin resistance, or serum LH pulsatility.[40–42]

In conclusion, decreased estrogen secretion is the main endocrine abnormality in relation to the occurrence of hot flushes.

REFERENCES

1. Neucarten BL, Kriner RG: Menopausal symptoms in women of various ages. *Psychosom Med J* 1965; 27:26–27.
2. Barr W: Problems related to postmenopausal women. *S Afr Med J* 1975; 49:437–439.
3. Thompson B, Hart SA, Durno D: Menopausal age and symptomatology in general practice. *J Biol Sci* 1973; 5:71–82.
4. Jaszmann L, Van Lith ND, Zaat YCA: The perimenopausal symptoms. *Med Gynecol Soc* 1969; 4:268–276.
5. Hannan JH: *The Flushings of the Menopause*. London, Bailliere, Tindal and Cox. 1927, pp 1–22.
6. Thomson Y, Oswald I: Effect of estrogen on the sleep, mood and anxiety of menopausal women. *Br Med J* 1977; 2:1317–1319.
7. Schiff I, Regestein Q, Tulchinsky D, et al: Effects of estrogen on sleep and psychological state of hypogonadal women. *JAMA* 1979; 242:2405–2407.
8. Erlik Y, Tataryn IV, Meldrum DR, et al: Association of waking episodes with menopausal hot flushes. *JAMA* 1981; 245:1741–4.
9. Molnar GW: Body temperatures during menopausal hot flushes. *J Appl Physiol* 1975; 38:499–503.
10. Chang RJ, Judd HL: Elevation of skin temperature of the finger as an objective index of postmenopausal hot flushes: Standardization of the techniques. *Am J Obstet Gynecol* 1979; 135:713–717.
11. Collet ME: Basal metabolism at the menopause. *J Appl Physiol* 1949; 1:629–639.
12. Reynolds SRM: Dermovascular action of estrogen, the ovarian follicular hormone. *J Invest Dermatol* 1941; 4:7–22.
13. Sturdee DW, Wilson KA, Pipili E, et al: Physiological aspects of menopausal hot flush. *Br Med J* 1978; 2:79–80.
14. Molnar GW: Investigation of hot flushes by ambulatory monitoring. *Am J Physiol* 1979; 237:R306–310.
15. Sturdee DW, Reece BL: Thermography of menopausal hot flushes. *Maturitas* 1979; 1:201–205.
16. Tataryn IV, Lomax P, Bajorer JG, et al: Postmenopausal hot flushes: A disorder of thermoregulation. *Maturitas* 1980; 2:101–107.

17. Tataryn IV, Lomax P, Meldrum DR, et al: Objective techniques for the assessment of post-menopausal hot flushes. *Obstet Gynecol* 1981; 57:340–344.
18. Mashchak CA, Kletzky OA, Artal R, et al: The relation of physiological changes to subjective symptoms in postmenopausal women with and without hot flushes. *Maturitas* 1985; 6:301–308.
19. Kronenberg F, Cote LJ, Linkie DM, et al: Menopausal hot flushes, thermoregulatory, cardio-vascular, and circulating catecholamines and LH changes. *Maturitas* 1984; 6:31–43.
20. Casper RF, Yen SSC: Menopausal flushes: Effect of pituitary gonadotropin desensitization by a potent luteinizing hormone-releasing factor agonist. *J Clin Endocrinol Metab* 1981; 53:1056–1058.
21. De Fazio J, Meldrum D, Laufer L, et al: Induction of hot flushes in premenopausal women treated with a long acting GnRH agonist. *J Clin Endocrinol Metab* 1983; 56:445–448.
22. Aitken JM, Davidson A, England P, et al: The relationship between menopausal vasomotor symptoms and gonadotropin excretion in urine after oophorectomy. *J Obstet Gynecol Br Common* 1974; 81:150–154.
23. Hunter DJS, Julier D, Franklin M, et al: Plasma levels of estrogen, LH, and FSH, following castration and estradiol implant. *Obstet Gynecol* 1977; 49:180–185.
24. Abe I, Furwhashi N, Yamaya Y, et al: Correlation between climacteric symptoms and serum levels of estradiol, progesterone, FSH, and LH. *Am J Obstet Gynecol* 1977; 129:65–67.
25. Tataryn IV, Meldrum DR, Lu KH et al: LH, FSH, and skin temperature during the menopausal hot flush. *J Clin Endocrinol Metab* 1979; 49:152–154.
26. Casper RF, Yen SSC, Wilkes MM: Menopausal flushes: A neuroendocrine link with pulsatile LH secretion. *Science* 1979; 205:823–825.
27. Larsen IF: Hot flushes after hypophysectomy. *Br Med J* 1977; 2:1356.
28. Meldrum DR, Erlik Y, Lu JHK, et al: Objectively recorded hot flushes in patients with pituitary insufficiency. *J Clin Endocrinol Metab* 1981; 52:684–687.
29. Elkind-Hirsh KE, Ravnikar V, Schiff I, et al: Determination of endogenous immunoreactive LHRH levels in the plasma of postmenopausal women. Proceedings of the 28th Annual Meeting of the Society of Gynecological Investigation (Abst. 20). St. Louis, March 18–21, 1981.
30. Gambone J, Meldrum DR, Laufer L, et al: Further delineation of hypothalamic dysfunction responsible for menopausal hot flushes. *J Clin Endocrinol Metab* 1984; 59:1097–1102.
31. Ausel S, Schomberg DW, Tyrey L, et al: Vasomotor symptoms, serum estrogen and gonadotropin levels in surgical menopause. *Am J Obstet Gynecol* 1976; 126:165–169.
32. Chakravarti S, Collins WP, Forecast JD, et al: Hormonal profiles after the menopause. *Br Med J* 1976; 2:784–787.
33. Erlik Y, Meldrum DR, Judd HL: Estrogen levels in postmenopausal women with hot flushes. *Obstet Gynecol* 1982; 59:403–407.
34. Meldrum DR, Tataryn IV, Frumar AM, et al: Gonadotropins, estrogens, and adrenal steroids during the menopausal hot flush. *J Clin Endocrinol Metab* 1980; 50:685–689.
35. Meldrum DR, DeFazio JD, Erlik Y, et al: Pituitary hormones during the menopausal hot flush. *Obstet Gynecol* 1984; 64:752–756.
36. Yen SSC: The biology of menopause. *J Reprod Med* 1977; 18:287.
37. Pardridge WM, Mietus LJ: Transport of steroid hormones through the rat blood-brain barrier. Primary role of albumin-bound hormone. *J Clin Invest* 1979; 64:145.
38. Gambone JC, Pardridge WM, Lagasse LD, et al: In vivo availability of circulating estradiol in menopausal women with and without endometrial cancer. *Obstet Gynecol* 1982; 59:416.
39. Illner P, Marques P, Williams DD, et al: Endocrine responses to *ruminal* cooling in goats, in *Proceedings of the Third Symposium on the Pharmacology of Thermoregulation*, Coopen KE, Lomax P (eds). Basel, Karger, pp 58–61.
40. Lightman SL, Jacobs HS, Maguire AK, et al: Climacteric flushing: Clinical and endocrine response to infusion of naloxone. *Br J Obstet Gynecol* 1981; 88:919–924.
41. DeFazio J, Verheugen C, Chetkowski R, et al: The effects of Naloxone on hot flushes and gonadotropin secretion in postmenopausal women. *J Clin Endocrinol Metab* 1984; 58:578–581.
42. Tulandi T, Kinch RA, Guyda H, et al: Effects of naloxone on menopausal flushes, skin temperature, and LH secretion. *Am J Obstet Gynecol* 1985; 151:277–280.

CHAPTER **5**

Alterations in the Urogenital System

ARIEH BERGMAN, M.D.
PAUL F. BRENNER, M.D.

THE MUCOSAL LININGS of the vagina and the urethra are extremely sensitive to alterations in the estrogen milieu. The squamous epithelial tissues respond to both increases and decreases in the endogenous estrogen levels as well as the administration of exogenous estrogen. The maturation of the vaginal and the urethral mucosa is dependent upon the presence of estrogen and can be altered either by the absence of estrogen or the presence of antiestrogenic factors, such as hormones, drugs, or diseases. Hypoestrogenism can also alter the relationship between intravesicular pressure and the urethral pressure.

The marked decline in ovarian estrogen secretion results in significant physical changes, particularly in those female tissues that are the most sensitive to either the presence or the deprivation of estrogen. The changes that occur in the vagina as the result of the menopause are the reflection of the withdrawal of hormonal support for a very estrogen-responsive tissue. The vaginal mucosa of postmenopausal women who do not receive supplemental estrogen therapy becomes attenuated and appears pale and almost transparent from a decrease in vascularity. It may be only three or four cells thick. The rugated appearance of the vaginal vault during a woman's reproductive years may disappear completely in the postmenopause. Marked atrophic changes in the vagina can result in atrophic vaginitis. In this condition, the vaginal epithelium is very thin, inflamed, and even ulcerated. Bleeding sites can be present in the vagina as the result of atrophic vaginitis.[1] The cervix, instead of protruding into the vagina, atrophies and retracts and eventually may become flush with the apex of the vault. The upper one third of the vagina has a tendency to constrict, and the entire vagina tends to become shorter in length and looses its elasticity. In extreme cases, the narrowing of the upper portion of the vagina and the retraction of the cervix present the physician with great difficulty in identifying the cervix in order to obtain the annual Pap smear. In the postmenopausal years, the ligaments supporting the uterus lose their tone. This may lead to partial uterine prolapse or total uterine procidentia. The elastic tissue of the vaginal wall also loses its tensile strength, and a cystocele and or rectocele may develop. In the postmenopausal years the vaginal pH increases, becoming either alkaline or slightly acidic. The change in the vaginal pH is often enough to permit the growth of bacteria that are otherwise not normally found in the vagina, and this may result in the development of a clinical vaginal infection with a copious purulent discharge.

Not only are there vaginal changes as the result of estrogen depletion in the postmenopause, but there are also atrophic changes of the external genitalia which may lead to pruritis vulvae. The changes in the external genitalia of postmenopausal women are the result of both the aging process and the decline in estrogen. There is a reduction in the amount of pubic hair. The loss of subcutaneous fat and elastic tissue creates a wrinkled appearance of the labia majora and minora. The atrophy of the labia majora is usually greater than that of the labia minora. The secretion of the Bartholin glands is reduced. The labia become less sensitive and are less likely to swell and separate in response to sexual stimulation.

The physical changes of the lower genital tract associated with the menopause vary widely from one individual to another. At one extreme is the woman whose vaginal changes, brought about by the decline in endogenous estrogen, proceed so slowly that they are barely perceptible to her. At the other extreme is the woman who experiences rapid atrophic changes over a relatively short period of time. In general, women who undergo a rather sudden menopause as the result of surgical castration, irradiation castration, or even certain diseases, such as a severe pelvic infection that has destroyed virtually all normal ovarian tissue, are those most likely to have the most rapid physical changes and the most pronounced symptomatology.

During a woman's reproductive years, the vagina is lined by a thick, stratified, squamous epithelium. In the well-estrogenized vaginal mucosa, each epithelial cell is rich in glycogen, and the lactobacillus is a normal inhabitant of the vagina. This microorganism metabolizes glycogen to produce an acidic vaginal environment. The low pH of the vagina normally found in the reproductive years is a deterrent to vaginal infections. The decline in estrogen concentrations in the peripheral circulation of the postmenopausal woman has a profound effect on the genitourinary system. The squamous epithelium atrophies, the glycogen content of the cells becomes quite low, and the vaginal pH increases.

ALTERATIONS IN VAGINAL CYTOLOGY

The surface cells of the vaginal epithelium are exfoliated and are found in the vaginal desquamate. This desquamate is normally composed of three different types of epithelial cells: the parabasal cell, the intermediate cell, and the superficial cell. The parabasal cell is the most immature of the three cells. Its presence in the vaginal desquamate usually indicates either a very low level of estrogen exposure to the vaginal mucosa or the presence in the hormonal environment of antiestrogens, such as progesterone or corticosteroids. A vaginal infection may also result in the exfoliation of parabasal cells. Estrogen stimulation causes a thickening of the vaginal mucosa and a maturation of the epithelium to intermediate and superficial cells. The superficial cell is the most mature of the three cell types and is indicative of an estrogen-dominant environment. In the well-estrogenized vaginal epithelium, the superficial cells are located on the surface, with the intermediate cells situated immediately below them. The maturity of the squamous epithelium of the vagina, and therefore, the cell type found in the vaginal desquamate, is a reflection of the woman's hormonal environment.

The cytologic examination of vaginal cells as an indicator of the hormonal environment is most accurate if the specimen is obtained from scraping the lateral wall of the vagina at the level of the external cervical os. The *maturation index* (MI) is the determination of the ratio of parabasal, intermediate, and superficial cells that are present in the vaginal specimen when 100 consecutive cells are studied. A shift of the MI (parabasal cells/intermediate cells/superficial cells) to the left indicates a decline in the maturity of the cells found in the vaginal desquamate. A shift of the MI to the right indicates an increase in the number of intermediate and superficial cells and, therefore, enhanced maturity of the exfoliated vaginal cells.[2]

The composition of the cells found in the vaginal pool may also be expressed as the *maturation value* (MV). Each cell in the specimen from the vagina is assigned a numerical score: parabasal cells, 0.0; intermediate cells, 0.5; and superficial cells, 1.0. The maturation value is the total score obtained when 100 consecutive cells are evaluated. Estrogen stimulation increases the maturation value, and estrogen deprivation decreases the maturation value.[3]

Another method of expressing the cytohormonal effect on the epithelial cells exfoliated from the vagina is the *karyopyknotic index* (KI). The KI is the percent of superficial cells found in the total population of the squamous cells examined. The presence of estrogen increases the KI, while a hormonal environment deficient in estrogen decreases the KI.[4]

The MI is influenced by many factors that may be either hormonal or nonhormonal. The presence of high levels of endogenous estrogen or the administration of exogenous estrogen causes the epithelial cells of the vaginal mucosa to mature to superficial cells prior to desquamation. This results in a shift of the MI to the right. The presence of progesterone in the hormonal milieu causes the epithelial cells to mature to intermediate cells before exfoliation. Progesterone from any source accentuates the midzone, intermediate cells, of the maturation index. Corticosteroids have an effect similar to progesterone on the vaginal epithelial cells and, again, produces an MI where the intermediate cells predominate. Androgens result in the appearance of all three epithelial cell types in the vaginal desquamate in equal numbers. In an androgen-dominant hormonal environment, parabasal cells, intermediate cells, and superficial cells may all be found on the surface of the vaginal mucosa, and this produces a spread pattern in the MI. The nonhormonal factors that influence the MI include the use of digitalis or tetracycline therapy, hypothyroidism, and the presence of a vaginal infection. Both digitalis and tetracycline treatment cause the epithelial cells to mature to the intermediate cell stage and, very much like progesterone and corticosteroids, produce a midzone shift in the MI.[5] Hypothyroidism may shift the MI to the left. A vaginal infection may result in all three epithelial cells appearing in the vaginal pool with an equal distribution, and this produces a spread pattern in the MI similar to that seen with androgens.

The MI changes throughout a woman's life, reflecting the changes in her own sex steroid levels. At birth there is an accentuation of the midzone of the MI (0-95-5) in response to the recent exposure of the fetus to the high maternal levels of progesterone and estrogen during pregnancy. Within the first few weeks of life, the steroid levels decline precipitously, and the MI (100-0-0 to 75-25-0) mirrors the low levels of endogenous sex steroids and the immaturity of the vaginal mucosa. During a woman's reproductive years, the MI responds to the presence of unopposed estrogen (0-40-60) and, in the luteal phase of the menstrual cycle, the presence of estrogen and progesterone in the peripheral circulation (0-70-30). During the postmenopausal years, in the absence of estrogen replacement therapy, the MI reflects the sharp reduction in ovarian estrogen production (0-95-5) and ultimately the lack of all hormonal stimulation (100-0-0). The former cytohormonal pattern has been referred to as estatrophy, and the latter, as teleatrophy.

While the MI may be a reflection of the hormonal environment, it is not very reliable clinically in predicting which postmenopausal women will experience vasomotor symptoms or what the response of these symptoms will be to therapy.[6] Stone and co-workers studied 29 women who were surgically castrated.[7] There was no correlation between the women's MI and the presence or absence of hot flushes. In a similar manner, the maturation index has not proven to be clinically useful in distinguishing the women who are destined to develop postmenopausal osteoporotic fractures from those women who will not sustain this devastating disease.

The maturation index is still used to determine the need for estrogen replacement. This practice is associated with several important problems. The use of the maturation index, a cytologic parameter, to assay the estrogen status of a specific patient, which is a hormonal parameter, is very difficult to standardize. The reliability of any assay depends on the criteria of precision, sensitivity, specificity, and accuracy. In order for the cytologic findings to be a precise index of a subject's estrogen environment, a linear relationship must exist between the maturation of the exfoliated vaginal cells and the amount of estrogen stimulation to the vagina. A linear relationship between these two parameters has never been demonstrated. The use of a cytologic index to assay endogenous estrogen levels accurately requires a monohormonal environment. Such an environment does not exist in postmenopausal women. Androgens are secreted from both the postmenopausal ovaries and the adrenal glands, and also present are low levels of progesterone and corticosteroids. The presence of these other steroids may inhibit the vaginal response to estrogen, or, depending on the initial cell pattern, they may have a synergistic effect with estrogen on the maturation of the vaginal mucosa. The sensitivity of the maturation index shows a wide range of individual differences. Under identical hormonal conditions, the type of cells found in the vaginal desquamate varies greatly from one individual to another. These differences may be partially due to individual threshold levels of estrogen that must be reached before the vaginal mucosa starts to mature. The refractoriness or decreased sensitivity of the lining of the vagina to estrogen stimulation in some women is a clinical reflection of a high threshold required for a response. The wide range of patient variation seen in the maturation index is a result of the poor specificity of this bioassay. Local factors, vaginal infections, and exogenous medications are all known to interfere with the interpretation of this cytologic index. Mechanical factors, uterine prolapse, or chemicals that cause a local irritation to the lining of the vagina may produce a differentiation of the superficial layer of the vagina. Vaginal infections are also known to promote maturation of the cells lining the vagina. Women with vaginal infections seem to be more responsive to estrogen stimulation of the vagina than women who do not have vaginal infections. Exogenous treatment with digitalis enhances the maturation of the vaginal mucosa. Similar vaginal smear patterns can be demonstrated in women who have markedly different endocrinologic environments. The presence of intermediate cells can be the result of a slight estrogen deficiency following a previously normal estrogen exposure, progestogen administration, the presence of estrogen and progesterone, or the presence of androgen. The accuracy of the maturation index is severely limited. The selection of the maturation index to determine the need for estrogen replacement is a poor choice. As an assay, the maturation index lacks precision, sensitivity, specificity, and accuracy. The criteria of reliability of the maturation index, while acceptable in the 1960s, is clearly unacceptable in the 1980s, with the superior methodology now available.

URODYNAMIC PRESSURE CHANGES

The urinary system undergoes marked alterations in the postmenopausal years that may result in a diminished capacity for effective urine control and, eventually, the appearance of urinary incontinence. There are three factors, all equally important, in the maintenance of urinary continence. These factors are urethral mucosa resistance, the intra-abdominal location of the proximal urethra, and the contraction of the periurethral striated muscle fibers at the time of stress.

The urethral mucosa and distal vagina have a common embryologic origin—the urogenital sinus.[8] The urethral mucosa cells are therefore estrogen-sensitive and contain estrogen receptors in a concentration similar to that of the vaginal epithelial cells.[9–11] In the premenopausal woman, one third of the total resistance, which is a key factor in maintaining urinary continence, is derived from the "urethral mucosa" factor.[12, 13] The urethral mucosa factor is comprised of the urethral mucosal thickness and the engorgement of the underlying blood vessels.[12] This factor diminishes in the postmenopausal years as the result of the atrophy of all estrogen-dependent tissues including the urethral mucosa. The urethral mucosa is composed of transitional cells proximally and squamous cells distally. In the premenopausal years, the squamous epithelium extends upwards towards the urethrovesical junction and increases the thickness of the urethral mucosa. In the postmenopausal years, the squamous epithelium regresses and becomes thinner, and the MI from the urethral mucosa reveals predominantly parabasal cells.[14] These atrophic changes are very similar to those that occur in the vagina. In 17 postmenopausal patients who were not receiving estrogen replacement therapy and who were seen for urinary tract symptomatology, urethral cytology was obtained by gentle scraping from the midurethra. Cytologic examination revealed the presence of mainly parabasal cells. Urethral cytology was obtained in 15 of these women after 6 weeks of estrogen therapy. Following treatment, there was a shift of the maturation index to the right in the urethral specimen (Fig 5–1).

The changes in the lower urinary tract in the postmenopausal years are manifested dynamically as a drop in urethral pressure. The urethral closure pressure is defined as the urethral pressure minus the vesical pressure. The urethral closure pressure is an important factor in the maintenance of urinary continence, and this pressure decreases significantly in the postmenopausal years. In studies using urodynamic testing, it has been demonstrated that a 30% drop in urethral closure pressure at rest and during stress occurs in postmenopausal women.[15] This drop in pressure is attributed mainly to the loss of the "urethral mucosa" factor.

There is a decrease in the support of the pelvic organs in the postmenopausal period, including diminished support of the urethrovesical unit. Various degrees of a cystocele usually accompany uterine descensus. The loss of the support to the base of the bladder and the urethra results in urodynamic alterations that affect the remaining two factors involved in the maintenance of urinary continence. Prolapse of the urethrovesical junction removes this unit from the intra-abdominal pressure sphere. The poorly supported urethra does not permit effective contraction of the striated periurethral muscle fibers at the time of stress.

When pelvic organs retain their normal support, the proximal urethra is in the intra-abdominal pressure sphere. The urethra is supported in this position by the two pubourethral ligaments as well as by the endopelvic fascia.[16] In the postmenopause, there is a decrease in the support of all the pelvic organs. The urethrovesical junction descends and is no longer in the intra-abdominal pressure sphere. As a result, a sudden increase in the abdominal pressure during stress, which should be equally transmitted to the bladder and proximal urethra, is now transmitted to the bladder only. This causes an increase in the intravesicular pressure without urethral compensation and the resultant

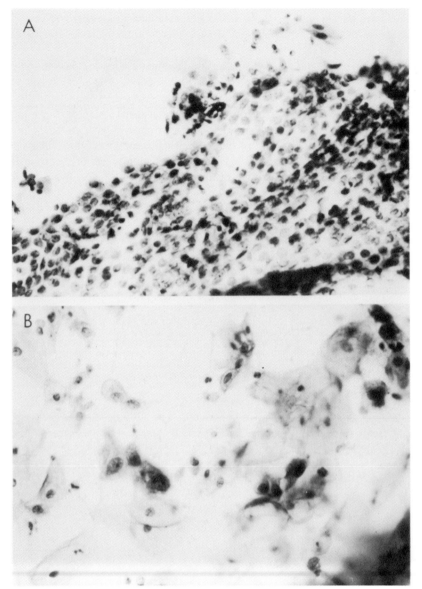

FIG 5–1.
Urethral cytology obtained from midurethra in a patient with good clinical response. Note abundance of transitional cells before treatment (**A**) and superificial squamous cells appearance after estrogen treatment (**B**).

loss of urine. Urodynamic measurements have demonstrated the poor transmission of abdominal pressure to the proximal urethra when varying degrees of prolapse of the bladder base occurs.[17]

Pelvic relaxation in the multiparous, postmenopausal woman usually is accompanied by the relaxation of periurethral striated muscle. This muscle is composed of 65% slow-twitched fibers and 35% fast-twitched fibers.[18] The fast-twitched fibers contract reflectory at the time of increased intra-abdominal pressure, which enables the urethra pressure to increase immediately to above the vesical pressure at the time of stress.[18] Urodynamic measurements demonstrate an increase in urethral pressure during stress which exceeds the resting pressure (Fig 5–2). The periurethral muscle fibers must be at an optimal tension in order to contract reflectory at the time of stress. This optimal tension is lost with urethral relaxation, which accompanies the pelvic relaxation typically found in parous postmenopausal women. The diminished support of the pelvic structures does not enable the muscle fibers to maintain the tension that is necessary for their reflectory contraction.

It is not surprising that various degrees of urinary incontinence are found in most postmenopausal women, and inadequate control of urination is one of the most troublesome conditions of women at this stage of their lives.

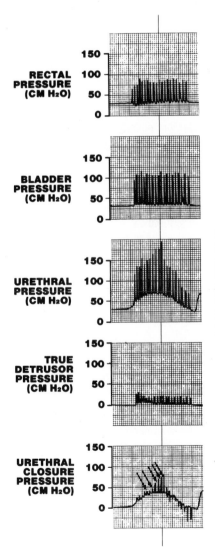

FIG 5–2.
Urethral pressure to cough profile in a continent patient. Arrows point urethral pressure increase at time of stress, due to reflectory contraction of periurethral striated muscle. (From Ostergard DR: *Gynecologic Urology and Urodynamics.* Baltimore, Williams & Wilkins Co, 1980. Used by permission.)

ATROPHIC URETHRITIS AND VOIDING DISORDERS

The thin and friable urethral mucosa that is frequently seen in postmenopausal women who are not receiving estrogen replacement therapy is responsible for diminished urethral resistance, a burning sensation while voiding, and dysuria. The attenuation of the trigone, which occurs from atrophy, is the cause of urinary urgency and frequency. These urinary symptoms of urgency, frequency, dysuria, and suprapubic pain in the absence of a urinary tract infection are known as the senile urethral syndrome.[19] In postmenopausal women, in whom the urethral syndrome is secondary to hypoestrogenism, the term *senile urethritis* or *atrophic urethritis* is used to describe this entity.[20, 21]

This syndrome is the result of the irritation of the thin urethral mucosa. The burning sensation is related to the urine coming into close contact with the urethral sensory nerves, which are branches of the pudendal nerve. Urinary urgency and frequency are symptoms related to the neurologic loop that coordinates urethral and detrusor sensory and motor activity. This loop was first described by Bradley et al.[22] It originates at the detrusor muscle, communicates with the lower micturition center (S_2–S_4 level) through the pelvic nerves and through the pudendal nerve. This neurologic loop is a center that coordinates bladder and urethral function. At the time of voiding, sensory impulses from the urethra, following urethral relaxation, reach the bladder, causing the sensation of urgency and detrusor contraction. Reduced urethral pressure and urethral relaxation cause the symptoms of urgency and frequency.[23–25] Postmenopausal women have a 30% drop in their urethral closure pressure, which is attributed mainly to the loss of the "urethra mucosa" factor. Estrogen therapy improves the "urethra mucosa" factor, and the symptoms of urgency, frequency, dysuria and suprapubic tenderness are alleviated. (See Chapter 12, Beneficial Effects of Pharmacologic Agents—Genitourinary.)

Commonly, postmenopausal women are unable to completely empty their bladders. Urine flow rates are characteristically reduced in postmenopausal women, and residual urine volumes are increased.[26] A normal effective voiding mechanism involves numerous neurologic reflexes.[22, 27] Voiding starts with urethral relaxation, which is activated by neuronal impulses originating at the cerebral cortex and terminating at the periurethral muscle.[22] Effective voiding is maintained by detrusor contraction with continuous urethral relaxation. Neurologic impulses for this phase are conducted through the loop originating in the detrusor and terminating at the urethral muscle. This neurologic loop is coordinated at the lower micturition center at the level of S_2–S_4.[22] Voiding is terminated by urethral contraction, which causes a reflectory detrusor inhibition through the same neurologic loop that coordinates urethral and detrusor functions. Any central or peripheral neuropathy may interrupt this sensitive neurologic mechanism and result in ineffective voiding. Various degrees of neuropathy are associated with advanced age. By 80 years of age, only a few people have intact ankle jerk reflexes or intact olfactory and auditory sensations.[28] It is not surprising that postmenopausal women have an impairment of the function of their voiding mechanisms and voiding disorders.

REFERENCES

1. Notelovitz M: Gynecologic problems of menopausal women: part 1. Changes in genital tissue. *Geriatrics* 1978; 33:24.
2. Budoff PW, Sommers SC: Estrogen-progesterone therapy in postmenopausal women. *J Reprod Med* 1979; 22:241.
3. Meisels A; The menopause: A cytohormonal study. *Acta Cytol* (Baltimore) 1966; 10:49.

4. McLennan MT, McLennan CE: Estrogenic status of menstruating and menopausal women assessed by cervicovaginal smears. *Obstet Gynecol* 1971; 37:325.
5. Stone DF, Sedlis A, Stone ML, et al: Estrogen-like effects in the vaginal smears of post-menopausal women. *Acta Cytol (Baltimore)* 1967; 11:349.
6. Kaufman SA: Limited relationship of maturation index to estrogen therapy for menopausal symptoms. An analysis of 200 patients. *Obstet Gynecol* 1967; 30:399.
7. Stone SC, Mickal A, Rye PH: Postmenopausal symptomatology, maturation index and plasma estrogen levels. *Obstet Gynecol* 1975; 45:625.
8. Ostergard DR: Embryology and anatomy of the female bladder and urethra, in Ostergard DR (ed): *Gynecologic Urology and Urodynamics*. Baltimore, Williams & Wilkins Co, 1980, p 3.
9. Batra S, Iosif S: Functional estrogen receptors in the female urethra. *Proceedings of Second Joint Meeting of ICS and Urodynamic Soc*. Aachen, 1983, p 548.
10. Ingleman-Sundberg A, Rosen J, Gustafsson SA, et al.: Cytosol estrogen receptors in the urogenital tissues in stress-incontinent women. *Acta Obstet Gynecol Scand* 1981; 60:585.
11. Iosif S, Batra S, Ek A, et al: Estrogen receptors in the human female lower urinary tract. *Am J Obstet Gynecol* 1981; 141:817.
12. Zinner NN, Sterling AM, Ritter RC: Role of urethral softness in urinary incontinence. *Urology* 1980; 16:115.
13. Raz S, Ziegler M, Caine M: The vascular component in the production in intraurethral pressure. *J Urol* 1972; 108:93.
14. Zuckerman S: Morphological and functional homologies of the male and female reproductive system. *Br Med J* 1936; 2:264.
15. Reed T: Urethral pressure profile in continent women from childhood to old age. *Acta Obstet Gynecol Scand* 1980; 59:331.
16. Zacharin RF: Abdominoperineal urethral suspension in the management of recurrent stress incontinence of urine: 15 years' experience. *Obstet Gynecol* 1983; 62:644.
17. Bhatia NN, Ostergard DR: Urodynamics in women with stress urinary incontinence. *Obstet Gynecol* 1982; 60:552.
18. Tanagho EA, Miller ER: Functional consideration of urethral sphincteric dynamics. *J Urol* 1973; 109:273.
19. Scotti RJ, Ostergard DR: The urethral syndrome. *Clin Obstet Gynecol* 1984; 27:515.
20. Cifuentes L: Epithelium of vaginal type in the female trigone: The clinical problem of trigonitis. *J Urol* 1947; 57:1028.
21. Youngblood VH, Tomlin EM, Davis JB: Senile urethritis in women. *J Urol* 1957; 78:150.
22. Bradley WE, Bockswold GL, Timm GW, et al: Neurology of micturition. *J Urol* 1976; 115:481.
23. Bergman A, Bhatia NN, Hasen J: Effect of thryoid-releasing hormone on bladder and urethral pressures. *Br J Urol* 1984; 56:397.
24. Bergman A, Bhatia NN, Hasen J: Urinary urgency and thyrotropin-releasing hormone. *Am J Obstet Gynecol* 1984; 148:106.
25. Ulmsten U, Henriksson L, Iosif S: The unstable female urethra. *Am J Obstet Gynecol* 1982; 144:93.
26. Abrams P, Torres M: Clinical urodynamics. *Urol Clin North Am* 1979; 6:71.
27. Blaines JG: The neurophysiology of micturition: A clinical study of 550 patients. *J Urol* 1982; 127:958.
28. Johnson W: *The Older Patient*. New York, Paul Hoeber Inc, 1960, pp 88–103.

CHAPTER 6

Alterations in Skeletal Homeostasis With Age and Menopause

ROBERT LINDSAY, M.B., Ch.B., Ph.D., F.R.C.P.
JACK F. TOHMÉ, M.D.

AT SKELETAL MATURITY, which usually is assumed to be about the end of the third decade of life, bone mass and density are lower in women than men. Subsequent bone loss with aging is a universal phenomenon, starting in the fourth and fifth decades in women and somewhat later in men. However, regardless of the age at which it occurs, the onset of the menopause heralds profound but subtle changes in skeletal homeostasis that, for most individuals, are reflected in an acceleration of this bone-loss phenomenon. Current evidence suggests that this period of exaggerated loss is exponential with time, and hence self-limiting. However, individual variation is marked, both in the degree of loss of skeletal tissue and the time over which it occurs. The process is asymptomatic and is of little clinical consequence until the patient presents to the physician with an osteoporotic fracture. Such fractures are exceedingly common among the aging female population, and they carry a significant associated morbidity and mortality. Vertebral crush fracture, hip fracture, and fractures of the distal radius are the most common, although fractures involving any bone may occur. From our current data, it appears likely that some 25%–50% of all women will have reached a bone mass below some theoretical fracture threshold by the time they are in their early 60s. While there is still some controversy about the exact pathophysiology involved in production of both the sexual dimorphism of bone loss and the osteoporotic fracture syndromes, it is nonetheless clear that the loss of ovarian function is a significant factor in osteoporosis among women. Indeed, if this phenomenon did not occur, it seems likely that fracture frequency among aging women would be no greater than that recorded for men. Thus, these menopausal changes in bone remodeling are superimposed on the phenomenon of aging that involves loss of lean body mass and skeletal mass, and exaggerate in some fashion the reduction in skeletal mass.

This chapter will be devoted mostly to a discussion of bone remodeling and its control in the adult. The factors involved in bone loss will be discussed, inasmuch as they are understood, as well as those changes that occur at the menopause and result in excessive bone loss. Also to be discussed will be the criteria used currently for early evaluation of the patient who may be at risk from osteoporosis.

THE IMPORTANCE OF THE PROBLEM

As indicated, bone loss is an asymptomatic process that is of clinical relevance only when the patient presents with a fracture. The frequency of such fractures rises with age, this increase occurring earlier and being of greater magnitude among women than among men[13] in most cultures. The problem is also greater among white and Asiatic races than among the black population. Epidemiologic data have been difficult to obtain for osteoporosis, but it has been suggested that 25% of women will in fact have radiologic evidence of osteoporosis by age 60 years. In the United States, by the end of the current decade, there will be 20 million women older than 65 years, and of these, 5 million will have, therefore, radiologic evidence of osteoporosis. Of women who attain the age of 80 years, one in four can expect to have suffered a hip fracture. The incidence of hip fractures among women doubles by each decade after 50 years.[15] The overall incidence of fractures of the proximal femur is approximately 1.3% per year for women over the age of 65 and about 0.3% per year for men over 65.[30] The real incidence of vertebral crush fractures, the most common osteoporotic fracture, is unknown, since this fracture, by itself, does not usually result in hospital admission.

Using fractures of the proximal femur as the benchmark, recent evidence indicates that the overall incidence of this disorder is increasing. Data from centers in the United Kingdom and the U.S.A. have suggested that hospital admissions and discharges as a result of fracture of the femoral neck are increasing every decade at a rate greater than would be expected from the rise in the median age of the population.[11, 29, 46] Data from our center, generated from discharge summaries obtained from a cross-sectional survey of United States hospitals, indicate a rise in incidence of both vertebral fractures and hip fractures. Between the years 1970 and 1980, there was an increase of 40% in the overall discharges reported for hip fracture, with no evidence of a similar increase among traumatic fractures (Fig 6–1). About 80% of the increment can be accounted for by the increasing median age of the population and, therefore, the increase of absolute numbers of individuals at risk.

In 1984, more than 300,000 hip fractures were expected to occur in the United States, both intertrochanteric and subcapital. By the end of the century, if the current trend continues, there will be approximately half a million fractures per year. The incidence rises exponentially among women, from 9/100,000 person years for women aged 35–44 years to a peak of 3,317/100,000 person years (or 3.3% per year) for women aged 85 or older. The peak incidence is half as great in men at 85 or older.[35]

Overall, however, about 85 percent of all hip fractures occur in women. Not only does this result in a considerable morbidity and mortality but also in significant health care costs. The total cost of health care for patients with osteoporosis in the United States exceeds 4 billion dollars a year currently and may quadruple by the end of this century. In most studies in which hip fracture patients have been observed, there is an associated mortality rate of approximately 10%.[23] Such mortality figures bring hip fractures (and secondarily, osteoporosis) into the top 12 most common causes of death in the United States. In addition, about 30% of the patients admitted to acute-care hospitals as a result of hip fractures are subsequently discharged to long-term care facilities, placing a further burden on the health care delivery systems.

The magnitude of this public health problem, which currently costs the country almost 6 billion dollars annually for all aspects of health care of osteoporotic patients, has resulted in a massive public awareness campaign and an explosion of interest among health care professionals. An understanding of the problem and its pathogenesis requires knowledge of the processes controlling skeletal homeostasis in the adult and of the changes that result in loss of bone tissue.

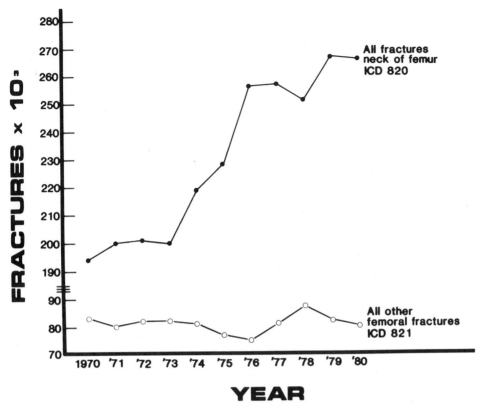

FIG 6–1.
Total estimated fractures of the femoral neck in the U.S.A. from 1970 through 1980 (ICD Code 820). All other femoral fractures (coded ICD 821) are shown for comparison and are assumed to be traumatic.

BONE REMODELING IN THE ADULT

Bone remodeling (Fig 6–2) is the process by which adult bone can renew the bone tissue in such a way that the overall composition, mass, and volume remain essentially unaffected. It is assumed that the mechanisms involved in the continuous loss of bone that occurs in the adult result from impairment of the bone remodeling sequence. In the adult human, the majority of bone remodeling takes place following a defined process that has been described in detail by Frost (see Fig 6–2). Remodeling appears to take place in small packets of bone, often referred to as *quanta*. The process is initiated when osteoclasts are recruited to begin resorption of the bone packet. The origin of these osteoclasts is unknown, as is the control of the activation process. Once begun, however, resorption continues until a cavity of some 50–60 μ in depth has been created. At this point, under influences as yet unknown, the osteoclasts cease to function, disappear, and are replaced by monocytic cells, which appear to prepare the surface of the cavity for the next phase of the remodeling cycle. This phase is sometimes called reversal. After the reversal phase, osteoblasts appear and begin to refill the cavity with new bone. Osteoblasts, under normal conditions, will only lay down new bone on a surface at which there has been resorption. If ideal homeostasis existed, then the amount

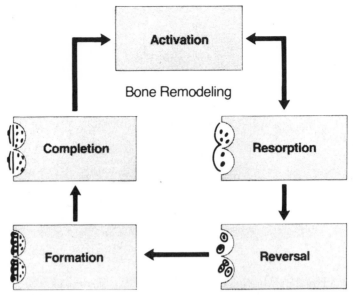

FIG 6-2.
The bone remodeling cycle as envisaged by Frost (1973). The initial activation step is followed by a period of bone resorption and then, after what has been called a reversal process, a period of bone formation ensues.

of new bone laid down would be exactly equal to that resorbed by the osteoclasts. For some reason that is poorly understood, in the adult the amount of bone laid down by the osteoblasts is somewhat less than that removed by the osteoclasts. This could result from either excessive osteoclast function or defective osteoblast function, or a combination of both.

Such bone remodeling cycles are activated throughout the adult human at the approximate rate of six to nine per minute. More frequent activation, by itself, would result in an initial *temporary* increase in the amount of bone that is lost. However, since there is a deficit between the amount of bone resorbed and new bone laid down, then more active remodeling must eventually result in a permanent loss of bone at an increased rate.

Many of the factors controlling bone turnover are not well understood. Activation is a process that must be controlled by a variety of local factors, both chemical and physical, as well as systemic factors, such as parathyroid hormone and 1,25 dihydroxyvitamin D. Local electrical currents generated by changes in physical enviroment are probably important in regulating activation frequency. It is equally clear that some local signaling mechanisms must exist. Osteoclasts may be attracted by chemotactic signals and must be able to sense in some way the size of the cavity, as must osteoblasts. The different lineages of osteoclasts and osteoblasts suggest that communication must exist between the adult cell populations and also with the monocytic cells of the reversal phase. These communication signals are assumed to be chemical, and they may include prostaglandins, various growth factors and other peptides, and perhaps also the group of peptides often known as lymphokines and monokines. General or systemic influences on these cell populations clearly include parathyroid hormone, calcitonin, and the vitamin D metabolites. Other endocrine influences may include insulin, glucocorticoids, growth hormone, and thyroxine. The mechanism by which the sex steroids influence these processes is not well understood but may be indirect.

PATHOGENESIS OF BONE LOSS

Of prime importance in the pathogenesis of bone loss is the imbalance between formation and resorption that starts during the fourth decade in the adult human. With such an imbalance, activation frequency also becomes important. Other modeling processes that occur in the adult, such as periosteal bone formation and endosteal bone resorption, which are primarily cortical bone phenomena, are thought to have only a minor importance in the genesis of the fractures of postmenopausal osteoporosis. However, changes in cortical bone mass produced by inequalities in those systems may significantly affect the strength of bone in the femoral neck. The resistance to the bending and twisting forces to which this region is submitted may require not only a critical mass of cortical bone but also young bone that has more elasticity than more highly calcified old bone.

While it seems likely that there is an intrinsic defect in the remodeling system in favor of resorption, it is equally evident that dramatic change in turnover occurs at the menopause or following oophorectomy. Cessation of ovarian function is accompanied by a small rise in serum calcium and phosphate and an increased urinary loss of calcium and hydroxyproline, all indicators of increased bone resorption (Fig 6–3). An increase in serum alkaline phosphatase and perhaps also BGP (bone gla-protein or osteocalcium) demonstrates the concomitant increment in bone formation. Parfitt (1979) has calculated that at least 50% of the bone loss in postmenopausal women can be accounted for by

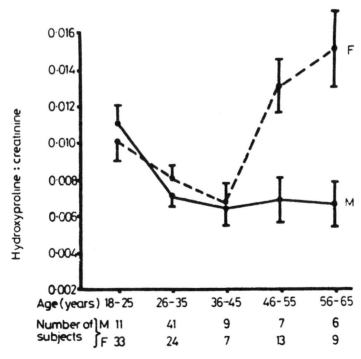

FIG 6–3.
The rise in excretion of hydroxyproline containing peptides, which occurs about the time of the menopause in women but does not occur in men (Hodgkinson & Thompson, 1982).

the imbalance between the osteoclast and osteoblast; the remainder results from more rapid activation of bone remodeling units. This phenomenon is particularly obvious in trabecular bone, where 80% of bone remodeling occurs. Estimates of bone loss in the spine, for example, where about 60% of the bone mass of the vertebrae consists of trabecular bone, suggest that the rate of loss of trabecular bone may be as great as 5%–15% per year[14] in the early years following menopause or oophorectomy. This, in all likelihood, accounts for the high incidence of vertebral crush fractures in women aged 55–65 years. The slower loss of cortical bone is accounted for, at least partially, by the high volume-to-surface area ratio and subsequent relatively low turnover, especially when considered in relation to trabecular bone.

There seems little doubt that the sexual dimorphism so evident in the clinical expression of osteoporosis results from this loss of ovarian function and the subsequent changes in skeletal remodeling. In prospective studies, the postmenopausal exaggeration of bone loss appears to be exponential, accounts for approximately 50% of the expected age-related bone loss (by age 80 years), and is prevented by estrogen treatment (Fig 6–4). Removal of estrogen therapy results in a rate of bone loss that is equivalent to the fast component of postoophorectomy bone loss (Fig 6–5)—further confirmation of the estrogen dependence of bone remodeling. In addition, it is noteworthy that loss of ovarian function among premenopausal women can also result in reduced bone mass, as, for example, in exercise-induced amenorrhea.[10]

These changes in skeletal performance can be measured as changes in women's calcium requirement and balance, using carefully controlled kinetic studies.[16–18] In a series of elegant studies conducted through the menopause, Heaney has demonstrated a significant deterioration in calcium homeostasis following menopause. Postmenopausal

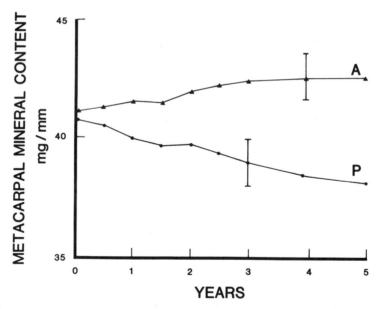

FIG 6–4.
Prevention of bone loss in oophorectomized women using estrogen therapy. *Line A* indicates mean bone mass during five-year follow-up of 64 patients treated with an average daily dose of Mestranol of 24–28 mg. *Line P* indicates mean bone mass during similar follow-up of control group randomly given matching placebo tablets.

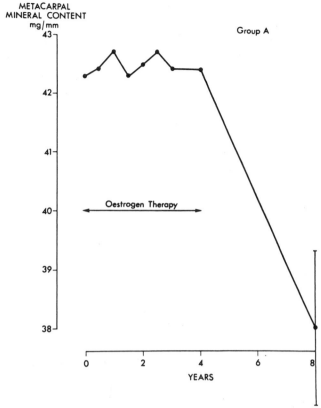

FIG 6–5.
Bone loss after removal of estrogen treatment. Patients were treated with 25 mcg Mestranol daily for four years. Therapy was discontinued and bone loss ensued. The rate of loss was equivalent to that observed in the immediate postmenopausal or postoophorectomy period.

women tend to absorb less calcium from their diet, perhaps due to reduced levels or activity of 1,25 dihydroxyvitamin D. Despite reduced absorption efficiency, urinary calcium losses are greater in postmenopausal women, leading to the assumption that this excessive urinary loss of calcium must come from the skeleton. The net result is a deterioration in calcium balance performance occurring across the menopause. It is as yet not completely clear which is the *primary* defect. Although circumstantial evidence suggests that the skeletal response may be the initial event, other postulates have suggested as primary defects both the malabsorption of calcium and renal loss of calcium.

RATE OF LOSS

Many models of age-related bone loss have been suggested, usually to attempt to identify those at greatest risk of developing clinical osteoporosis. As bone mass appears to be normally distributed, so is rate of loss. In addition, there is a correlation between maximum bone mass and subsequent rate of loss, so that those with the greatest mass lose fastest. It is important to realize that more information is needed on the relationships between bone mass at maturity and rate of loss before assessments of risk can be made for individual patients. It is possible, for example, that individuals who acquire osteoporotic fractures, expecially vertebral crush fractures, could represent a subpopulation of individuals who exhibit a particularly rapid rate of bone loss.[7] However, our own studies as well as those of others,[22] have not been able to identify such a group and suggest that bone loss is normally distributed, as is bone mass.

EXTRINSIC FACTORS AFFECTING BONE LOSS

Many factors may influence loss of skeletal mass with aging, in addition to the changes occurring at the menopause. Most of the so-called "risk factors" apply equally to both sexes and hence cannot, by themselves, account for the sexual dichotomy of clinical osteoporosis. However, clearly, by skeletal maturity there is a sex and race difference, in both the total amount of bone present and its density, in favor of men and blacks. These differences will aggravate the effects of subsequent bone loss among white and Asian women. Not only do such women lose bone faster, they start with less. The inequality between the sexes that is observed at maturity does not become evident until the male growth spurt. Therefore, perhaps there may be some value in examining the control of growth and its effects on skeletal mass to determine if it is possible to increase maximum bone mass in young women, an area in which there is as yet little information.

In addition, many other factors affect the skeleton (Table 6–1). The most important are nutrition and lifestyle, but endocrine status and intercurrent disease processes must not be forgotten.

TABLE 6–1.

Risk Factors Associated With
Postmenopausal and Age-Related
Osteoporosis

GENETIC FACTORS

Female sex
Caucasian or Asian race
Positive family history
Small build

ENDOCRINE FACTORS

Female sex
Early menopause (or oophorectomy)
Nulliparity
Small build

ENVIRONMENTAL FACTORS

Lifelong low calcium intake
Sedentary lifestyle
Alcohol abuse
Cigarette smoking
High protein intake
High caffeine intake
High sodium intake
High phosphate intake
Low vitamin D intake

Nutrition

The common view dictates that calcium intake is an important determinant of bone loss. Indeed, there is significant circumstantial evidence to suggest that view. However, definitive evidence is more difficult to find. The most convincing data suggesting a role for calcium intake as a causative factor come from a Yugoslavian study.[33] In this study, fracture frequency as a function of age was compared in two villages, apparently different only in terms of calcium intake. The expected rise in hip fracture with age was significantly less in the village in which the life-long average of calcium intake was almost 1 gm/day than in the district with low calcium intake (approximately 450 mg/day average). Curiously, other types of fractures were not affected by calcium intake, and bone mass differences between the villages appeared greater among the young, suggesting that bone *loss* was not affected by dietary calcium. Heaney's data (1977) suggest that, on average, premenopausal women will be in calcium balance with an intake of around 1 gm/day, whereas postmenopausal women will require an extra intake of 500 mg. In this context, it is worth noting that the average intake of calcium in the U.S.A. is 400–600 mg/day. Extrapolating from Heaney's data, it is not surprising therefore that most adults are in negative calcium balance. However, one might then reasonably expect a slower loss of bone mass in the high calcium intake population in the Yugoslavian study, a finding which is not evident from the data.

Studies designed to demonstrate that calcium supplementation can prevent deterioration in the skeleton have produced somewhat mixed results. Decrease in bone loss was evident in at least two studies, while at least two more have produced negative results. However, these studies have involved calcium in the form of a carbonate supplement, and few data allow us to compare calcium from that source with the calcium supplied by food. The two types of calcium potentially could differ in bioavailability and pharmacokinetic behavior, and there may be differences due to the anion. When dietary sources of calcium are considered, there is, additionally, a close relationship between intakes of calcium, phosphorus, and protein; potentially, all could have a significant effect on bone loss or mineral homeostasis. Increases in protein intake are associated with a proportionate increase in calcium loss through the kidney (Johnson et al., 1970; Margen et al., 1974). A doubling of protein intake acutely results (by increasing liquid protein) in a 50% increase in urinary calcium. Balance studies have produced essentially similar data in middle-aged women. Thus, an increase in protein intake equivalent to 4 oz of meat per day would result in a deterioration of calcium balance of about 30 mg. Curiously, since phosphorus intake would also increase under such circumstances and since phosphorus lowers urinary calcium, the net effect might be significantly less than that postulated from the liquid protein or balance studies. Other dietary factors that potentially, at least, can exacerbate bone loss include alcohol and caffeine. Both could have direct and indirect effects on the skeleton and calcium homeostasis, impacting negatively on the capacity of the organism to maintain skeletal status.

Lifestyle

Recent studies have indicated that abnormal inactivity, such as prolonged bed rest or space flight, will result in excessive loss of bone. Additionally, the high activity pattern of athletes tends to be accompanied by skeletal hypertrophy. Marathon runners have been shown to have higher skeletal mass,[2] and among other athletes, local skeletal mass is greater in the most frequently used limb.[36] However, it does not follow necessarily from these observations that large or small increases in exercise for the so-called "normally active" population will be necessarily beneficial.

Several studies have now suggested, however, that simple exercise programs of short duration can influence bone mineral mass. Walking and running exercises (one hour, twice weekly) significantly increased the bone mass of the lumbar spine;[24] and somewhat similar programs have also been shown to be effective[3, 43] in the peripheral skeleton. However, in our own preliminary observations, physical activity appears important as a determinant of bone mass only when there is a sufficiently high calcium intake to produce a positive calcium balance. Also, exercise programs that are severe enough to cause amenorrhea in women may be detrimental to skeletal health.[10] Presumably, the loss of ovarian function can override any potential benefit of activity.

Associations between osteoporosis and cigarette consumption have been reported,[8] and this may also be mediated at an early age prior to skeletal maturity.[28]

Nulliparity, if that can be called a lifestyle risk factor, is important in determining bone mass at menopause. Repeated pregnancies (within limits) appear to increase mineral mass, or at least maintain it, through any period of premenopausal loss. That the use of the oral contraceptive results in a similar effect suggests that the mechanism may be related to exposure to sex steroids, presumably estrogens.

Finally, the existence of intercurrent disease processes affecting mineral metabolism, such as thyrotoxicosis, hyperparathyroidism, Cushing's syndrome, and Type I diabetes, will also interfere with the capability of the organism to maintain the skeleton.

Despite the ready description of such associations, it is difficult to know the weight that should be given to each of these "risk" factors. In addition, the possible additive or even synergistic effects of these factors, when several are present in one individual, are not understood.

Sex Steroids

As we have discussed, ovarian failure is one of the most significant factors influencing bone loss in women. Elegant and rigidly controlled studies have shown that estrogen therapy for the oophorectomized or postmenopausal woman significantly retards bone loss for at least as long as the treatment is provided.[1, 21, 25, 27, 39] In our long-term study, we have demonstrated that mestranol (average daily dose 24.8 μg) prevented bone loss, whereas a matching placebo failed (see Fig 6–4). After about 10 years of therapy, height loss was evident among some members of the placebo-treated group, whereas no height loss was seen in the estrogen-treated group. Radiographs confirmed the presence of vertebral deformities in a significant number of the placebo-treated patients, whereas such changes were generally absent in the estrogen-treated group. The minimum effective dose of estrogen appears to be about 0.625 mg conjugated equine estrogens per day.[31] When estrogen therapy is discontinued, bone mass declines at a rate comparable to the immediate postmenopausal period.[20, 26]

MODE OF ACTION OF ESTROGENS

There is currently no evidence that estrogens in physiologic amounts can influence the skeleton directly. Estrogen receptors have not been found in bone,[6] and it is generally assumed that estrogens must function indirectly, perhaps by interacting with the three hormones primarily involved in the control of calcium metabolism: parathyroid hormone, calcitonin, and the vitamin D system. The exact mechanism of interaction has

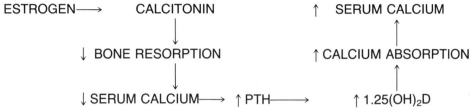

FIG 6–6.

yet to be elucidated. Currently, however, the most convenient hypothesis for the action of estrogens assumes that estrogens stimulate the production of endogenous calcitonin. Calcitonin levels and the responses of calcitonin to calcium appear to be lower in women than in men at all ages. Pregnancy has been shown, in some studies but not all, to stimulate calcitonin levels in women to at least those that occur in men.[5, 45] It has also been suggested that ovulation, when estrogen levels are highest during the menstrual cycle, is associated with higher calcitonin levels, although this remains disputed.[4, 38] Therapy with estrogens has been reported to increase plasma calcitonin in women.[45] Since the only important biologic action of calcitonin appears to be osteoclast inhibition and reduction of bone resorption, such increments in circulating calcitonin might reduce the flow of calcium from bone to blood. The subsequent biochemical events that could be postulated in this circumstance, namely, a fall in serum calcium and a rise in PTH and 1,25 dihydroxyvitamin D, could account for the other known biochemical events that follow estrogen administration (Fig 6–6). What data is available, therefore, is in the main consistent with this hypothesis for estrogen action. However, more detailed studies are still required, and a nongenome-dependent action of estrogen directly on bone is still a possibility.

IDENTIFICATION OF HIGH RISK INDIVIDUALS

By early or mid adult life, it is already evident that women, as a class, are more liable to be at risk from osteoporosis than men. Those factors that increase the risk among women have already been outlined. Although it appears that estrogen treatment is the most effective preventive therapy, it is not yet appropriate to offer such treatment to the large segment of the female population that will have one or more clinical risk factors. Thus, there is increasing use of bone mass measurements to screen individuals who may be at risk. These techniques vary in accuracy, reproducibility, expense, and amount of radiation exposure (Table 6–2). Most have been described in detail in recent literature.[9, 34]

Currently, our laboratory utilizes both dual- and single-beam photon absorptiometry. The combination of these techniques allows us to estimate both peripheral (mid or distal radius) and central (lumbar vertebrae, or neck of femur) sites. The bone measured is primarily cortical at the peripheral sites and is a combination of both trabecular and cortical bone at the central sites. Whichever techniques are adopted, it is critical to obtain not only normative data but also good estimates of the accuracy and precision of the technique appropriate to the particular clinic setting, since estimates, particularly of precision, may vary significantly for each technique and are often operator-dependent.

The most common technique available at present is single-photon absorptiometry. However, recent evidence suggesting that changes occurring centrally may differ from

TABLE 6–2.

Noninvasive Techniques for Measurement of Bone Mass

TECHNIQUE	SITE	CORTICAL TRABECULAR RATIO	ACCURACY	PRECISION	RADIATION
Radiogrammetry	Metacarpal	99:1	?	±2%	5–8 mrem
Radiodensity	Metacarpal	99:1	?	2%– 15%	5–8 mrem
Single-photon absorptiometry	Mid-radius	95:5	4%	2%–4%	5 mrem
	Distal radius	75:25	5%	2%–4%	5 mrem
Dual-photon absorptiometry	LV 2–4	40:60	5%–7%	2%–5%	5–15 mrem
	Femur neck	75:25	?	?	5–15 mrem
	Total skeleton	80:20	2%–4%	2%–4%	10–40 mrem
Computerized tomography (CT)	Vertebral body	5:95	?*	?*	200 mrem
Neutron activation analysis	Total body	80:20	3%–5%	2%–3%	1 mrem
	Trunk	30:70	±10%	5%	400 mrem

*Precision and accuracy of CT vary depending on methodology. Dual energy scanning improves accuracy (by some correction for marrow fat), but precision does not appear to change. Radiation dosage doubles, however.

those occurring at the periphery[40] makes it imperative for those who wish to use such techniques to have available both a central and a peripheral estimate. A combination of techniques involving measurements of radial and lumbar vertebral mineral content using single- and dual-photon techniques produces a radiation exposure equal to or less than that obtained from a single chest x-ray, and it may be, under well-controlled circumstances, both accurate and sufficiently reproducible to allow follow-up of individual patients. Relatively modest capital investment and running costs also make this combination of techniques attractive. For those who have access to computerized axial tomography (CAT scan), this technique provides, with appropriate software, accurate estimates of trabecular bone unobtainable by other techniques.[14]

In most clinics, the use of bone mass measuring techniques should be limited to those who are in a high-risk category and be offered initially around the time of menopause. The presence of two of five major clinical associations is sufficient to recommend a measurement of bone mass. However, as we have noted, the measurement of mass and loss are continuous variables within the population, and it is somewhat difficult to make clinical judgements on mass measurements alone. Hence, one must also consider these clinical ''risk factors'': (1) a strong family history of osteoporosis; (2) a poor diet, as shown by a calcium intake of less than 500 mg/day and a high alcohol intake; (3) a poor lifestyle, marked by inactivity, cigarette smoking, and alcohol abuse; (4) a low sex steroid load, caused by early menopause or oophorectomy, prolonged amenorrhea, or nulliparity; and (5) intercurrent illness or drug use, such as glucocorticoid excess or thyrotoxicosis.

If a bone mass measurement is made and found to be low, preventive steps are instituted. On this single estimate of mass, these steps may be no more than the removal of risk factors which can be achieved by alterations in lifestyle. If bone mass is normal, it may be repeated in one year to evaluate rate of bone loss. Excessive loss also requires preventive measures. Excessive loss and reduced mass (below 50th percentile) probably require the introduction of pharmacologic methods of prevention. Prevention and treatment of osteoporosis are reviewed in detail in Chapter 13, Prevention of Postmenopausal Osteoporosis.

REFERENCES

1. Aitken JM, Hart DM, Lindsay R: Oestrogen replacement therapy for prevention of osteoporosis after oophorectomy. *Br Med J* 1973; 3:515-518.
2. Aloia JF, Cohn SH, Ostuni JA, et al: Prevention of involutional bone loss by exercise. *Ann Intern Med* 1978; 89:356-358.
3. Aloia JF, Cohn SH, Babu T, et al: Skeletal mass and body composition in marathon runners. *Metabolism* 1978; 27:1793-1796.
4. Barran DT, Whyte MP, Haussler MR, et al: Effect of the menstrual cycle on calcium in regulating hormones. *J Clin Endocrinol Metab* 1980; 50:377-379.
5. Body JJ, Heath H III: Estimates of circulating monomeric calcitonin: Physiological studies in normal and thyroidectomized man. *J Clin Endocrinol Metab* 1983; 57:897-903.
6. Chen TL, Feldman D: Distinction between alpha-fetoprotein and intracellular estrogen receptors: Evidence against presence of estradiol receptors in rat bone. *Endocrinology* 1978; 102:236-244.
7. Christiansen C: Prophylactic treatment for age-related bone loss in women, in Christiansen C, et al (eds): *Osteoporosis*. Denmark, Aalborg Stiftsbogtrykkeri, 1984, pp 587-593.
8. Daniell HW: Osteoporosis and the slender smoker. *Arch Intern Med* 1976; 136:298-304.
9. Dequeker JV, Johnston CC: *Non-Invasive Bone Measurements*. Oxford, IRL Press, 1981.
10. Drinkwater BL, Nilson K, Chesnut CH III, et al: Bone mineral content of amenorrheic and eumenorrheic athletes. *N Engl J Med* 1984; 311:277-280.
11. Fenton-Lewis A: Fracture of neck of the femur: Changing incidence. *Br Med J* 1981; 283:1217-1220.
12. Frost HM: *Bone Remodeling and Its Relation to Metabolic Bone Disease*. Springfield, Ill, Charles C Thomas, 1973.
13. Gallagher JC, Melton LJ, Riggs BL, et al: Epidemiology of fractures of the proximal femur in Rochester, Minnesota. *Clin Orthop* 1980; 150:168-171.
14. Genant HK, Cann CE: Clinical impact of quantitative computed tomography for vertebral mineral assessment, in Margulis AR, Gooding CA (eds): *Diagnostic Radiology: 26th Postgraduate Course*. San Francisco, University of California Printing Office, 1983, pp 445-448.
15. Gordan G, Vaughan C: *Clinical management of the Osteoporoses*. Acton, Mass, Publishing Sciences Group, 1976.
16. Heaney RP, Recker RR, Saville PD: Calcium balance and calcium requirements in middle-aged women. *Am J Clin Nutr* 1977; 30:1603-1611.
17. Heaney RP, Recker RR, Saville PD: Menopausal changes in bone remodelling. *J Lab Clin Med* 1978, 92:964-970.
18. Heaney RP, Recker RR, Saville PD: Menopausal changes in calcium balance performance. *J Lab Clin Med* 1978; 92:953-963.
19. Hodgkinson A, Thompson T: Measurement of the fasting urinary hydroxyproline: Creatinine ratio in normal adults and its variation with age and sex. *J Clin Pathol* 1982; 35(8): 807-811.
20. Horsman A, Nordin BEC, Crilly RG: Effect on bone of withdrawal of oestrogen therapy. *Lancet* 1979; ii:33.
21. Horsman A, Gallagher JC, Simpson M, et al: Prospective trial of oestrogen and calcium in postmenopausal women. *Br Med J* 1977; 2:789-792.
22. Hui SL, Berger JO: Emperical bayes estimation of rates in longitudinal studies. *J Amer Stat Assn* 1983; 78:753-760.
23. Jensen JS, Tondevold E: Mortality after hip fractures. *Acta Orthop Scand* 1979; 50:161-167.
24. Krolner B, Toft B, Nielsen SP, et al: Physical exercise as prophylaxis against involutional bone loss: A controlled trial. *Clin Sci* 1983; 64:541-546.
25. Lindsay R, Hart DM, Aitken JM, et al: Long-term prevention of postmenopausal osteoporosis by oestrogen. *Lancet* 1976; i:1038-1041.
26. Lindsay R, Hart DM, MacLean A, et al: Bone response to termination of oestrogen treatment. *Lancet* 1978; i:1325-1327.
27. Lindsay R, Hart DM, Forrest C, et al: Prevention of spinal osteoporosis in oophorectomized women. *Lancet* 1980; ii:1151-1154.
28. Lindsay R: The influence of cigarette smoking on bone mass and bone loss, in DeLuca HF, Frost HM, Jee WSS, et al: (eds): *Osteoporosis: Recent Advances in Pathogenesis and Treatment*. Baltimore, University Park Press, 1981; p 477.

29. Lindsay R, Herrington BS: Osteoporotic fractures in the United States of America: *Seminars in Reproductive Endocrinology* 1983; 1(1):55-67.
30. Lindsay R, Dempster DW, Clemens T, et al: Incidence, cost, and risk factors of fracture of the proximal femur in the U.S.A., in Christiansen C, et al (eds): *Osteoporosis*. Denmark, Aalborg Stiftsbogtrykkeri, 1984, pp 311-315.
31. Lindsay R, Hart DM, Clark DM: The minimum effective dose of estrogen for prevention of postmenopausal bone loss. *Obstet Gynecol* 1984; 63:759-763.
32. Margen S, Chu J-Y, Kaufman NA, et al: Studies in calcium metabolism I: The calciuric effect of dietary protein. *Am J Clin Nutr* 1974; 27:584-589.
33. Matkovic V, Kostial K, Simonovic I, et al: Bone status and fracture rates in two regions of Yugoslavia. *Am J Clin Nutr* 1979; 32:540-549.
34. Mazess RB: Non-invasive measurement of bone, in Barzel U (ed): *Osteoporosis II*. New York, Grune & Stratton, 1979, pp 5-26.
35. Melton LJ III, Riggs BL: Epidemiology of age-related fractures, in Avioli LV (ed): *The Osteoporotic Syndrome*. New York, Grune & Stratton, 1983, p 54.
36. Montoye HJ, Smith EL, Fardon DF, et al: Bone mineral in senior tennis players. *Scandinavian Journal Sports Science* 1980; 2:26-32.
37. Parfitt AM: Quantum concept of bone remodeling and turnover: implications for the pathogenesis of osteoporosis. *Calcified Tissue Int* 1979; 28(1):1-5.
38. Pitkin RM, Reynolds WA, Williams GA, et al: Calcium regulating hormones during the menstrual cycle. *J Clin Endocrinol Metab* 1978; 47:626-632.
39. Recker RR, Saville SD, Heaney RP, et al: Effect of estrogens and calcium carbonate on bone loss in postmenopausal women. *Ann Intern Med* 1977; 87:649-655.
40. Riggs BL, Wahner HW, Dunn WL, et al: Differential changes in bone mineral density of the appendicular and axial skeleton with aging: relationship to spinal osteoporosis. *J Clin Invest* 1981; 67:328-335.
41. Samaan NA, Anderson GD, Adam-Mayne ME: Immunoreactive calcitonin in the mother, neonate, child, and adult. *Am J Obstet Gynecol* 1975; 121:622-625.
42. Saville PD: Observation of 80 women with osteoporotic spine fractures, in Barzel US (ed): *Osteoporosis*. New York, Grune & Stratton, 1970, pp 38-46.
43. Smith EL, Reddan W, Smith PE: Physical activity and calcium modalities for bone mineral increase in aged women. *Med Sci Sports Exerc* 1981; 13:60-64.
44. Stevenson JC, Hillyard CJ, MacIntyre I: A physiological role for calcitonin: protection of the maternal skeleton. *Lancet* 1979; ii:769-770
45. Stevenson JC, Abeyasekera G, Hillyard CJ: Calcitonin and the calcium regulating hormones in postmenopausal women: Effect of oestrogens. *Lancet* 1981; i:693-695.
46. Wallace WA: The increasing incidence of fractures of the proximal femur: an orthopaedic epidemic. *Lancet* 1983, i:1413-1414.
47. Whitehead M, Lane G, Young O, et al: Interrelations of calcium-regulating hormones during normal pregnancy. *Br Med J* 1981; 283:10.

CHAPTER **7**

Cardiovascular Effects of the Menopause

WILLIAM B. KANNEL, M.D.
TAVIA GORDON

THE LARGEST COMPONENT of adult mortality in western countries is the part attributable to the cardiovascular diseases. Of these the two major causes are coronary heart disease (CHD) and stroke. However, the impact of these two diseases is not the same for men as for women. In young women, mortality from CHD is substantially lower than it is in young men. With increasing age, CHD mortality rises in both groups, but the rate of rise is greater for women than men. If we calculate the mortality sex ratio (the death rate for men divided by the death rate for women), that ratio for CHD decreases with age. For stroke mortality, the picture is quite different. In the United States the stroke death rate for young women is currently about the same as that for young men, but with increasing age, stroke mortality for men increasingly exceeds that for women. Table 7–1 gives the data for the United States in 1979. In a general way, a similar picture is presented by mortality statistics for other western countries.[1]

It is natural to inquire whether these changes in the mortality sex ratio are in any way related to the menopause. That is the question addressed in this chapter. We shall review the available information, focusing on coronary heart disease and on the few identified cardiovascular risk factors about which usable information is available. The reader is forewarned, however, that good information on this subject is rather scanty, despite the fact that all women who survive to age 60 will have entered the menopause, most of them within a relatively narrow age band.

TABLE 7–1.

Death Rates for Coronary Heart Disease and Stroke for Men and Women, ages 30–59, in the United States, 1979

AGE (IN YEARS)	CORONARY HEART DISEASE		STROKE	
	MEN	WOMEN	MEN	WOMEN
	ANNUAL RATE/100,000			
30–34	9.4	2.2	3.4	3.4
35–39	29.4	6.5	6.9	6.2
40–44	74.4	16.3	12.5	12.6
45–49	160.6	34.8	21.1	19.8
50–54	288.0	70.0	35.5	29.1
55–59	468.1	131.9	57.8	44.3

NATURAL HISTORY

The incidence rate by age for the natural menopause appears to be biologically determined, although subject to minor variation under the influence of environmental factors. The median age of natural menopause given by various studies is between 50 and 51 years.[2-7] In the United States, about 1% of those women who have not become menopausal by surgical means will have a spontaneous menopause before age 40 and about 95 percent will be menopausal by age 55 years. Essentially all women will be menopausal by age 58 years.

On the other hand, the incidence rate by age for surgical menopause is culturally and medically determined. In the Framingham Study population, 29% of adult women had a surgical procedure that brought on the menopause.[2] However, of women born between 1890 and 1894, only 17% had a surgical menopause. The percentage increased with successive birth cohorts, reaching a peak with the Framingham Study cohort born between 1905 and 1909, of whom 34% entered the menopause by surgical means (Table 7–2). There was some variation in the percentage by ethnicity, nativity, and education, as well. In particular, only 21% of women who had been to college had a surgical menopause, as contrasted with 30% for women with less schooling.

The incrementing percentage of women who are menopausal by either a surgical or natural process makes it difficult to infer the effect of the menopause simply by examining age-specific data for men and women, whether these data are average values for some characteristic or the incidence rates for some disease. Even if the menopause leads to an abrupt change in the level of some characteristic, the gradually increasing percentage of menopausal women would produce the appearance of a smoothly altering average value with increasing age. Since there are other changes that occur with increasing age, it is hopeless to attempt to discern a menopausal effect without actually identifying which women are menopausal at any age and which are not. The subject is complicated further by the use of steroid therapy following oophorectomy and in some instances following the natural menopause.

BLOOD PRESSURE

In cross-sectional data from a variety of populations, the average blood pressure for young women is lower than that for young men, but with increasing age the differential decreases. In data from the 1960–1962 Health Examination Survey,[8] the crossover both for systolic and diastolic pressures occurs at about age 50 years, the average pressure

TABLE 7–2.

Framingham Study: Proportion of Women Having
Surgical Menopause by Year of Birth

YEAR OF BIRTH	POPULATION AT RISK	PERCENT SURGICAL
1890–94	349	17.2
1895–99	424	23.4
1900–04	435	32.2
1905–09	495	34.1
1910–14	507	30.6
1915–19	488	31.6
Total	2698	28.9

TABLE 7–3.

Framingham Study: Averages of Some Cardiovascular Risk Factors for Men and
Women, Ages 30–59, Exam 2

| | BLOOD PRESSURE | | | | SERUM CHOLESTEROL | | BLOOD GLUCOSE | |
| | SYSTOLIC | | DIASTOLIC | | | | | |
AGE	MEN	WOMEN	MEN	WOMEN	MEN	WOMEN	MEN	WOMEN
30–34	125.2	116.7	79.3	73.5	218.0	198.0	80.0	78.1
35–39	127.6	119.6	81.6	76.0	223.8	204.8	79.2	79.7
40–44	131.1	125.6	84.0	79.7	228.6	219.2	81.5	80.6
45–49	130.9	133.9	84.2	83.2	229.7	230.4	84.7	82.4
50–54	135.6	144.7	85.7	87.5	229.9	247.4	84.9	84.1
55–59	140.7	151.5	85.3	88.0	229.2	257.1	84.1	86.8

being lower for women than men at younger ages and higher at older ages. Cross-sectional data from the Framingham Study follows a similar pattern (Table 7–3). However, when the cohort is followed longitudinally, it appears that the crossover is largely due to the greater mortality associated with elevated blood pressure in men[9] (Figs 7–1 and 7–2).

When menopausal and premenopausal Framingham women of the same age were compared, there was no indication that the menopause led to a blood pressure change, either for systolic or diastolic pressure.[10] This accords with the findings of Taylor et al.[11] However the limited available data are ambivalent. One prospective study reported that there was a temporary abatement of the rise in blood pressure at the time of the menopause, although this effect was statistically significant only for systolic pressure.[12] On the other hand, a cross-sectional study based on the 1960–1962 Health Examination Survey suggested that diastolic blood pressure rose with the onset of the menopause.[13]

Blood pressures and the prevalence of hypertension in the Framingham Study cohort was found to be distinctly higher in women whose hemoglobin or hematocrit is at the upper end of the normal distribution. Given the fact that the menopause leads to an

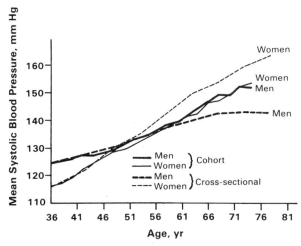

FIG 7–1.
Average age trends in systolic blood pressure levels for cross-sectional and cohort data examinations 3 to 10, Framingham Study.

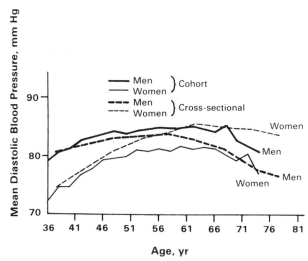

FIG 7–2.
Average age trends in diastolic blood pressure levels for cross-sectional and cohort data examinations 3 to 10, Framingham Study

increase in blood hemoglobin concentrations, an increase in blood pressure would be anticipated; but the available data do not seem to accord with this expectation.

BLOOD LIPIDS

Available data for the United States indicate that within the age range of 35 to 64 years there is a considerable increase in the serum cholesterol level of women.[14] In the age group of 35 to 44 years, the average level was higher for men than women. A crossover occurred in the age range of 45 to 54 years, and by age 55–64 years, average serum cholesterol levels for women were distinctly greater than those for men. Cross-sectional data from the Framingham Study show a similar crossover (see Table 7–3).

In the Framingham Study series, average serum cholesterol levels rose after a woman underwent either a natural or a surgical menopause. Evidence of a rise following surgical menopause without bilateral oopherectomy was, however, not statistically significant (Table 7–4). A more searching analysis disclosed that the rise after natural menopause is greater than appears in this table. The study rule was to designate a women as having had a natural menopause only after she had had 12 months without menses. Examinations, however, were at two-year intervals. Thus, a woman who had been menopausal for 11 months would go 35 months before she had an examination at which she was designated menopausal. Using the examination two periods before the menopausal examination as the premenopausal baseline, the average rise in serum cholesterol level after a spontaneous menopause was 12.2 mg/dl, similar to that for surgical menopause.

Other studies agree that the menopause leads to an average increase of serum cholesterol level. In the Goteborg study of women, a group of 387 women aged exactly 46 years in 1968–1969 were reexamined six years later.[12] Those who passed through the menopause in the intervening period had a larger rise in their serum cholesterol levels than those who did not. This has also been concluded from case-control studies.[15–18]

TABLE 7–4.

Average Change in Blood Pressure, Serum Cholesterol, and Relative Weight After
Menopause in Women, Ages 40–51, Framingham Study*†

| | | SURGICAL MENOPAUSE | |
CHARACTERISTIC	NATURAL MENOPAUSE	W/O BILATERAL OOPHORECTOMY	WITH BILATERAL OOPHORECTOMY
Systolic blood pressure			
One exam after menopause	−0.4	−2.7	0.7
Two exams after menopause	−0.8	−0.3	−0.1
Diastolic blood pressure			
One exam after menopause	−0.3	+0.9	−0.4
Two exams after menopause	−0.2	1.5	−0.6
Serum cholesterol			
One exam after menopause	6.5	5.9	12.4
Two exams after menopause	8.0	12.4	17.3
Relative weight			
One exam after menopause	−0.3	0.1	−1.2
Two exams after menopause	−0.2	−0.4	−0.7
Number of cases	480	77	137

*From Hjortland MC, et al: *Am J Epidemiol* 1976; 103:304–311. Used by permission.
†Data adjusted for age and measurement standards.

A number of studies have noted a rise in serum triglyceride levels following the menopause.[12, 15–18] The rise was not always statistically significant, but this is probably attributable to the small numbers involved in the studies, combined with the large inter-individual variation of triglyceride levels.

There are few data on the effect of the menopause on individual lipoproteins. Lipo-protein determinations made early in the Framingham Study indicate that there was a rise in the high density, low-density, and very-low-density lipoproteins (HDL, LDL, VLDL) at the time of menopause.[19] The rise in VLDL cholesterol is consistent with the rise in triglyceride levels already noted. The rise in HDL with the menopause that was estimated from the earlier Framingham lipid and lipoprotein data must be considered moot. Notelovitz et al.[16] compared 19 oophorectomized young women with 21 pre-menopausal, age-matched controls. Although both serum cholesterol and triglyceride levels were significantly higher in the oophorectomized women than in the controls, there was no difference between the groups with respect to low-density or very-low-density lipoproteins, while the high-density lipoproteins were significantly lower in the oophorectomized group. Robinson et al.[20] compared 112 women aged 40–59 years who had been oophorectomized before age 45 with 104 age-matched women who had only had a hysterectomy. While the oophorectomized group had higher levels of serum cho-lesterol and phospholipids, as well as higher levels of beta (LDL) cholesterol, and these differences were statistically significant, there was no clear difference between the two groups in their levels of alpha (HDL) cholesterol. More information on this subject is clearly needed.

WEIGHT

Among the fundamental cardiovascular risk factors is weight. With increasing weight comes increasing blood pressure and serum cholesterol levels, an increase in LDL, a decrease in HDL, and an increase in blood sugar levels—all of which are associated with greater cardiovascular risk.[21] However, the Framingham experience does not indicate that the menopause leads to a weight change.[10] Rather, it shows that at any given age, women who enter the menopause spontaneously are leaner than their premenopausal counterparts. This accords with inferences drawn from skinfold measurements made on American women during the 1960–1962 Health Examination Survey.[13] It was concluded on the basis of these data that leaner women tended to have an earlier menopause than fatter women.

In large part the relation of leanness to earlier natural menopause is probably secondary to the effect of cigarette smoking. In the Framingham Study it was noted that the natural menopause occurred earlier in women who smoked than in nonsmokers. Since smokers weigh less on the average than nonsmokers, this appeared as an association of leanness with early menopause. This observation is consistent with reports from other studies.[12, 22–24] Willett et al.[25] followed a group of 66,663 premenopausal women for two years. In that period, 5,004 became menopausal. Cigarette smokers were more likely to become menopausal than nonsmokers. Moreover, the more a woman smoked, the greater the chances of becoming menopausal. In multivariate analysis, there was a weak inverse relation of relative weight to the chances of a spontaneous menopause for smokers, even after taking the amount they smoked into account. There was no comparable relation demonstrable among nonsmokers.

CARDIOVASCULAR RISK FACTORS: SUMMARY

There is surprisingly little evidence of alterations in the standard cardiovascular risk factors consequent to the menopause. The only distinct effect appears to be an increase in blood lipids and lipoproteins. These are primarily risk factors for coronary heart disease. Blood pressure, which is heavily implicated in the risk of stroke, does not appear to be affected by the menopause, nor does the menopause appear to lead to a weight change. Cigarette smoking appears to speed up slightly the onset of natural menopause, and since women who smoke are leaner than nonsmokers, leanness is also associated with a slightly earlier menopause. There is no good evidence that the menopause has a discernible effect on glucose intolerance, which is an especially important risk factor for women, predisposing them to coronary heart disease and congestive heart failure.[26]

Given the profound hormonal alterations produced by the menopause, a much more general alteration in cardiovascular risk factors might well have been anticipated. On the other hand, as we shall see, the menopause—presumably through the hormonal changes associated with it—is itself a major coronary risk factor for women.

CORONARY HEART DISEASE

Of the various cardiovascular diseases, the one that has a substantial body of evidence linking it to the menopause is coronary heart disease. Stroke, which is the other major cause of cardiovascular mortality, is primarily a disease of old age and hence is unlikely to be an immediate direct consequence of the menopause. Furthermore, the apparent absence of a link between the menopause and blood pressure means that the menopause has little indirect effect on stroke, since hypertension is the major risk factor for stroke.

The relation between CHD and the menopause was studied in 1,598 women in the Framingham Study who were premenopausal at the time they enrolled in the study and were followed either through the menopause or to death.[27] Of these, 1,181 had a natural menopause and 365 a surgical menopause. A natural menopause was considered to have occurred only after the woman had failed to menstruate for 12 successive months. This was, of course, a retrospective designation. Routine examinations occurred at two-year intervals. If a woman was still premenopausal at one examination and menopausal at the next, the intervening two-year interval was designated as menopausal. No effort was made to divide that interval into pre- and postmenopausal portions, since it would have been impossible to date every disease event exactly, relative to the onset date. The interval preceding the menopausal interval was considered premenopausal, the intervals following the menopausal interval were designated postmenopausal.

When the premenopausal cardiovascular experience was compared with postmenopausal experience, the rate for the latter was 2.8 times that for the former in the age range of 45–49 years and 2.6 times for the age interval of 50–54 years. When these data are combined using the method of Mantel-Haenszel, the relative odds were 2.7. For the surgical menopause the comparable figure was also 2.7. There was no obvious difference in CHD risk between women having a surgical menopause with bilateral oophorectomy and women having a surgical menopause without bilateral oophorectomy (Fig 7–3). Estrogen therapy following surgical menopause was relatively uncommon in this series and did not play a significant role in the results.

In the age interval of 40–54 years, more than a third of the cases occurring after menopause presented as myocardial infarction or CHD death. For natural menopause the ratio was 11/31; for surgical menopause it was 10/26. By contrast, none of the 13 cases appearing among premenopausal women took this severe form, all but one presenting in the form of angina pectoris. In short, the menopause tripled the risk of CHD and greatly increased the proportion of severe cases.

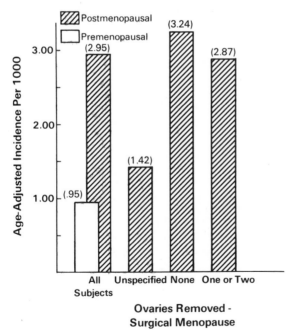

FIG 7–3.
Coronary heart disease incidence according to surgical menopause, 24-year follow-up, Framingham Study, women, aged 45–54.

The Framingham Study used a straightforward prospective approach to examine the risk associated with the menopause. An alternative approach was used for a study conducted in Goteborg, Sweden.[28] A representative group of women aged 50 years was examined in 1968–1969. Women who had menstruated in the preceding month were designated as premenopausal. Women who had had a bilateral oophorectomy or had not menstruated in the preceding six months were designated as postmenopausal. There were about the same number in each group. These women were used to characterize CHD risk factors associated with the menopause. On the average, postmenopausal women had higher serum cholesterol and triglyceride levels and lower levels of systolic pressure and included more cigarette smokers than the premenopausal women of the same age. There was no significant difference between the two groups in their average diastolic pressures.

The 1968–1969 cohort was reexamined in 1974–1975. In the interval, myocardial infarction had developed in nine women and de novo angina pectoris had developed in 42. These CHD incidence cases had a larger proportion of women with menopause before age 45 years than did a comparable reference population. This prospective finding was confirmed by a case-control study. The investigators concluded that the risk associated with early menopause was largely accounted for by the effect of increased lipids and an excess of cigarette smoking, although no formal basis for this conclusion was advanced. In the Framingham Study neither of these factors "explained" more than a small part of the excess risk associated with the menopause.

Oliver[29] examined the characteristics of 150 women who had developed coronary heart disease before age 45 years. Of these, 81 had presented with myocardial infarction and 64 with angina pectoris. In this series 20% (29 women) were found to be menopausal; 11 women entered menopause spontaneously, the remainder had it surgically induced. He noted that this was well in excess of the expected prevalence of menopausal women for this age group.

A number of studies that are either case-control or case history have concluded that surgical menopause with bilateral oophorectomy enhanced the risk of coronary heart disease,[17, 20, 30–34] but this is not a universal finding.[35–37] Rosenberg et al.[33] found the relative odds of nonfatal myocardial infarction to be 2.9 when young women with bilateral oophorectomy were compared with still menstruating women of the same age. This figure is remarkably similar to the relative odds of 2.7 reported by the Framingham Study.

As previously noted, the Framingham Study found the CHD risk to be the same whether a hysterectomy was accompanied by bilateral oophorectomy or not. This was also found by Ritterband et al.[38] After reviewing some of the available evidence, Centerwall[39] also concluded that hysterectomy without bilateral oophorectomy enhanced the risk of an early myocardial infarction in young women. He noted that the reason for this effect was not understood at present. However, Higano et al.[40] found that angina pectoris occurred more frequently in hysterectomized young women with bilateral oophorectomy than in hysterectomized women without bilateral oophorectomy, even when those receiving estrogen were excluded from the series.

In summary, despite some modest dissent, the conclusion appears firm that the menopause substantially increases the risk of CHD in young women, whether the menopause was spontaneous or surgically induced. While the evidence is less voluminous for hysterectomy without bilateral oophorectomy than for surgical menopause with bilateral oophorectomy, it seems likely that both increase CHD risk. In light of that, the mechanisms at work to increase risk remain to be elucidated.

ESTROGEN USE

Because of a variety of theoretical benefits, estrogen supplementation is commonly prescribed following the menopause. In the 1970s it was estimated that more than 30% of postmenopausal women were prescribed estrogen.[41] A commonly accepted use of estrogen is to minimize menopausal symptoms. In order to treat complaints such as perimenopausal flushing, estrogen use is often extended for six to twelve months and even to as long as three years.[42]

An increase in vascular disease with long-term use of estrogen-containing oral contraceptives has been extensively reported.[43] The risks associated with postmenopausal estrogen use are more difficult to evaluate. Estrogen therapy is believed to promote gynecologic cancer.[44, 45] The potential detrimental effects as well as the benefits of such medication on the cardiovascular system have been reported. A case-control study in Boston, a mail survey of nurses, and a retirement community study could find no evidence of an excess of nonfatal myocardial infarction in postmenopausal estrogen users.[45–47] The Lipid Research Clinics program reported the all-cause mortality in estrogen users to be only one half that of nonusers.[44] There has also been a report of decreased CHD mortality in estrogen users.[48]

The findings from the Framingham Study do not suggest any such cardiovascular benefits. Neither all-cause nor cardiovascular mortality were lower in postmenopausal women who used estrogens. Furthermore, prospective investigation of postmenopausal morbidity found that estrogen use was associated with an increased incidence of stroke and coronary heart disease.[49] This was true despite a more favorable cardiovascular risk profile in the postmenopausal estrogen users. There was an apparent interaction between cigarette smoking and postmenopausal estrogen use, such that cigarette smoking seemed to enhance the additional coronary risk associated with estrogen use. This interaction was not evident for stroke. The finding of an especially high coronary risk among women who both smoke cigarettes and use estrogen is consistent with what has been reported for oral contraceptives.[43, 46]

Short of a clinical trial, it will be difficult to resolve these apparently inconsistent findings. The fact that the cardiovascular risk profile for postmenopausal women may differ between women using estrogens and those who do not, as is suggested by the Framingham experience, will make it difficult to distinguish between biologic effects and selective bias. Since estrogen use has been recommended as a means of diminishing the risk of osteoporosis,[50] the effects of such use on cardiovascular risk needs to be more definitely determined. For the moment, the question is moot.

SUMMARY

Women are less vulnerable to cardiovascular disease than men, particularly to coronary disease and to its more severe manifestations of myocardial infarction and sudden death. This relative immunity wanes with advancing age, and on undergoing the menopause, women are more prone to cardiovascular disease and its more severe manifestations. This escalation of risk is not discernible from an inspection of the curve of cardiovascular incidence and mortality, which fails to show an abrupt change in rates at menopausal ages.

There is a narrowing of the gap in incidence with advancing age, which is related to the menopause. The menopause itself, presumably because of associated hormonal changes, is a major coronary risk factor for women. A substantial body of evidence links the menopause with CHD, substantially increasing the risk in young women, regardless of whether the menopause is spontaneous or surgically induced. Hysterectomy without, as well as with oophorectomy, predisposes to CHD; hence, the precise feature of reproductive physiology involved remains to be elucidated. Postmenopausal estrogen administration for osteoporosis and menopausal symptoms is not of demonstrated efficacy as prophylaxis against CHD, and may be detrimental, particularly in cigarette smokers.

There is a paucity of evidence for the worsening of standard cardiovascular risk factors on undergoing the menopause. The only distinct effect demonstrated is on blood lipoproteins, prime risk factors for CHD. Blood pressure and weight do not seem to be affected. No discernible effect on glucose intolerance, a powerful cardiovascular risk factor in women, has been shown to occur. Hence, the menopause itself, through some ill-defined mechanism, is a major independent risk factor for coronary disease.

REFERENCES

1. Johansson S, Vedin A, Wilhelmsson C: Myocardial infarction in women. *Epidemiol Rev* 1983; 5:67–95.
2. McNamara PM, Hjortland MC, Gordon T, et al: Natural history of menopause: The Framingham Study. *Obstet Gynecol* 1978; 27–35.
3. MacMahon B, Worcester J: Age at menopause: United States, 1960–1962. *Vital Health Stat* [*11*] no. 19. US Govt Printing Office, Washington DC, 1966.
4. Treloar AE: Menarche, menopause and intervening fecundability. *Human Biol* 1974; 46:89–107.
5. Burch PR, Gunz FW: The distribution of menopausal age in New Zealand: An exploratory study. *NZ Med J* 1967; 66:6–10.
6. Frommer DJ: Changing age at menopause. *Br Med J* 1964; 2:349–51.
7. McKinlay S, Jeffreys M, Thompson B: An investigation of the age at menopause. *J Biosoc Sci* 1972; 4:161–73.
8. Gordon T: Blood pressure of adults by age and sex: United States, 1960–1962. *Vital Health Stat* [*11*], no. 4. US Govt Printing Office, Washington DC, 1964.
9. Gordon T, Shurtleff D: Means at each examination and interexamination variation of specified characteristics: Framingham Study, Exam 1 to Exam 10, in Kannel WB, Gordon T (eds): *The Framingham Study: An Epidemiological Investigation of Cardiovascular Disease*. Section 29. DHEW Publ No. (NIH) 74–478. US Govt Printing Office, Washington DC, 1973.
10. Hjortland MC, McNamara PM, Kannel WB: Some atherogenic concomitants of menopause: The Framingham Study. *Am J Epidemiol* 1976; 103:304–11.
11. Taylor RD, Corcoran AC, Page IH: Menopausal hypertension: A critical study. *Am J Med Sci* 1947; 213:475–6.
12. Lindquist O: Influence of the menopause on ischemic heart disease and its risk factors on bone mineral content: Results from a longitudinal population study of women in Goteborg, Sweden. *Acta Obstet Gynecol Scand* [*Suppl*] 1982; 110:1–21.
13. Weiss NS: Relationship of menopause to serum cholesterol and arterial blood pressure: The United States' health examination survey of adults. *Am J Epidemiol* 1972; 96:237–41.
14. Moore FE, Gordon T: Serum cholesterol levels in adults: United States, 1960–1962. *Vital Health Stat* [*11*], no. 22. US Govt Printing Office, Washington DC, 1967.
15. Paterson MEL, Sturdee DW, Moore B: The effect of menopausal status and sequential mestranol and norethisterone on serum cholesterol, triglycerides and electrophoretic lipoprotein patterns. *Br J Obstet Gynaecol* 1979; 86:810–5.
16. Notelovitz M, Gudat JC, Ware MD, et al: Lipids and lipoproteins in women after oophorectomy and the response to estrogen therapy. *Br J Obstet Gynaecol* 1983; 90:171–77.
17. Johansson BW, Kaij L, Kullander S, et al: On some late effects of bilateral oophorectomy in the age range 15–30 years. *Acta Obstet Gynecol Scand* 1975; 54:449–61.
18. Hallberg L, Svanborg A: Cholesterol, phospholipids and triglycerides in plasma in 50-year old women. *Acta Med Scand* 1967; 181:185–94.
19. Kannel WB, Hjortland MC, McNamara PM, et al: Menopause and the risk of cardiovascular disease: The Framingham Study. *Ann Intern Med* 1976; 85:447–52.

20. Robinson RW, Higano N, Cohen WD: Increased incidence of coronary heart disease in women castrated prior to menopause. *Arch Intern Med* 1959; 104:908–13.
21. Kannel WB, Gordon T: Obesity and cardiovascular disease: The Framingham Study, in Burland WL, Samuel PD, Yudkin J (eds): *Obesity Symposium*. New York, Churchill Livingstone, Inc, 1974, pp 24–51.
22. Wald NJ: Cigarette smoking and coronary heart disease in young women, in Oliver MF (ed): *Coronary Heart Disease in Young Women*. New York, Churchill Livingstone, Inc, 1978, pp 43–53.
23. Daniell HW: Osteoporosis of the slender smoker: Vertebral compression fractures and loss of metacarpal cortex in relation to postmenopausal cigarette smoking and lack of obesity. *Arch Intern Med* 1976; 136:298–304.
24. Jick H, Porter J, Morrison AS: Relation of smoking and age and natural menopause: Report from Boston Collaborative Drug Surveillance Program, Boston University Medical Center. *Lancet* 1977; 1:1354–5.
25. Willett W, Stampfer MJ, Bain C, et al: Cigarette smoking, relative weight, and menopause. *Am J Epidemiol* 1983; 117:651–8.
26. Gordon T, Castelli WP, Hjortland MC, et al: Diabetes, blood lipids and the role of obesity in CHD risk for women: The Framingham Study. *Ann Intern Med* 1977; 87:393–7.
27. Gordon T, Kannel WB, Hjortland MC, et al: Menopause and coronary heart disease: The Framingham Study. *Ann Intern Med* 1978; 89:157–61.
28. Bengtsson C, Lindquist O: CHD during the menopause, in Oliver MF (ed): *Coronary Heart Disease in Young Women*. New York, Churchill Livingstone, Inc, 1978, pp 234–9.
29. Oliver MF: Clinical characteristics and prognosis of angina and myocardial infarction in young women, in Oliver MF (ed): *Coronary Heart Disease in Young Women*. New York, Churchill Livingstone, Inc, 1978, pp 221–32.
30. Cochran R, Gwinnip G: Coronary artery disease in young females. Possibility of oophorectomy as an etiologic aspect. *Arch Intern Med* 1962; 110:162–5.
31. Wuest JH, Dry TJ, Edwards JE: The degree of coronary atherosclerosis in bilaterally oophorectomized women. *Circulation* 1953; 7:801–8.
32. Rivin AV, Dimitroff SP: The incidence and severity of atherosclerosis in estrogen-treated males and in females with hypoestrogenic or a hyperestrogenic state. *Circulation* 1954; 19:533–9.
33. Rosenberg L, Hennekens CH, Rosner B, et al: Early menopause and the risk of myocardial infarction. *Am J Obstet Gynecol* 1981; 139:47–51.
34. Parrish HM, Carr CA, Hall DG, et al: Time interval from castration in premenopausal women to development of excessive coronary atherosclerosis. *Am J Obstet Gynecol* 1967; 2:155–62.
35. Novak ER, Williams TJ: Autopsy comparison of cardiovascular changes in castrated and normal women. *Am J Obstet Gynecol* 1960; 80:863–9.
36. Manchester JH, Herman HV, Gorlin R: Premenopausal castration and documented coronary atherosclerosis. *Am J Cardiol* 1971; 28:33–7.
37. Blanc JJ, Boschat J, Morin JF, et al: Menopause and myocardial infarction. *Am J Obstet Gynecol* 1977; 127:353–5.
38. Ritterband AB, Jaffe IA, Densen PM, et al: Gonadal function and the development of coronary heart disease. *Circulation* 1963; 27:235–51.
39. Centerwall BS: Premenopausal hysterectomy and cardiovascular disease. *Am J Obstet Gynecol* 1981; 139:58–61.
40. Higano N, Robinson RW, Cohen WD: Increased incidence of cardiovascular disease in castrated women. *N Engl J Med* 1963; 268:1123–4.
41. Stadel BV, Weiss N: Characteristics of menopausal women: A survey of King and Pierce counties in Washington, 1973–1974. *Am J Epidemiol* 1975; 102:209–16.
42. Rosenberg L, Shapiro S, Kaufman DW, et al: Patterns and determinants of conjugated estrogen use. *Am J Epidemiol* 1979; 109:676–86.
43. Stadel BV: Oral contraceptives and cardiovascular disease. *N Engl J Med* 1981; 305:612–18.
44. Bush TL, Cowan LD, Barrett-Connor E, et al: Estrogen use and all-cause mortality. *JAMA* 1983; 249:903–6.
45. Bain C, Willett W, Hennekens CH, et al: Use of postmenopausal hormones and risk of myocardial infarction. *Circulation* 1981; 64:42–6.

46. Rosenberg L, Armstrong B, Jick H: Myocardial infarction and estrogen therapy in post-menopausal women. *N Engl J Med* 1976; 194:1256–9.

47. Pfeffer RI, Whipple GH, Kurosak TT, et al: Coronary risk and estrogen use in postmeno-pausal women. *Am J Epidemiol* 1978; 107:479–87.

48. Ross RK, Paganini-Hill A, Mack TM, et al: Menopausal oestrogen therapy and protection from death from ischemic heart disease. *Lancet* 1981; 1:858–60.

49. Wilson WF, Garrison RJ, Castelli WP: Postmenopausal estrogen use and cardiovascular mor-bidity, abstract. *Cardiovasc Dis Epidemiol* Newsletter. AMA, January, 1984; 35:35.

50. Horsman A, Jones M, Francis R, et al: The effect of estrogen dose on postmenopausal bone loss. *N Engl J Med* 1983; 309:1405–7.

CHAPTER **8**

Skin and the Menopause

MARK BRINCAT Ph.D., M.R.C.O.G.
JOHN STUDD, M.D., F.R.C.O.G.

THE SKIN, one of the largest organs of the body, undergoes changes after the menopause in women. Many of these changes have previously been described simply as part of the 'aging' process. This explanation, however, fails to explain how the skin of women who are maintained on hormone therapy looks healthier than the skin of women of similar age who are not. After the menopause, women start to complain of generalized dry, flaky skin and of easy bruising. These symptoms are almost always reversible with appropriate sex hormone replacement within a very short space of time, usually within the first six months. It is evident, therefore, that the sex hormones and, in particular, estrogens play an important part in the maintenance of skin quality in women. This chapter discusses how the sex hormones affect skin and examines the possible similarities between the relationship of the connective tissue in the skin and sex hormones and the relationship of the connective tissue in the bone and sex hormones.

GENERAL ANATOMY OF THE SKIN

The human skin forms a sheet, like a single organ, composed of a population of cells of diverse embryonic origin. The contiguous groups of cells at times reveal their origin and their potentialities, although under normal conditions, cells exist side by side in complete harmony as a complex mosaic (Fig 8–1).

A thin outer layer, the epidermis, is composed of keratinocytes (keratin-producing cells) of ectodermal origin, intermingled with melanin-producing cells, the melanocytes, which arise from a specialized embryonic ectodermal tissue, the neural crest. The dermis, which is most pertinent to this discussion, is a stroma that forms the main bulk of the skin and is intimately bound with the overlaying epidermis; finger-like processes, or dermal papillae, project upwards into corresponding recesses in the epidermis. In contrast with the epidermis, the dermis is relatively cellular and predominantly fibrous, containing blood vessels. It is of mesodermal origin, like all connective tissue (including bone). It also contains several structures derived from the embryonic ectoderm, such as sweat glands and hair follicles.

Fibers of two main types are seen in the dermis; both are fibrous protein. By far the largest amount by weight is collagen (97.5%) with elastin fibers (2.5%) making up the rest.[35, 5] Collagen fibers are responsible for the main mass and resilience of the dermis. Collagen is disposed mainly parallel to the skin surface, whereas elastin fibers form a subepidermal network and are only thinly distributed elsewhere in the dermis.

The dermis and the epidermis are nourished by blood vessels that pass upwards from

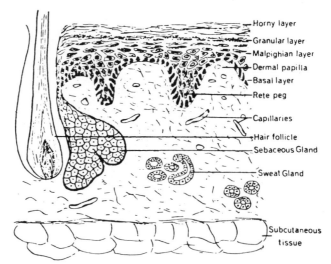

FIG 8–1.
A cross-section of the human skin, demonstrating its normal structure.

the subcutaneous layer. In the dermis, they form relatively small channels (arterioles) that pass towards the undersurface of the epidermis forming a rich capillary network in the dermal papillae. It is these vessels that are responsible for the menopausal flush, the most characteristic symptom of the menopause, affecting some 75% of all women in their first postmenopausal year[33] and still affecting 25% five years later.[52] Photoplethysmograph studies have shown that women suffering from postmenopausal flushes not only had abnormal peripheral (dermal) vascular behavior during a flush,[51] but also always had abnormal peripheral (dermal) vascular response to stimuli even when not flushing.[13] This abnormal control could be reversed with estrogen therapy. Other structures found in the dermis include veins, lymph vessels, sensory corpuscles, and autonomic and sensory nerves. Hair follicles and their attendant hair muscles and cutaneous glands are also situated in this deeper layer of the skin. In this region, cells are scanty, although representatives of the reticuloendothelial system, including histocytes, fibrocytes, and mast cells, are found.

THE EFFECTS OF ESTROGEN ON ANIMAL AND HUMAN SKIN

Little work has been done to investigate the effect of estrogen on the skin. Estradiol is concentrated in the basal cell layers of the epidermis.[44] Both estrogen and androgen receptors have been identified on fibroblasts in the skin.[8, 50]

In animals, estrogens appear to alter the vascularization of the skin,[25] and resultant change in the connective tissue of the dermis occurs, as reflected by increased mucopolysaccharide incorporation, hydroxyproline turnover, and alterations in ground substance.[25] In addition to increased dermal turnover of hyaluronic acid, the dermal water content is enhanced with estradiol therapy.[26, 27] Atrophy of the epidermis disappeared after treatment lasting six weeks, with the number of capillaries increasing and collagenous fibers appearing less fragmented. Both testosterone and estrogen ointments had similar effects on the skin of both sexes.[22–24] Rauramo[40] observed that oral estrogen therapy in castrated women caused thickening of the epidermis for three months, and this persisted for six months after therapy.

Punnonen[39] used two different strengths of estrogens in castrated women, estriol succinate and the stronger estradiol valerate. Both caused statistically significant thickening of the epidermis after three months, but whereas this thickness persisted with the estradiol succinate, 34% of the patients on estradiol valerate started to have significant thinning of their epidermis. It was postulated that this was happening because the dosage and treatment were too strong.

Mitotic Activity in the Epidermis.—The effects of estrogens on mitotic activity in the epidermis are conflicting. Punnonen[39] claimed that significantly higher mitotic activity exists in the epidermis in studies carried out using 3H-Thymidine labeling in-vitro, while Shahrad,[44] using the same labeling agent in his in-vitro studies, claimed that estrogen had a depressor effect on thymidine incorporation in the human epidermis. However, Shahrad used pharmacologically high concentrations of estrone, so there might be an optimum dose of estrogen to give the maximum beneficial results.

Collagen in the Dermis.—(This will be discussed more fully below.) Collagenous fibrils were less fragmented in the dermis of women treated with estrogens.[52] He also noted an increase in the number of capillaries in the dermis of these women.

Estrogens and Amorphous Ground Substance.—The production of mucopolysaccharides is another fibroblast function. Estrogen could increase the rate of collagen production[11] by altering the polymerization of mucopolysaccharides. Estrogens increase the hydroscopic qualities and reduce the adhesion of collagen fibers in connective tissues.[20] The dermis is one such site where estrogens work in this way. Due to enhanced synthesis of dermal hyaluronic acid, the dermal water content increases (Grosman, 1971, 1973).

In mice, hyaluronic acid content was shown to increase dramatically with estrogen administration with a close linear relationship existing between the increase in high molecular weight hyaluronic acid and the increase in tissue water.[26, 27] Uzuka, also working with mice had similar findings and suggested that the stimulation of hyaluronic acid synthesis in mouse skin in response to estrogens is mediated through estrogen receptors and involves the induction of the enzyme, hyaluronic acid synthetase.[54, 55]

SKIN THICKNESS, COLLAGEN CONTENT AND DISEASE

Relationship Between Skin Thickness and Skin Collagen

The skin is known to be affected by various systemic and endocrine disorders. Studies have been carried out on skin changes in various connective tissue and endocrine disorders. A brief review is presented below.

Black et al.[8, 9] and Shuster et al.[47] looked at the relationship between skin thickness and amount of skin collagen in patients with systemic sclerosis, patients with osteoporosis of mixed etiology, and hirsute women and found a good correlation between the two. In a small study, Black et al.[9] demonstrated changes in the collagen content and thickness of the skin in persons with osteoporosis of mixed etiology who were treated with androgens, when compared to osteoporotics who had not been on this treatment. Shuster et al.[47] found an increase in skin collagen in women with hirsutism, but the increase was not statistically significant. In scleroderma, Black[8] demonstrated a decrease in total collagen content and skin thickness in affected areas. In clinically normal areas, the skin thickness was decreased, but the collagen content was not significantly altered. Arho[4] did not show any difference between skin thickness and collagen content in patients with scleroderma when compared to normal patients. He also found a good correlation between skin thickness and collagen content in a number of patients with a variety of endocrine and collagen disorders. The conditions looked at by Arho, apart from normal skin, were acromegaly, rheumatoid arthritis, lupus erythematosus, scleroderma, Besnier's prurigo, psoriasis, and Cushing's syndrome. Patients with Besnier's prurigo and scleroderma had normal skin collagen contents. Acromegaly produced both thicker skin and higher skin collagen content, while patients with Cushing's syndrome and those who had been treated with corticosteroids had thinner skin and lower skin collagen content than normal.[4]

Skin Collagen Changes With Age

Reports on the skin collagen changes with age are conflicting. Shuster[45, 46] showed that the best way of expressing skin collagen content was by measuring the collagen content of a skin biopsy per square millimeter, of skin surface. This method takes into account the possibility of changes in the total mass of the dermis. Shuster and Bottoms[45] reported a reduction in total skin collagen with age, but this was not confirmed by Reed and Hall.[41] Shuster and Bottoms[48] found that the amount of collagen present in skin was at all ages higher in men than in women. Hall et al.[38] confirmed that skin collagen was higher in men than in women, but, once again, they could not significantly confirm the decline of skin collagen content with age. The effects of the menopause and of hypoestrogenism on skin collagen content has, however, not received any attention.

Effects of Corticosteroids on Skin Collagen and Skin Thickness

Several studies confirm that corticosteroid therapy or the presence of excess endogenous corticosteroids, such as occurs in Cushing's disease, reduces both skin collagen content and skin thickness in humans[19, 4, 28, 30, 21] and in rats and mice.[49, 30]

FIBROBLASTS

The fibroblast (*fibra,* fiber and *blastos,* germ) is the most numerous cell encountered in loose connective tissue. Fibroblasts are responsible for the production of fibers and for most of the amorphous components of the intercellular substance (ground substance, glycosaminoglycans). The loose connective tissue of the dermis develops from mesenchyma, with the mesenchymal cells differentiating into various cell types, including the fibroblast.

Fibroblasts and Sex Hormones

As has already been mentioned, both estrogen and testosterone receptors have been identified on fibroblasts in the skin.[8, 50]

Estrogens affect connective tissue by increasing the intercellular fluid content and rendering the ground substance more metachromatic and the fibroblasts more 'succulent' in appearance.[7] Testosterone causes fibroblastic proliferation; the cells are larger than in control experiments, with abundant and strongly basophilic and pyroninophilic cytoplasm.[7]

The effect of sex hormones has been determined by examining the histologic changes of ground substance and collagen. Estrogen administration, although producing little morphological effect on fibroblasts, resulted in the formation of metachromatic ground substance rich in hyaluronic acid (HA) and containing, due to the increased HA, an increased intercellular fluid content. Testosterone causes more definite morphological changes with increased metachromatic ground substance which is also rich in hyaluronic acid.[10]

That sex hormones can influence fibroblast function has been shown by studying collagen formation and degradation by the sponge-implant biopsy technique. Using this method, Boucek et al.[11] have shown a fundamental sex difference in collagen turnover. Collagen synthesis and accumulation proceed at comparable rates in male and female rat tissues up to a certain time (approximately 40 days in this study); thereafter, in male rats, although the rate of collagen accumulation slows, the total amount of collagen persists. In female rats, however, after this particular time, the collagen formed is reduced. This suggests that once a certain collagen level is achieved in the female, the collagen degradation exceeds collagen synthesis. This finding is associated with morphological changes in the related fibroblasts, which become narrower and show decreased cytoplasmic content and increased nuclear thinning during this period.

The sponge-implant biopsy technique is used as an assessment of fibroblast activity as determined by their healing activities (the invasion of implanted sponge by fibroblasts and subsequent collagen formation). Boucek[11] also looked at the difference between intact and oophorectomized female rats and observed that the oophorectomized rats had depressed fibroblast activity.

COLLAGEN

Collagen is the most abundant protein in mammals, constituting 25% of their total protein.[1] In the dermis, as has been indicated, collagen accounts for 97.5% by weight of the fibrous protein present. Studies on collagen from various sites have indicated the presence of two basic α-chains, α_1 and α_2. These alpha chains consist of just over 1,000 amino acid residues, arranged in groups of three, in the basic collagen triple helix configuration. This very stable structure forms the basic building unit of collagenous structures. Proline and hydroxyproline constitute 20%–25% of the total number of amino acids in collagen.

Collagen Types

So far, seven genetically different collagen α-chains, each about 1,000 amino acid residues, long have been well defined. The seven different α-chains are designated α_1 (I) through α_1 (V), α_2 (I) and α_2 (V). Fewer than a dozen types of collagen molecules have been described. The major types are referred to as types I, II, III, IV, and V (Table 8–1.)

TABLE 8–1.

Structurally and Genetically Distinct Collagens*

TYPE	MOLECULAR FORMULA†	TISSUE DISTRIBUTION
I	$[\alpha_1(I)\alpha_2(I)]$	Bone, skin, tendon, ligament, fascia, arteries, uterus, and dentin; accounts for 90% of body collagen.
II	$[\alpha_1(II)]$	Hyaline, cartilage
III	$[\alpha_1(III)]$	Skin, uterus, and arteries
IV	$[\alpha_1(IV)]$	Basement membranes
V	$[\alpha_1(V)\alpha_2(V)]$	Basement membranes and other tissues (similar to Type IV)

*Modified from Prockop D, et al,[37] and Hall DA, et al.[28]
†The seven different alpha chains are designated α_1(I) through α_1(V), α_2(I) and α_2(V).

Location of Different Collagen Types

The type and various combinations of alpha chains determines the type of collagen. Type I collagen is the major connective tissue protein of skin, bone, tendon, dentin, and a number of other tissues. This type accounts for 90% of body collagen.[1] It corresponds to $(\alpha_1[1])2\ \alpha_2(1)$, that is, two identical polypeptide chains and one slightly different chain, the $\alpha_2(1)$. A small amount of collagen containing three $\alpha_1(1)$ chains has been detected in experimental conditions and in embryonic-chick tendons and calvaria.

Hyaline cartilage contains Type II collagen. This consists of three identical α-chains called α_I (II). It was initially assumed that cartilage was the only tissue that contained Type II collagen, but it has recently been found in the cornea, vitreous body, and neural retinal tissues. The collagen known as Type III also consists of three identical alpha chains, called α_I (III). Type III collagen accounts for some 10% of the total collagen in adult tissues such as skin, uterus, muscle, large arteries, lung, and liver (see Table 8–1).

In summary, therefore, skin and bone share a common collagen Type I, skin also contains an amount of Type III collagen in addition. Table 8–1 shows the various types of collagen and the site of their occurrence. In addition to the types already mentioned, there are other, less important types.

The Effects of Growth, Development, and Aging on Collagen

Growth, development, and aging involve major changes in collagen biosynthesis and metabolism. For example, the amount of Type III collagen, frequently measured as the ratio of Type III to Type I collagen, is greater in the skin from young animals than in the skin of old animals (Miller, 1976). The basis for this observation is not fully understood, but it indicates "gene switching" similar to, though less complete than, the switch from embryonic and fetal hemoglobins to hemoglobin A. Growth of connective tissue involves increased rate of collagen biosynthesis, and the increased rates of the pro-α-chain translation are generally accompanied by increased tissue levels of intracellular posttranslational enzymes. Conversely, both the rates of translation and the levels of these enzymes decrease with age.[37, 18, 53, 42, 23] The hydroxylysyl glycosyltransferases[42, 3] tend to decrease less with age than do prolyl[53] and lysyl[42, 2] hydroxylases, but levels of these enzymes generally change in a parallel manner. In addition, collagen degradation parallels the decrease in collagen synthesis that, according to some authors, occurs with age.[31]

Although the bulk of body collagen in adults is remarkably stable, a fraction of the collagen in all tissues is continuously degraded and replaced, even in old age. Such changes in overall collagen metabolism can be (roughly) followed by assaying the excretion of peptide-bound hydroxyproline or hydroxylysine in urine,[31, 32] since excretion of these substances is largely caused by collagen degradation.[31]

In addition to changes in the genetic type and the amount of collagen, changes in the quality of collagen accompany growth and aging. The amounts of hydroxylysine[6, 43] and glycosylated hydroxylysine[43, 34] in Type I collagen and the amount of immature and reducible cross-links tend to reduce with age.[42] These observations indicate that the chemical characteristics, and perhaps the function, of collagen change with age. To what extent these changes are fundamental to the aging process is still unknown. The role of the sex hormones, which changes dramatically with age, is likewise unknown.[37, 38]

Studies on Postmenopausal Women

Brincat et al.[12] looked at the skin collagen content of a number of postmenopausal women who had been receiving the same estrogen and testosterone implant combinations as hormone replacement for at least two years and not more than ten years, and they compared this to an untreated age-matched group of postmenopausal women. The treated group had a highly significant greater skin collagen content than the untreated group (Fig 8–2). In later studies,[14–16] it was shown that in the treated group of women, no correlation existed between the skin collagen content and the duration of therapy, suggesting that after a certain period (less than two years) the skin collagen content equilibrated and did not continue to increase indefinitely (Fig 8–3). These same authors[15, 16] showed highly significant correlations between the years since menopause and skin collagen content in the untreated group of women, with the skin collagen content declining in an exponential manner.

Using a radiologic method for measuring skin thickness, skin was also shown to be significantly thicker in postmenopausal women who had been on hormone treatment than those age-matched women who had not (Fig 8–4).[15]

These studies showed that skin collagen and skin thickness are affected by the sex hormone status of a woman. Skin collagen has been shown to decline after the menopause at an average rate of 2.1% per postmenopausal year. This was unrelated to the actual chronologic age of the woman. The rate of decrease in collagen content was higher in the initial postmenopausal years than in the latter ones, the decline being exponential in nature.

In prospective studies carried out on postmenopausal women[17] it has also been shown that skin collagen content can actually be improved with estrogen or estrogen and testosterone hormone replacement. This improvement is self-limiting. There seems to be an optimum collagen content that a women achieves, beyond which no further collagen

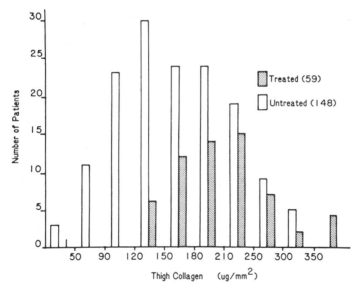

FIG 8–2.
Histogram showing the distribution of thigh skin collagen content in 148 untreated postmenopausal women and 59 treated postmenopausal women.

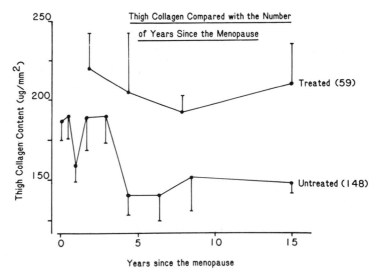

FIG 8–3.
Thigh skin collagen content (M ± SE) with years since menopause in 148 untreated postmenopausal women and in 59 postmenopausal women who had been on sex hormone treatment for between two and ten years.

increase occurs. This is shown as the '0' collagen value in Figure 8–5. A very strong correlation exists between the original collagen content that the woman has at the start of her treatment and the change in collagen that occurs after six months of treatment.[17] In those women with a low skin-collagen content who are several years postmenopausal, estrogens are of therapeutic and later of prophylactic value, while in those who have a

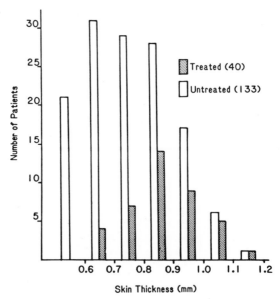

FIG 8–4.
Histogram showing the distribution of forearm skin thickness in 133 untreated postmenopausal women and 40 treated postmenopausal women.

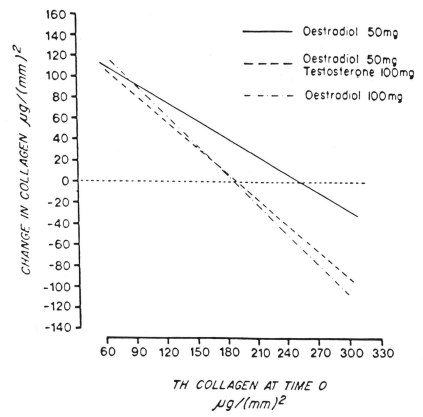

FIG 8–5.
Diagram shows the relationship between the change in thigh skin collagen content that occurred in postmenopausal women after six months of receiving 50 mg estradiol, 50 mg estradiol and 100 mg testosterone, and 100 mg estradiol implant, and their original baseline thigh skin collagen content.

high skin-collagen content and who are in their early postmenopausal years, estrogens are of prophylactic value only. Thus, a deficiency in skin collagen can be corrected but not overcorrected. Similarly, as has been noted above, there seems to be an optimum physiologic, estrogen dose for the epidermis also beyond which thinning rather than thickening of the epidermis occurs.[39, 44]

After six months of therapy with various physiologic regimens of estrogens and one regimen that included a small dose of testosterone, skin collagen levels were restored to levels similar to those in the treated group of postmenopausal women discussed above and to those in premenopausal women.[17]

Skin thickness, measured radiologically, represents dermal connective tissue as a whole, rather than collagen only (i.e., it also represents the amorphous ground substance). This has however been shown to have a highly significant correlation with skin collagen content, both in the treated and in the untreated group of postmenopausal women.[14] Skin thickness has been shown to become thinner after the menopause.[15, 16] It has been shown to decline at an average rate of 1.2% in the initial 10–15 postmenopausal years, a decrease that is not as high as that of the skin collagen content.

In summary, from the retrospective studies quoted above, there is evidence that skin collagen content and skin thickness can be restored and/or be prevented from declining in less than two years of sex hormone treatment. From the prospective studies described, the skin collagen content has been shown to be reconstituted after six months of physiologic sex hormone replacement.

Finally, no correlation was found between skin thickness and skin collagen content and the actual chronologic age of a woman, suggesting that actual age is not as important a factor in determining these parameters as the years since the menopause are.[14]

SEX HORMONES, SKIN, AND BONE

Apart from indicating the relationship of skin with the sex hormones, studies on the dermis and the menopause suggest the possible relationship between the behavior of connective tissue in general with the sex hormones. This suggestion is important because it might be possible to predict the behavior of the connective tissue element, the organic matrix in bone mass, in a particular individual from the state of the skin and thus be able to predict who is most at risk of having a bone mass that is sufficiently decreased so as to risk an osteoporotic fracture.

REFERENCES

1. Alberts B, Bray D, Lewis J, et al: Cell-cell adhesion and the extracellular matrix, in Alberts B, et al. (eds): *Molecular Biology of the Cell,* ed 12. New York, Garland Publishing Inc, 1983, pp 673–715.
2. Anttinen H, Orava S, Ryhanen L, et al: Assay of protocollagen lysyl hydroxylase activity in the skin of human subjects and changes in the activities with age. *Clin Chim Acta* 1973; 47:289–94.
3. Anttinen H, Oikarinin A, Kivviriko KI: Age related changes in human skin collagen galactosyltransferase and collagen glucosyl transferase activity. *Clin Chim Acta* 1977; 76:95–101.
4. Arho P: Skin thickness and collagen content in some endocrine connective tissue and skin diseases. *Acta Derm Venereol [Suppl] (Stockh)* 1972; 69:1–48.
5. Bailey AJ, Etherington DJ: Metabolism of collagen and elastin, in Florkin M, Neuberger A, Van Dienen LLM (eds): *Comprehensive Biochemistry.* New York, Elsevier North-Holland, Inc, 1980, 19B1; 5:408–431.
6. Barnes MJ, Constable BJ, Morton LF, et al: Age related variations in hydroxylation of lysine and proline in collagen. *Biochem J* 1974; 139:461–68.
7. Barnwood AW: The fibroblast. *Int Rev Connect Tissue Res* 1963; 1:1–28.
8. Black MM, Bottoms E, Shuster S: Skin collagen content and thickness in systemic sclerosis. *Br J Dermatol* 1970; 83:552–55.
9. Black MM, Shuster S, Bottoms E: Osteoporosis, skin collagen and androgen. *Br Med J* 1970; 4:773–4.
10. Boas NF: Isolation of hyaluronic acid from the cock's comb. *J Biol Chem* 1949; 181:573.
11. Boucek RJ, Noble NL, Woessner JF Jr: Properties of fibroblasts, in Page IH (ed): *Connective Tissue Thrombosis and Atherosclerosis.* New York, Academic Press, 1959, 193–211.
12. Brincat M, Moniz CF, Studd JWW, et al: Sex hormones and skin collagen content in postmenopausal women. *Br Med J* 1983; 287:1337–8.
13. Brincat M, De Trafford JC, Lafferty K, et al: Peripheral vasomotor control and menopausal flushing: A preliminary report. *Br J Obstet Gynaecol* 1984; 91:1107–1110.
14. Brincat M, Moniz CF, Studd JWW, et al: The long term effects of the menopause and of administration of sex hormones on skin collagen and skin thickness. *Br J Obstet Gynaecol* 1985; 92:256–59.
15. Brincat M, Studd JWW, Moniz CJ, et al: Skin thickness and skin collagen mimic an index of osteoporosis in the postmenopausal woman, in Christiansen C, et al (eds): *Osteoporosis,* Proceedings of the Copenhagen International Symposium on Osteoporosis, 1984; pp 353–355.
16. Brincat M, Studd JWW, Moniz CF, et al: Skin thickness measurement. A simple screening

method for determining patients at risk of developing postmenopausal osteoporosis, in Christiansen C, et al (eds): *Osteoporosis,* Proceedings of the Copenhagen International Symposium on Osteoporosis 1984; 1:323–326.

17. Brincat M: Skin collagen, skin thickness and metacarpal index in the diagnosis of women at risk of developing postmenopausal osteoporosis. *Drug Ther* 1985, in press.
18. Cardinale GJ, Udenfriend SB: Prolyl hydroxylase, *Adv Enzymol* 1974; 41:245–300.
19. Castor CW, Baker BL: The local action of adrenocortical steroids on epidermis and connective tissue of the skin. *Endocrinology* 1950; 47:234–241.
20. Danforth DN, Veis A, Breen M, et al: The effect of pregnancy and labour on the human cervix: Changes in collagen, glycoproteins and glycosaminoglycans. *Am J Obstet Gynecol* 1974; 120:641–651.
21. Ferguson JK, Donald RA, Weston TS, et al: Skin thickness in patients with acromegaly and Cushing's syndrome and response to treatment. *Clin Endocrinol* 1983; 18:347–53.
22. Goldzieher MA: The effects of Oestrogens on the senile skin. *J Gerontol* 1946; 1:196.
23. Goldzieher JW: The direct effect of steroids on the senile human skin. *J Gerontol* 1949; 4:104.
24. Goldzieher JW, Roberts IS, Rasols WB, et al: Local action of steroids on senile human skin. *Arch Dermatol* 1952; 66:304.
25. Goodrich SM, Wood JE: The effect of Oestradiol-17B on peripheral venous distensibility and velocity of venous blood flow. *Am J Obstet Gynecol* 1966; 96:407–410.
26. Grosman N, Hirdberg JE, Schon J: The effect of Oestrogenic Treatment on the Acid Mucopolysaccharide Pattern in Skin of Mice. *Acta Pharmacol Toxicol (Copenh)* 1971; 30:458–464.
27. Grosman N: Studies on the hyaluronic acid protein complex, the molecular size of hyaluronic acid and the exchangeability of chloride in skin of mice before and after oestrogen treatment. *Acta Pharmacol Toxicol (Copenh)* 1973; 33:201–208.
28. Hall DA, Reed FB, Nuki G, et al: The relative effects of age and corticosteroid therapy on the collagen profiles of dermis from subjects with rheumatoid arthritis. *Age Ageing* 1974; 3:15–22.
29. Hall DA: Chemical and biochemical changes in ageing connective tissues, in Hall DA (ed): *The Ageing of Connective Tissues.* New York, Academic Press, 1976, pp 79–144.
30. Kirby JD, Munro DD: Steroid-induced atrophy in an animal and human model. *Br J Dermatol* 1976; 94:111–119.
31. Kivirikko KI: Urinary excretion of hydroxyproline in health and disease. *Int Rev Connect Tissue Res* 1973; 5:93–163.
32. Krane SM, Kantrowitz FG, Byrne M, et al: Urinary excretion of hydroxylysine and its glycosides as an index of collagen degradation. *J Clin Invest* 1977; 59:819–827.
33. McKinlay SM, Jeffreys M: The menopausal syndrome. *Br J Prev Med Soc Med* 1974; 28:108–115.
34. Murai A, Miyahara T, Shiozawa S: Age related variations in glycosylation of hydroxylysine in human and rat skin collagens. *Biochem Biophys Acta* 1975; 404:345–348.
35. Neuman RE, Logan MA: The determination of collagen and elastin in tissues. *J Biol Chem* 1950; 186:549–556.
36. Neuman RE, Logan MA: The determination of hydroxyproline. *J Biol Chem* 1950; 184:299–306.
37. Prockop DJ, Kivirikko KI, Tuderman L, et al: The biosynthesis of collagen and its disorders. *N Engl J Med* 1979; 301(1):13–23.
38. Prockop DJ, Kivirikko KI, Tuderman L, et al: The biosynthesis of collagen and its disorders. *N Engl J Med* 1979; 301(2):77–85.
39. Punnonen R: Effect of castration and peroral therapy on skin. *Acta Obstet Gynecol Scand* 1973; 21(Suppl):1–44.
40. Rauramo L, Punnonen R: Wirkung einer oralen Ostnogentherapie mit oestriolsuccinat auf die haut kastierter Frauen. *Z Hant Gerchlects Kr* 1969; 44,13:463–470.
41. Reed FB, Hall DA: in Fricke R, Hartmann F (eds): *Connective Tissues—Biochemistry and Pathophysiology.* New York, Springer-Verlag, 1974, p 290.
42. Risteli J, Kivirikko KI: Intracellular enzymes of collagen biosynthesis in rat liver as a function of age and in hepatic injury induced by dimethylnitrosamine: Changes in prolyl hydrox-

ylase, lysyl hydroxylase, collagen galactosyltransferase and collagen glucosyltransferase activities. *Biochem J* 1976; 158:361–367.

43. Royce PM, Barnes MJ: Comparative studies on collagen glycosylation in chick skin and bone. *Biochim Biophys Acta* 1977; 498:132–142.
44. Shahrad P, Marks R: A pharmacological effect of oestrone on human epidermis. *Br J Dermatol* 1977; 97:383–386.
45. Shuster S, Bottoms E: Senile degeneration of skin collagen. *Clin Sci* 1963; 25:487–491.
46. Shuster S, Bottoms E: Effect of ultraviolet light on skin collagen. *Nature* 1963; 199:192–193.
47. Shuster S, Black MM, Bottoms E: Skin collagen and thickness in women with hirsutes. *Br Med J* 1970; 4:772.
48. Shuster S, Black MM, McVitie E: The influence of age and sex on skin thickness, skin collagen and density. *Br J Dermatol* 1975; 93:639.
49. Smith QT: Quantitative studies on cutaneous collagen, procollagen and hexosamine in normal and cortisone treated rats. *Br J Dermatol* 1962; 38:65–68.
50. Stumpf WE, Sur M, Joshi SE: Estrogen target cells in the skin. *Experientia* 1976; 30:196.
51. Sturdee DW, Wilson KA, Papili E, et al: Physiological aspects of the menopausal hot flush. *Br Med J* 1978; 2:79–80.
52. Thompson B, Hart SA, Durno D: Menopausal age and symptomatology in a general practice. *J Biosoc Sci* 1973; 5:71–72.
53. Tuderman L, Kivirikko KI: Immunoreactive prolyl hydroxylase in human skin, serum and synovial fluid: Changes in the content and components with age. *Eur J Clin Invest* 1977; 7:295–299.
54. Uzuka M, Nakamiza K, Ohta S, et al: The mechanism of oestrogen-induced increase in hyaluronic acid biosynthesis with special reference to oestrogen receptors in the mouse skin. *Biochem Biophys Acta* 1980; 627:199–206.
55. Uzuka M, Nakamiza K, Ohta S, et al: Induction of hyaluronic acid synthetase by oestrogen in the mouse skin. *Biochim Biophys Acta* 1981; 673:387–393.

CHAPTER 9

Psychologic Changes

LORRAINE DENNERSTEIN, M.B., B.S., Ph.D., D.P.M., F.R.A.N.Z.C.P.

THE ASSOCIATION between psychologic symptoms and the menopause has been one of the most contentious issues in menopause research. Opinions have varied widely and often reflect the discipline of the investigator. Gynecologists have swung from declaring all such symptoms as the "ills" arising from an estrogen-deficient state[42] to maintaining that only vasomotor symptoms and vaginal atrophy were "true" symptoms of the menopause.[36] Social scientists have maintained the view that psychologic symptomatology occurring in midlife is not related causally to underlying biologic changes but rather reflects expectations and attitudes of the particular sociocultural group.[14] More recently, a common meeting ground for disciplines seems to have been found, with a recognition of the interactive effects of endocrine changes with sociocultural and psychologic factors in any individual.[17]

This is good news for the clinician, who no longer has to determine whether symptoms are due solely to estrogen deficiency or result from coincidental socio-domestic-economic crises.[41] Instead, the clinician can utilize a broader integrative model in which the relative roles of each factor are considered and a total approach to therapy planned.

In so doing, the clinician needs full knowledge of the type of psychologic complaints that do relate to the menopause and the ways in which biologic, psychologic, and sociocultural factors may influence these symptoms.

This chapter will describe the symptomatology, epidemiology, and etiology of psychologic complaints at the menopause. (Chapter 16 will discuss in detail the effects of hormones on psychologic complaints in the context of a total approach to therapy.)

PSYCHOLOGIC SYMPTOMATOLOGY

Psychologic symptoms of the menopause are reported to include diminished energy and drive, difficulty with concentration, irritability, aggressiveness, nervous exhaustion, fluctuations in mood, tension, depression, introversion, and sense of internal frustration and inadequacy, intolerance of loneliness, marital troubles, and antisocial behavior patterns,[21] as well as anxiety, headache, and insomnia.[20] These symptoms are multiplicative, ill-defined, and nonspecific. All may occur at any age and in either sex. Such symptoms also occur in certain major psychiatric disorders, especially those of generalized anxiety and depression. As these disorders are important differential diagnoses, a short description of each follows.

Generalized Anxiety Disorder

In this condition, anxiety is the primary and dominant part of the clinical picture. The severity, frequency, or duration of the anxiety interferes with the individual's well-being, occupation, or interpersonal relationships. Anxiety is a complex emotion elaborated from an underlying feeling or fear or apprehension. The woman in an anxiety state looks tense and may be restless during the interview or show other signs of motor tension. She may complain of autonomic concomitants of anxiety such as dry mouth, sweating, aches and pains, headaches, tachycardia, palpitations, difficulty breathing, nausea, and diarrhea. The anxiety may be "free-floating" or attached to specific situations (phobic anxiety).

The clinician needs to distinguish such symptoms from other psychiatric disorders in which anxiety is frequently present (such as depression or schizophrenia) and from physical disorders that may present in this way (hyperthyroidism, hypoglycemia, or, very uncommonly, pheochromocytoma).

Mayer-Gross et al.[27] state that the clinical presentation seen at the menopause is similar to that of an anxiety neurosis, with predominantly somatic symptoms and a strong but fluctuating depressive coloring. The new criteria for diagnosis of anxiety disorder (neurosis) in the *Diagnostic and Statistical Manual of Mental Disorders*, ed. 3 (DSM-III), demand symptoms from three of four categories (motor tension, autonomic hyperactivity, apprehensive expectation, and vigilance, and scanning). These must be present continuously for at least one month. In contrast, the severity of the psychologic complaints of the menopausal years are less, and the symptomatology is not continuous, but fluctuating.

Depression

Depression is a disorder in which there is a persistent lowering of mood as the primary feature. Nearly half the patients with depression report complaints suggesting physical illness. Such accompaniments of depression include fatigue, decreased energy, appetite disturbance, weight loss, constipation, bodily aches and pains, headaches, difficulty breathing, dry mouth, and unusual sensations in the abdomen, chest, or head. In addition to feelings of sadness, depressed patients often suffer anxiety, loss of interest, difficulty in concentration, painful thoughts, and suicidal ideation.

It is important to note that depression symptoms may occur in other physical and psychiatric illnesses, such as schizophrenia, and the presence of such illnesses must be excluded. The diagnosis of depression is made on the basis of persistent and prominent lowering of mood, combined with the presence of at least four of the accompanying symptoms every day for at least two weeks (DSM-III).

Traditional Kraepelin psychiatry described the existence of the specific nosologic entity of involutional melancholia. This was said to differ from other depressions in the following respects: the patient has no prior history of affective illness; there is longer duration of the disease (seven to nine months); there is characteristic phenomenology (with hysterical traits); the patient's behavior is agitated; and diurnal fluctuation is not present.[27] Modern classifications have regarded involutional melancholia as a subtype of unipolar (endogenous) depression.[32] (There is no description of involutional melancholia in the latest list of DSM.) Winokur[43] studied psychiatric admissions and found no significantly greater risk of developing depression at the menopause when compared with other phases. Both Weissman[40] and Krupinski and Stoller[22] report the peak incidence of depressive states to be in the 30s.

Menopausal Psychologic Complaints

The psychologic complaints presented by women of menopausal age may be severe and persistent enough to meet the diagnosis of a major psychiatric illness. In most cases the disorder is less severe, and it is not continuous, but fluctuating. This chapter will focus on these minor psychologic symptoms. Prior to considering the prevalence and etiology of these symptoms, some of the methodologic difficulties inherent in menopause research will be briefly described.

METHODOLOGIC PROBLEMS

Some of the conflicting views adopted by investigators of different ideologies have been fueled by methodologic problems. A major difficulty has been the inadequate description and definition of the endocrine status of the women investigated, making comparison of results almost impossible. Many studies mention chronologic age only, deducing a relationship to endocrine status that may not be accurate. There has also been the added difficulty arising from the recognition that although the cessation of menses is a discrete event (the menopause), endocrine changes occur over a much longer and more ill-defined period of time—the climacteric years. Studd et al.[35] contended that the climacteric may extend from the late 30s to the early 50s.

Epidemiologically, there are the problems of inadequate population sampling and retrospectivity. Some samples are derived from menopause clinic populations, whereas others are general population studies. Not surprisingly, results from such disparate sources are often inconsistent. Age groups studied also differ. Other difficulties include inter- and intracultural differences in the recognition and definition of, and response to, symptoms. Few studies attempted to "cover" the interest in the menopause, so bias may have been introduced into responses. There are also the problems of defining and measuring the psychologic symptoms of the menopause. Varying measures of psychologic symptoms may have produced differing results.

Finally, a major problem in epidemiologic research has been that almost all studies have been cross-sectional rather than longitudinal. Cross-sectional studies obscure individual differences in response to changing levels of endogenous (or exogenous) hormones. Yet these differences have been shown to be highly significant.[9]

PREVALENCE

Population studies have attempted to examine the relationship of psychologic symptoms to chronologic age and menopausal status. Many of these studies were reviewed previously.[8] A number of studies[31, 19, 38, 24, 1] reported evidence that suggested that many minor psychologic changes (such as nervousness, irritability, headaches, depression, and decreased social adaptation) do occur in greater frequency in women whose menstrual cycles have changed recently (Fig 9–1). These results have been confirmed in more recent studies. Bungay et al.[3] studied, by postal questionnaire, a representative sample of the Oxford population. Menopausal status was not assessed; the authors assumed a mean age of menopause of 50 years with a standard deviation of three years. A peak incidence of hot flushes and night sweats occurred with the mean age of meno-

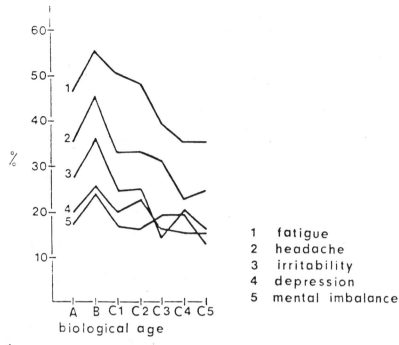

FIG 9–1.
Complaints in women whose menstrual pattern had altered within 1 year. (From Jaszman LJ: Epidemiology of the climacteric syndrome, in Van Keep PA, Lauritzen C (eds): *Ageing and Estrogens.* Basel, S Karger AG, 1972, p 17. Used by permission.)

pause. Rising in the fifth decade and peaking in the years just prior to 50 were such symptoms as loss of confidence, difficulty making decisions, anxiety, forgetfulness, difficulty in concentration, feelings of unworthiness, tiredness, dizzy spells, and palpitations. A different pattern was observed for the symptoms of irritability, low backache, and aching breasts. These symptoms had a high prevalence through the years of 30 through 50 and then began to decline.

Cooke[5] studied a population of Scottish women. Menopausal status was enquired about as well as chronologic age. They found that the severity of psychologic complaints began to rise in the late 30s, reaching a peak in the early 40s, and began to decline in the late 40s.

ETIOLOGY

Biologic Factors

Aging.—One explanation for the symptomatology of menopause is that it is due to increasing chronologic age. Two studies[31, 19] found that insomnia was unrelated to menopause but, rather, increased with increasing chronologic age (Fig 9–2). Bungay et al.[3] also found an increase in insomnia with age, but also a decline beginning at 55 years. The only symptom investigated in this latter study that steadily increased with age was difficulty with intercourse. A similar pattern of difficulty with intercourse was also experienced by male respondents in this study.

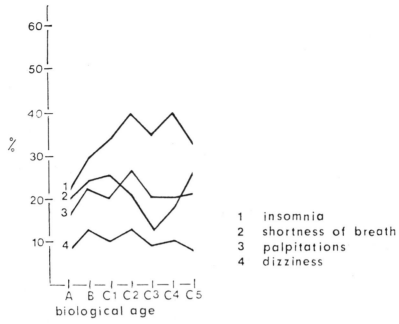

1   insomnia
2   shortness of breath
3   palpitations
4   dizziness

FIG 9–2.
Complaints during early postmenopause. (From Jaszman LJ: Epidemiology of the climacteric syndrome, in Van Keep PA, Lauritzen C (eds): *Ageing and Estrogens*. Basel, S Karger AG, 1972, p 19. Used by permission.)

Neuroendocrine Status.—This view ascribes symptomatology to declining ovarian function. Psychologic symptoms may reflect a change in the brain and, in particular, hypothalamic function, with the changing levels of steroids. The endocrine changes that are responsible for the symptoms may be lowered levels of estrogens, progesterone, or both, or raised levels of follicle-stimulating hormone (FSH) and luteinizing hormone (LH). Alternatively, symptoms could reflect an imbalance elsewhere in the hypothalamic pituitary-gonadal axis. Evidence is accumulating that amine metabolism may be affected by levels of endogenous and exogenous steroid hormones. Altered amine metabolism may be responsible for affective disorders.[33]

Psychologic symptoms are sometimes claimed to be secondary manifestations of disabling vasomotor symptoms, such as hot flushes and sweating.[23] The vasomotor symptoms and those of atrophic vaginitis are held by some to be the only "true" symptoms of ovarian failure.[36] Psychologic complaints are then explained by a "domino-theory." That is, if the flushes cause the woman to stay awake and the night sweats cause her to change the bed linen, she will report insomnia and fatigue, which may lead to irritability and nervousness.[37]

Epidemiologic studies reviewed have demonstrated an increase in psychologic complaints in the climacteric years, premenopausally. While some have argued that the failure to find a direct link with the occurrence of the menopause excludes biologic factors as causative,[5] it is evident that endocrine changes do not begin with the cessation of menses but many years earlier (see Chapter 3). The finding of an association between such increased psychologic complaints and the years of changed ovarian activity could also then be equally interpreted as indicating possible causative links.

The lack of longitudinal studies of women through the climacteric years was mentioned earlier. The results of a longitudinal study of sexual behavior were reported recently by McCoy.[7] She found a decline in the sexual interest, responsiveness, and activity of women when premenopausal and postmenopausal levels were compared. Most interesting was the finding that the decline in sexual functioning predated the menopause and occurred during a phase in which endocrinologic change was also occurring. Changes in mood were not reported, but a similar longitudinal study, in which both psychologic and endocrinologic variables are measured simultaneously, is needed.

Another way of examining the possible role played by hormonal factors is to study the effects of replacement hormone therapies. These studies are reviewed more extensively in Chapter 11. In summary, double-blind, placebo-controlled studies have found that there are measurable beneficial effects of estrogen on mood (Fig 9–3). Response to the addition of progestins is variable, and the reasons for this are discussed. The large placebo response and the highly significant differences between patients suggest that many factors may be important in determining response. While biologic factors, such as individual vulnerability to hormonal effect, may be important, psychologic and sociologic factors also have major roles.

Psychologic Factors

Earlier writers, of the psychoanalytic school, had negative views of the menopause. Freud[15] observed that sudden increases in the quantity of "libido" are habitually

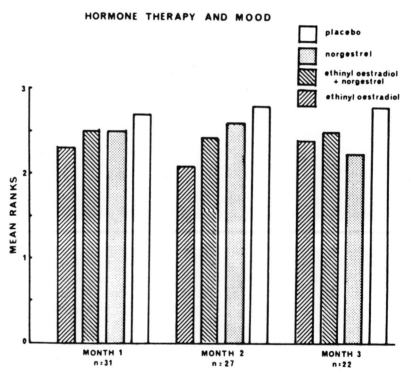

FIG 9–3.
Hormone therapy and mood. (From Dennerstein L, Burrows GD, Hyman GJ, et al: Hormone therapy and effect. *Maturitas* 1979; 1:247. Used by permission.)

associated with puberty and the menopause. The menopause was seen as a model of a physical disorder affecting the instinctual life in the "id" and increasing the strength of the instincts beyond the limit up to which the "ego" was capable of coping with them. This generated a neurosis.

Deutsch[10] referred to the loss of reproductive capacity as "a partial death." The menopause was a time of disappointment and mortification. The depletion and decline in sexual attractiveness, usefulness, and biologic function was experienced by some women intrapsychically as an object loss.[12] Depression resulted when the object lost was invested with the loser's self-esteem. The affects of giving up were helplessness and hopelessness. Oral and narcissistic needs were intensified.

Fessler[13] claimed that climacteric depression was the continuation into the period of the menopause of the patient's preclimacteric condition—essentially an "hysteric" one. As climacteric depression was said to have a marked resemblance to hysteria, ego defense mechanisms similar to those in the phallic stage were presumed to operate. Fessler claimed that the woman overcame her penis envy by the ability to bear a child. The menopause caused her to relive castration anxiety.

Benedek[2] introduced the concept of a developmental phase in which "the internal physiological changes and the psychological processes stimulated by them were integrated (or responded to) in a way that enabled the individual to master further, and anew environmental stimulations." No other period except puberty puts the individual's capacity to master internal changes to such a test. The lack of hormones at the menopause diminished the "ego's integrative strength" in a way similar to the premenstrual phase of the cycle. "Ego-alien" emotional responses created disappointment in the self and a reactive depression followed. It was emphasized that the reaction that became manifest in the climacterium existed previously. The climacteric diminished that part of the integrative strength of the personality dependent upon stimulation by gonadal hormones.

More recent writers (such as Collins et al.[4]) conceptualized menopause as a stage in the life cycle of a woman. Her individual reactions to the cessation of menstruation and the accompanying hormonal changes may be determined by underlying personality factors or previous coping styles.[37] Four different coping patterns were described by Van Keep and Prill.[39] These were:

The Adequate Behavioral Pattern.—These women experienced physical and psychic symptoms but were able to cope. Sixty to seventy percent of women were estimated to show this pattern. Such women were said to cope because of their introspective abilities, a harmonious family life, good integration within their environment, and a satisfying career or strongly held religious beliefs.

The A-Personal Way of Coping.—This was most evident in the lower socioeconomic groups. These women accepted any physical inconvenience as well as climacteric complaints, as unavoidable disturbances, which were registered without being considered very bothersome (15%–25%).

The Neurotic Way of Coping.—This method was most often seen in women who had similar neurotic reactions to problems earlier in life. Psychologic problems during the climacteric phase centered around the significance of their bodies. Menstruation, fertility, and sexual functions have given and still give their bodies a feminine significance. The loss of menstruation and fertility was not easily tolerated and a neurotic protest followed (8%–15%).

The Hyperactive Coping Mechanism.—The woman with this coping mechanism refused to allow her biologic functions to interfere with her life. She did not acknowledge the existence of climacteric complaints either in herself or in others, and did not ask for medical help for her complaints (5%–10%).

Such views suggest that women who present for therapy of psychologic complaints at the menopause are necessarily neurotic; this suggestion may lead to dangerous stereotyping by the clinician.

More recently, Collins et al.,[4] in a small Swedish study of women seeking help at a menopause clinic, explored the relationship between underlying personality variables and psychologic complaints. They found that vasomotor and sleep-related symptoms were not associated with any personality variable other than that of feminine interest. Psychosomatic and psychologic symptoms were significantly correlated with personality variables said to relate to anxiety proneness. Psychological symptoms were also correlated with an external locus of control or the feeling that external factors determined one's life.

While more studies are needed, important aspects for the clinician are that underlying personality factors may play a role in an individual's response to hormonal changes.

Sociologic Factors

The sociologic view is that menopausal symptomatology may be socioculturally defined and engendered. Within this general framework, investigators have proceeded in the following areas:

Cross-Cultural Differences.—The hypothesis of cross-cultural studies is that the norms and values of a particular culture determine the significance attached to concepts such as youth, menstruation, fertility, sexuality, sterility, menopause, and aging. Thus, more menopausal complaints are expected from women living in cultures (such as those of western nations) that are youth-oriented, where fertility is valued and aging is feared.

Flint[14] reported on her studies of 483 Rajput caste women in India. These women were well-nourished and wealthy. They reported few symptoms other than that of menstrual cycle change, and they said they eagerly awaited the menopause. The lack of symptomatology was interpreted as due to the positive changes in the woman's life following menopause. Prior to menopause, she either lived in purdah (veiled and secluded) or was not allowed the company of men. After menopause, Rajput women were released from purdah and were allowed to talk and, in some areas, to drink with men. Older people in this culture were revered as models of wisdom and experience, so aging itself was not to be feared so much as signs of impending senility.

Maoz[25] reported similar findings in a study in which Arabian women were compared with women from Iran and Africa. The Arabian women reported little or no menopausal symptomatology. In their culture, menopause was not viewed negatively and not seen as a crisis. Wilbush[18] described how women in Arabian and Zulu societies were able to find a number of ways of overcoming the loss of status associated with being unable to bear children. These ways included acquiring social children through a surrogate "womb," emphasizing the positive aspects of being worthless (no one would bother to harm them), appreciating that they were no longer being contaminated by menstrual blood, and attempting to influence their husbands through the manipulation of his choice of a younger second wife.

Davis[6] studied 38 women aged 35–65 years in a Newfoundland fishing village. Although these women maintained high status through midlife, the majority reported hot flushes, tension headaches, anxiety, and tiredness in association with the menopause. Davis concluded that the biologic changes of the perimenopause may elicit a common negative response cross-culturally, regardless of women's status. This study was unique in exploring the cognitions of the women concerned and seeking to understand how they conceptualized the changes experienced. A folk explanation for the changes provided a female support system for those who experienced difficulty.

There are obviously many problems in such cross-cultural research. These include possible bias introduced by the investigators, language problems, and the possibility that some cultures express emotional changes in masked ways. An incidence of climacteric complaints similar to that reported in western cultures was found by Moore[28] in a study of 50 rural women in Southeast Zimbabwe. Women were interviewed by a bilingual nursing sister in the hospital. It was not clear whether cultural attitudes toward menopause in this society differed from those reported by Wilbush, who also studied Zulus. No studies appear to have compared the endocrine status of women from different cultures, on the presumption that the duration and severity of endocrine changes is similar in different cultures. This may not be the case. Nevertheless, there is some evidence to suggest that cultural factors may be important in determining an individual's response to biologic changes and the expression of perceived changes.

Life Transitions.—Dominian[11] described the climacteric as a period of major "psychosocial transition." This term refers to changes in life that are lasting in their effects, take place over a relatively short period of time, and affect large numbers of people in the world. Some authors have argued for the "empty nest" as the major psychosocial transition of this period of life.[38] Neugarten[29, 30] failed to find evidence to support the view that the "empty nest" period was a time of crisis. To the contrary, Glen[16] found that women whose children had left home were generally more satisfied than women whose children remained. Other psychosocial transitions that occur at this phase of life include: loss of parents and/or spouse, transition of parents from a supporting role to being supported, physical ill-health and forced acknowledgement of one's own mortality, loss of youth and attractiveness in a youth-oriented society, and transition from mother to grandmother. Few studies have attempted to verify these constructs, but they are important in helping us understand the adjustments that women in midlife must make.

Sociodemographic Variables.—Factors such as employment status, social class, marital status, and social network have been the subject of a number of studies, with interesting and, at times, disparate findings. McKinlay and Jefferys[24] failed to find any association between symptoms and employment status, age at leaving school, social class, domestic workload, marital status, and parity. Two European studies reported conflicting results. Van Keep and Kellerhals[38] studied Swiss women according to menopausal status and found that women in lower social classes had higher symptom scores, with the exception of women in the perimenopausal group, in which women in the higher social class had the highest score. Severne[14] studied Belgian women. She found that, during the climacteric, the effect of work was socially differentiated. For the upper socioeconomic group work outside the home almost always had a favorable effect. This was not true for women of the lower socioeconomic group. Van Keep also reported that women who were well-integrated into their environment and surrounded by friends reported less climacteric symptoms than those who were lonely.

Holt and Mikkelsen[17] reported that women in their Norwegian study who had a good social network tended not to suffer climacteric problems of a psychologic nature. The presence of a personal income, rather than socioeconomic status, was associated with fewer vasomotor complaints.

Stressful Life Events.—Many of the elements of the psychosocial transition can be described as stressful life events. These include exit events, such as the death of the husband or a close relative or friend, and the departure of children from the home, as well as entrance events, such as becoming a grandparent. Procedures for measuring stressful life events have been developed over the last decade and are now being utilized by menopause researchers. Bungay et al.[3] found no evidence in their study that "life events" cluster about the mean age of menopause. Worrying events were reported more often by women in their 40s and 50s. These events were positively associated with the reporting of symptoms. The authors did note that symptoms also occurred in women who did not report such events.

Cooke[5] investigated the relationships between climacteric complaints, psychosocial vulnerability factors, and life events. He found an increase in such events during the climacteric years. Cooke also found that nonexit stress was associated with psychologic complaints (such as depression, crying spells, panic attacks, and worrying), whereas exit stress was not. Both exit and nonexit stress were required to produce elevation in "somatic" symptomatology (faintness and dizziness, headaches, and tingling or numbness in the body). Using a hierarchical regression analysis, Cooke found that the loss of one's mother before age 11 and employment status act as vulnerability factors for life event stress, influencing the occurrence of psychologic complaints. The degree of involvement with children was directly associated with the occurrence of psychologic complaints. The number of confidants available to the patient was directly associated with the lessening of psychologic symptomatology and had a synergistic effect with life-event stress. Thus, the availability of confidants may help to diffuse life stress. Neither the level of confiding in the spouse, the number of children at home, nor the quality of communication with children had any effect. Similar results were found for the "somatic" complaints, except that the degree of involvement with the children no longer had any effect.

Personal interpretation of events as stressful may vary between individuals, sexes, age groups, and cultures. Resnick[34] reported that U.S. women in the 35–45-year age group mentioned intrapersonal events such as work and mastery experiences as the most significant life events.

Ballinger[34] compared patient and nonpatient groups in an Australian study. The most important measures that distinguished between groups were psychologic symptoms, total life distress, metabolic symptoms, and, lastly, Hamilton depression and anxiety scores. Patients were more likely to have experienced a depression previously and been treated by a psychiatrist. Hot flushes did not distinguish groups when their frequency was considered (80% in both groups reported hot flushes), but did when their severity was considered.

Thus, in summary, it would appear that many psychosocial variables may be important in determining women's experience of the menopause. These factors include the meaning of changes produced by the climacteric process within a particular culture, the woman's social class, whether or not she works outside the home, the adequacy of her social network, the degree of her involvement with her children, and the occurrence of undesirable life events. The loss of her mother at an early age and a past history of depression may also make the woman more vulnerable to life stress.

CONCLUSIONS

Studies reviewed in this chapter demonstrate that premenopausal women report more minor psychologic complaints than do women in other age groups. Biologic, psychologic, and sociologic factors are probably all important in these complaints. Underlying endocrinologic changes may in themselves be sufficient to trigger emotional changes leading to distress. In other women these changes may lead only to psychologic complaints when other factors are present. Such vulnerability factors include low socioeconomic class especially when combined with work outside the home, lack of a supportive social network, undesirable life events, great degree of involvement with children, loss of mother before age 11, and previous history of depression or treatment by a psychiatrist. Personality factors of anxiety proneness have also been found to be associated with more psychologic complaints.

These findings support an interactive biopsychosocial model of the psychologic complaints experienced in the climacteric years.

REFERENCES

1. Ballinger CB: Psychiatric morbidity and the menopause: Screening of a general population sample. *Br Med J* 1975; 3:344–346.
2. Benedek T: Climacterium: A development phase. *Psychoanal Q* 1950; 19:1–27.
3. Bungay GT, Vessey MP, McPherson CK: Study of symptoms in middle life with special reference to the menopause. *Br Med J* 1980; 2:181–183.
4. Collins A, Hansson U, Eneroth P: Postmenopausal symptoms and response to hormonal replacement therapy: Influence of psychological factors. *J Psychosom Obstet Gynaecol* 1983; 2:227–233.
5. Cooke DJ: A psychosocial study of the climacteric, in Broome A., Wallace L. (eds): *Psychology and Gynaecological Problems.* London, Tavistock Publications, 1984, pp 243–265.
6. Davis DL: Women's status and experience of the menopause in a Newfoundland fishing village. *Maturitas* 1982; 4:207–216.
7. Dennerstein L: Sexuality in the climacteric, in Notelovitz M, van Keep PA (eds): Proceedings of the 4th International Congress on the Menopause. Lancaster, England, MTP Press Ltd, in press.
8. Dennerstein L, Burrows GD: A review of studies of the psychological symptoms found at the menopause. *Maturitas* 1978; 1:55–64.
9. Dennerstein L, Burrows GD, Hyman GJ, et al: Hormone therapy and affect. *Maturitas* 1979; 1:247–259.
10. Deutsch H: *The Psychology of Women, vol 2: Motherhood.* New York, Grune & Stratton, 1945, pp 456–485.
11. Dominian J: The role of psychiatry in the menopause. *Clin Obstet Gynecol* 1977; 4:3–29.
12. Engel GL: *Psychological Development in Health and Disease.* Philadephia, WB Saunders Co, 1962, pp 208–209, 294–301.
13. Fessler L: The psychopathology of climacteric depression. *Psychoanal Q* 1950; 19:28–42.
14. Flint MP: Sociology and anthropology of the menopause, in van Keep PA, Serr DM (eds): *Female and Male Climacteric.* Lancaster, England, MTP Press Ltd, 1979; pp 1–8.
15. Freud S: *The Standard Edition of the Complete Psychological Works of Sigmund Freud,* Strachey J (ed). London, Hogarth Press and the Institute of Psycho-Analysis, vol 12, p 236; vol. 20, p 242.
16. Glen ND: Psychological well-being in the postparental stage. Some evidence from national surveys. *J Marriage Family* 37:105–110.
17. Haspels AA, Musaph H: Psychosexual aspects of mid-life, in van Keep PA, Utian WH, Vermeulen A (eds): *The Controversial Climacteric.* Lancaster, England, MTP Press Ltd, 1981, pp 39–50.
18. Hepworth M: Sociological aspects of mid-life, in van Keep PA, Utian WH, Vermeulen A

(eds): *The Controversial Climacteric*. Lancaster, England, MTP Press Ltd, 1981, 19–28.

19. Jaszman L: Epidemiology of climacteric syndrome, in van Keep PA, Lauritzen C (eds): *Ageing and Estrogens*. Basel, S Karger AG, 1972, pp 11–23.
20. Jern HZ: Hormone therapy of the menopause. *J Am Med Wom Assoc* 1975; 30:491–493.
21. Kopera H: Estrogens and psychic functions, in Van Keep PA, Lauritzen C (eds): *Ageing and Estrogens*. Basel, S Karger AG, 1973, pp 118–133.
22. Krupinsksi J, Stoller A: Psychological disorders, in Krupinski J, Stoller A (eds): *The Health of a Metropolis*. Australia, Melbourne, Heinemann Educational, 1971, pp 44–51.
23. Lauritzen C: The management of the pre-menopausal and the post-menopausal patient, in van Keep PA, Lauritzen C (eds): *Ageing and Oestrogens*. Basel, S Karger AG, 1973, pp 2–22.
24. McKinlay SM, Jefferys M: The menopausal syndrome. *Br J Prev Soc Med* 1974; 28:108–115.
25. Maoz B: The perception of menopause in five ethnic groups in Israel. Thesis, Leiden, the Netherlands, 1973.
26. Maoz B, Durst N: Psychology of the menopause, in van Keep PA, Serr DM, Greenblatt RB (eds): *Female and Male Climacteric*. Lancaster, England, MTP Press Ltd, 1979, pp 9–16.
27. Mayer-Gross W, Slater E, Roth M: Exogenous reactions and symptomatic psychoses, in Slater E, Roth M (eds): *Clinical Psychiatry,* ed 3. London, Bailliere, Tindall and Cassell, 1969, pp 342–387.
28. Moore B: Climacteric symptoms in an African community. *Maturitas* 1981; 3:25–29.
29. Neugarten B: The awareness of middle age, in Neugarten B (ed): *Middle Age and Ageing*. Chicago, University of Chicago Press, 1968.
30. Neugarten B: Age groups in American society and the rise of the young-old. *Ann Am Acad Pol Soc Sci* 1974; 415:187–198.
31. Neugarten B, Kraines RJ: Menopausal symptoms in women of various ages. *Psychosom Med* 1965; 27:266–273.
32. Rosenthal SR: Involutional depression, in Ariele S (ed): *American Handbook of Psychiatry,* ed 2. New York, Basic Books, 1974, vol 3, pp 694–709.
33. Schildkraut JJ: The catecholamine hypothesis of affective disorders: A review of supporting evidence. *Am J Psychiatry* 1965; 122:509–522.
34. Severne L: Coping with life events and stress at the climacteric, in Notelovitz M, van Keep PA (eds): *Proceedings of 4th International Congress on the Menopause*. Lancaster, England, MTP Press Ltd., 1986.
35. Studd JWW, Chakravarti S, Okram D: *Clinics in Obstetrics and Gynaecology, vol 4, No. 1: The Menopause,* Greenblatt RB, Studd JWW (eds). Philadelphia, WB Saunders Co, 1977, pp 3–29.
36. Utian WH: The true clinical features of post-menopause and oophorectomy and their response to oestrogen therapy. *S Afr Med J* 1972; 46:732–737.
37. Van Keep PA: The menopause, Part B: Psychosomatic aspects of the menopause, in Dennerstein L, Burrows G (eds): *Handbook of Psychosomatic Obstetrics and Gynaecology*. New York, Elsevier North-Holland, Inc, 1983, pp 483–490.
38. Van Keep PA, Kellerhals JM: The impact of socio-cultural factors on symptom formation. *Psychother Psychosom Med Psychol* 1974;
39. Van Keep PA, Prill HJ: Psycho-sociology of menopause and post-menopause, in van Keep PA, Lauritzen C (eds): *Estrogens in the Post-Menopause. Front. Hormone Res*. Basel, S Karger AG, 1975, pp 32–39.
40. Weissman MM: The myth of involutional melancholia. *JAMA* 1979; 242:742–744.
41. Whitehead MI: The menopause, Part A: Hormone 'replacement' therapy—the controversies, in Dennerstein L, Burrows G (eds): *Handbook of Psychosomatic Obstetrics and Gynaecology*. New York, Elsevier North-Holland, Inc, 1983, pp 445–481.
42. Wilson RA, Wilson TA: The fate of the nontreated post-menopausal woman: A plea for the maintenance of adequate oestrogen from puberty to the grave. *J Am Geriatr Soc* 1963; 11:347–362.
43. Winokur G: Depression in the menopause. *Am J Psychiatry* 1973; 130:92–93.

CHAPTER **10**

Sexuality in the Menopause

RUTH B. WEG, Ph.D.

THE CONVENTIONAL SCRIPT for the American woman who is now menopausal and/or postmenopausal in her 50s, 60s and 70s is singular, but not consistent with today's changing roles and behaviors. Although the stereotype regarding the postmenopausal woman's sexuality is often negative, what few data that do exist have begun to indicate the variety of sensual, sexual, and intimacy needs and behaviors after menopause. Western societies have come to regard the middle-aged peri- and postmenopausal woman as relatively asexual, not by accident or insidious malice, but consequent to the vagaries of a menopausal heritage that is based on the sexual philosophies and practices of nearly 2,000 generations of human history. A reasonable summary statement regarding the sexuality of the human family through the centuries is that marital, procreative sexuality has had primacy above all other dimensions of sexual behavior. The corollary to this is that the asexual label is assigned to the later, barren years of the female, whose womb is the incubator for the future.[8]

THE STUDY OF SEXUALITY AS SCIENCE: THE OLDER FEMALE AS SUBJECT

The early 1900s and the years immediately after World War I were the beginnings of the scientific investigation of human sexuality. Women not only participated more fully in the economic and political life of the West they became part of an emerging sexual revolution. The birth control movement, explicit marriage manuals, and a survey of the sexual lives of 2,200 women appeared in 1929. Women were increasingly recognized as sexual persons, though not yet unconditionally.[38, 52]

Kinsey and colleagues were the first scientists to publish an extensive survey of American sexual behavior.[29, 30] It was the beginning of public realization of the wide range of human sexual expression. Some middle-aged and older women were among the interviewees. Postmenopausal women were reported to retain sexual capacity, interest, and satisfaction; for some, greater pleasure developed as the fear of pregnancy disappeared. This research effort, designed to make inquiry into sexuality acceptable to the scientific community, was marked by quantification, to satisfy the objectivity of the scientific method. Researchers counted the number of orgasms achieved by interviewees from all possible sexual behaviors, including intercourse (heterosexual/homosexual), fellatio/cunnilingus, and self-stimulation. A significant omission, however, was an investigation into the nature, quality, and meaning of human relationships—an omission that for a long time kept the study of sexuality confined to analysis of genital encounters and responsivity. The Masters and Johnson[35, 36] investigation into the physiology of sexual arousal and response freed women from the feelings of inadequacy engendered by the Freudian edict that vaginal orgasm only is the response of the "mature" woman.[20] Kinsey's findings concerning the older woman were confirmed in the Masters and Johnson study, which stated, "there is no time limit drawn by the advancing years of female sexuality."[35(223)]

Continuing the emphasis on the physical aspect of sexuality, a longitudinal study on many aspects of aging performed by the Duke Center for the Study of Aging and Human Development also gathered sexual activity information.[56] An active sex life in the earlier years (interest, frequency, enjoyment) was found to be the most accurate predictor of later life sexuality. Interest in sex was greater than activity for a variety of reasons, such as illness, lack of a partner, boredom, or living situation. Although older women appeared to become less sexually active at a faster rate than men did, this was usually due to their mates' lack of desire or to severe illness. Married women had greater sexual activity than single women. After 78 years of age, women showed more interest in sex than men did. A major variable for the continued sexual expression of the older woman was the availability of a sanctioned (marriage) partner; the relative scarcity of such partners is a frequent barrier to later-life sexuality.

It would appear that what began as an attempt to open the door to the scientific study of human sexuality had temporarily shut out dimensions of human sexuality other than the genital aspect; the reportable data remained largely focused on the physical acts of intercourse and orgasm. Friendship, companionship, and the affective and psychologic meanings of relationships (same sex, opposite sex) remained unexamined. This lack of data is disadvantageous for the study of sexuality as experienced by those of all ages and both sexes, but particularly so in the case of the middle-aged and older woman.

SEXUALITY: GENITAL AND WHOLE-PERSON FOCI

Human sensuality and sexuality encompass more than the anatomy and physiology of sexual intercourse, the levels of hormones, the frequency of orgasm, more than the interaction of genital systems; it is an integral part of the human being at any age. As one form of connection to other persons and as a symbol of reaffirmation of self, the freedom and opportunity for sexual expression are basic to mental and physical well-being, and both become at risk with increasing age.[62] Human beings remember and desire the pleasure and pain of affectional relationships, in which intercourse/orgasm may or may not be involved. Affectional relationships include intimacy, love, friendship, play, caring, and touching.[13, 22, 61] The need for these experiences exists independently of age, and they do not require the lineless, curvaceous bodies of youth to be exciting and fulfilling. The long-held notion that lovemaking and the "sex act" are the prerogatives only of the passionate young is losing adherents, as new information about the sexual lives of middle-aged and older persons comes to light.

Human sexuality is normally lifelong, beginning soon after birth, changing in nature and expression, but staying relatively intact until life is over. More middle-aged and older women are resisting the sexless stereotype and acknowledging sexual needs in themselves and others.[31] Still too prevalent in the society at large and among health professionals is the tendency to disregard the sexual needs of the middle-aged and older woman. But such women, especially the widowed, divorced, and never married are those who know best the ache of frustration and the hunger for affection, love, and the human touch.

The menopausal woman's heritage is poignantly summarized in a piece written in 1850:

"Compelled to yield to the power of time, women now cease to exist as the species and hence forward live only for themselves. Their features are stamped with the impress of age, and their genital organs are sealed with a signet of sterility. The first advice they ought to receive is to reject all sorts of drugs and receipts that are loudly proclaimed by ignorance and puffed by charlatanism. They ought not to sleep upon featherbeds nor in any bed that is too soft and too warm—for such are attended with the disadvantage of exciting the generative organs, which should henceforth, be left, as far as possible, in a state of inaction."[44(532)]

In 1978, the premenopausal woman continued to be described (albeit in contemporary language) as lacking in feminine qualities, as distressed and insecure:

"The premenopausal decade (roughly age 40–50) may be a difficult obstacle for many women. During this time, the symptoms revolve about a deterioration of feminine physical attributes frequently flavored by an intense distaste for aging . . . patients begin to notice dry or flabby skin, sagging breasts, increased skin pigmentation of the hands, chest or face and flabby musculature. . . ."[32(551)]

In the treatment of the perimenopausal women, Kistner states, ". . . the basic concept of management includes psychotherapy to educate, reassure, and support the patient, together with the relief of distressing symptoms and correction of estrogen insufficiency."[32]

With these "gifts" from the past, the middle-aged woman has had to struggle to maintain a positive self-image as a lovable and loving human being despite negative images and messages from a society that has assigned her to the dehumanizing, painful category of neuterdom.

THE MENOPAUSAL WOMAN: NORMAL OR DISEASED?

Madness, depression, and disease as inevitable accompaniments of menopause was the 1850 characterization of menopause in "Dr. Chase's *Last Receipt Book and Household Physician.*"[59] Though it was based on no scientific evidence, this description is understandable, since Dr. Chase's 19th-century practice may have included the most severely suffering menopausal women, from whom he extrapolated to all menopausal women. But late 20th century gynecologic texts are also guilty of the disease image of menopause, portraying it as a time of defeminization, depression, instability, and *in fine,* asexuality.[46]

To many in society (and to herself), the middle-aged menopausal woman becomes the dumpy matron or the "old bag," while the climacteric man is seen as graying, attractive, mature. "That old women are repulsive is one of the most profound esthetic and erotic feelings in our culture."[48] This double standard of aging is what makes the first wrinkles so frightening to middle-aged women, who may feel impelled to buy "rejuvenating" cosmetics or to visit the plastic surgeon. The societal imperative that women be decorative and procreative is so strong that they may see menopause as an end to love and life. But what evidence is there that menopause is a disease?

There are visible changes in the majority of perimenopausal and menopausal women: Gradually, the body contours become less round and full, and they are rarely as they were 20 years earlier. For most, muscle tone and skin elasticity do diminish; wrinkles and sagging appear where none were present before in arms, legs, breasts, and abdomen; and vulval tissue is diminished. The facts of physiologic change during the climacteric and the menopause are discussed elsewhere in this volume—this chapter will concentrate on the impact that these facts and the perceptions concerning menopause have on the sexual behavior and the emotional and psychosocial milieu of the menopausal woman. It should be emphasized that not one of these changes has any significant effect on the capacity of the menopausal woman to be an adequate, loving sex partner.

Menopause has both objective and subjective dimensions. Objectively, it is an event (or series of events) measurable and susceptible to analysis. Subjectively, it is a unique individual experience, related to the countless variables within each individual and her physical and psychosocial environment. As one point in the climacteric, menopause is, after all, only the end of the menstrual phase of a woman's life; it is not a disease and not a basis for the end of libido and sexual expression.[57, 62] Various reports attribute a variety of subjective symptoms to menopausal women, ranging from few or no symptoms to one or more of a long list: hot flashes, sweating, headaches, dizziness, hypertension, palpitations, appetite loss, insomnia, anxiety, and "nervousness."[3, 60] It is apparent that most of these symptoms and signs could have other origins apart from menopause, particularly since they have also been complaints of younger women.[40] There is increasing agreement "that no constellation of symptoms exists that is identifiable as a 'menopausal syndrome.'"[39]

Furthermore, ongoing research into women's views regarding these largely emotional and psychologic symptoms point increasingly to the significance of a hostile psychosocial environment for menopausal women in contemporary societies.[1, 17, 42, 53, 58] It is instructive to know that women in some non-Western societies who are rewarded for the end of their fertility show few symptoms at menopause,[9, 19, 64] whereas those women in Western societies who are considered to have outlived their youth and productivity experience more of the aforementioned symptoms.[50] At a recent British medical symposium on the medical problems of middle-aged women, physicians argued that some psychiatric and psychosexual problems are attributable to societal attitudes, which assign so much positive significance to the sexual attractiveness of youth.[7] Women who have been able to function in multiple roles (mother, wife, and worker) appear to have minimal or no symptoms.[42]

Statements regarding the normality of menopause are missing from most medical literature, so that a more representative research base is necessary for an accurate understanding. In medical articles and books that discuss the menopause, there is a frequent discrepancy between the particular experience of the woman and the physician's observation and interpretation. Kaufert[26] reports from a recent Canadian study that 44% of women participants beween 40 and 60 years of age had never discussed menopause with their physicians, and 83% relied on magazines and books for answers to their questions. Yet, the questions asked by most women of female investigators suggest that women are eager for information about their bodies, and want to know what to expect so that they may be better able to foresee and adapt to the normal changes of the climacteric and menopause.[57] Unfortunately, there has been little medical interest in the fairly smooth transition into menopause and beyond. The usual methodology in medical studies of the disturbed or aberrant menopause is to gather general data and analyze blood samples obtained once or twice from a random population for comparison purposes. These techniques are therefore inadequate for the identification of any long-range events and/or changes.

In a survey undertaken to examine the perceptions of women aged 40–60 years regarding the menopause, women reported a variety of symptoms, and there was a range of concern about these symptoms, but even with symptoms, the women generally did not see the menopause as an illness. The survey's author suggests, "support techniques and assisting women to cope with problems encountered during menopause. . . . may be much more appropriate for some women than 'treatment' programs using drugs and surgery."[21]

Margaret Mead found the menopause "an energetic, creative time" for women, a period of zest.[57] The perception that the menopausal woman is deficient may be only the function of a male perspective.[24] The woman-oriented, sensitive, and supportive health professional should avoid overemphasis on the problems of the natural (or even surgical) ending of fertile life, should assure the woman of the separation of libido and fertility, and should encourage discussion of menopause and any emotional/physical concerns which may exist.

Pathology.—The climacteric and the menopause do not inevitably lead to illness and disease. Rather, the myth of the menace of menopause and societal's image of the middle-aged woman may increase her vulnerability to physical and psychologic symptoms. The excesses in eating, drinking, drug use, the systemic disorders, and the increase in depression associated with menopause can occur at any age and may indeed affect sexual libido and activity. Malnutrition, fatigue, anemia, untreated diabetes also are known to "inhibit desire and abort arousal and sexual climax."[61(168)]

Men and women alike may think that pelvic surgery makes a middle-aged woman "less than a woman," so this surgery is often a major determinant for the end of sexual activity. Although there is no evidence that hysterectomy depresses libido and orgasmic response, the fear and belief that it does are often parent to the deadening reality.[58, 62] In a retrospective study of women who had experienced surgical menopause, Cosper et al.[12] found that psychosocial factors (e.g., concern with loss of femininity) are the major determinants in subsequent altered libido and activity, not the changing physiology or anatomy.

Another serious threat to a woman's self-confidence and self image is the mastectomy, which requires a number of difficult adjustments. The first is the loss of her body integrity, the second is the fear that the love of her partner will be lost, or if she is unattached, that she will be no longer lovable. Both feelings compound the deep-seated fear of cancer and death. More effective pre- and postsurgical counseling and guidance by peers and health professionals for the patient and her family can defuse some of the fears, create a more positive outlook, and provide accurate information.[66]

Illness, even terminal disease, does not destroy the human need for caring, loving, and sexual relationships. Not only may this need be heightened, but such relationships help the patient to cope and to maintain a hopeful struggle. Studies suggest that even institutionalization among middle-aged and elderly individuals does not eliminate the importance of sexual desire and physical love.[25, 65]

SEXUAL/SENSUAL EXPRESSION AND RESPONSIVITY

Many peri- and premenopausal women have believed the myth that the drying up of the "elan vital" means the end of sexual function, and they question the meaning of life. The acceptance of this mythology may be a precursor to illness, it may modify interpersonal exchanges, and it can effectively turn off sexual activity as well as the inner sense of one's own sexuality.[23]

Extremist authorities in the past often predicted menopausal women would exhibit either nymphomania or frigidity, in contrast to more recent studies, which indicate that many women are generally positive about menopause and find a new excitement in their sexual lives with long-term or new mates.[14, 42] In middle-aged and older women (as in men) continued sexual activity is correlated, in part, with the degree of enjoyment of sexual experience earlier in life.[2, 43] With women who are older today, the sanctioned partner and his/her continued activity are major determinants.

Kinsey[30] and Kaplan[27] describe female sexual development as being slower than the male's: a woman reaches sexual maturity in her early 20s and continues to grow and peak with the years. It is difficult to identify how much of the apparently slower female development is because of learned cultural inhibitions. These inhibitions are often finally rejected by 40–50-year-old women approaching menopause, which may account for part of the resurgence of sexual activity in the middle years and the reports of heightened libido in today's menopausal and postmenopausal woman. In addition, the absence of fear of pregnancy and the lack of the need for birth control devices can make sexual expression more spontaneous. The man during this climacterium period is frequently at a low ebb in sexual activity and interest and is more concerned with changes in his responsivity and performance. Thus, these men and women are often out of phase sexually, so that millions of heterosexual women frequently feel unloved and unlovable, starved for affection and emotional support, confirming the societal stereotype of asexuality.

In one sense, the middle-aged woman is sexually advantaged compared to most mid-life and older men, for, despite the continued hormonal depletion and the consequent anatomical and functional changes, she remains responsive. Although decreased circulatory efficiency and lower hormonal levels eventually lead to diminution of vulval tissue, and reduction of the size of the cervix, ovaries, and uterus, she is no less the interested, capable sexual partner. Although the uterus will at times during intercourse contract spasmodically rather than rhythmically, which may be painful, there is little alteration in the clitoris, and its function as sensate focus remains.[38] Although the vaginal mucosa grows thinner, less elastic, and more friable, the rugal pattern smooths out, and there are more complaints of vaginitis and reduced lubrication, most of these changes may be diminished with careful hormonal replacement therapy, thus enhancing the potential for sexual desire and pleasurable interaction.[37, 62]

Responsivity patterns, the timing and extent of phases in sexual stimulation and response, change because of age-related neuroendocrine and circulatory changes. Vasocongestion diminishes, skin flush is less, and the time for labial and vaginal lubrication may increase from the 15–30 seconds of the earlier years to as long as five minutes.[35, 36] The time needed to excite and elevate clitoral tissue is prolonged, but as noted earlier, the response is intact. Uterine contractions are reduced in number from three to five to one or two more likely increasingly arrhythmic. Between the ages of 50 and 70 years, orgasmic duration is gradually decreased and resolution is more rapid, as in the middle-aged and older man.

Sexual activity can be emotional and communicative, not just physical. The quiet talk, the humor, the sensuous joy of holding another and being held are a large part of the pleasure. The sex act itself may or may not be part of the lovemaking. What is so often discussed by middle-aged women is the importance of sensual, intimate, and sexual activity for the renewal of self recommitment to life's motivations and the release of emotional and physical tensions.[63] The menopause is a most inappropriate time to deprive more than half of humankind of the wholeness of her life.

Health professionals should remember not only that a woman's sexual needs do not necessarily diminish in the postmenopausal years but her sexuality may be expressed in ways other than heterosexual intercourse.

Masturbation.—Self pleasuring for women as an acceptable dimension of sexual expression awaited the growth of the women's movement.[61] The act of masturbation starts early in life and continues into old age. Both the taboos about masturbation, learned in childhood, which may be overcome in the later years, and the guilt surrounding this practice and its condemnation by various religions are fading. Self-stimulation can help maintain responsivity of the genitalia, "release tensions, stimulate sexual appetite, and contribute to well-being."[58] However, loneliness for the middle-aged woman who is without a partner is not so easily eliminated. Masturbation is no substitute for sharing with a loving, caring partner.

Homosexuality.—It is clear that homosexuality and bisexuality are part of the range of human sexual behavior. Recent studies are slowly destroying the ignorance and stereotypes associated with gay and lesbian communities.[5] Lesbians in their late middle and older years, who generally have long-term relationships, may even have an advantage over nonlesbians, since the number of eligible partners is potentially larger than for heterosexual women.[33]

RESURGENCE AND/OR REJECTION OF ACTIVITY

More middle-aged and older women are discovering their need to acknowledge sexual expression. They seek a more active sexual role and take the first step in the development of different kinds of intimate relationships.[4, 63] The menopausal woman can be sexually competent and vigorous; she can be orgasmic and multiorgasmic, provided there is effective stimulation. Lovemaking may become more gentle, prolonged, and caring, and is increasingly more oriented toward personal intimacy than the passion of earlier years. Difficulty in reaching a sense of intimacy in the sex act is the most frequent complaint of women, rather than the decrease in frequency of the explosive, passionate orgasm.[31, 63]

Some middle-aged and older women withdraw from coitus or any physical expression of sexuality. This behavior is most often related to lifelong unsatisfactory experiences and early negative socialization. Although investigations and therapists' reports[6, 35, 36, 37, 43, 49] have found libido among a majority of midlife and postmenopausal women to be at higher levels than among many older men, some perimenopausal, menopausal, and postmenopausal women—often, married women—develop a lack of interest in sexual activity. Furthermore, this behavior complicates the marital relationship.

Because of the widespread societal attitudes already discussed and their own personal attitudes, some menopausal and postmenopausal women willingly relinquish an active sex role. It is reasonable to perceive a decrease in libido and sexual behavior as multifactorial: the decrease in sexual hormones may cause genital atrophy, a noticeable difficulty with vaginal lubrication, and an extension of the time needed to become sexually excited. These physical difficulties may be compounded by a sexually ignorant partner, inappropriate stimulation, a lifelong or more recent lack of sexual enjoyment and satisfaction with her partner, a lack of self esteem, and a misunderstanding of the role of sexuality in the middle and later years. Societal expectations that older people marry for companionship only suggest that the interest and capacity for sexual expression are at an end.[47] In response to past miseducation, unpleasant sexual experiences, hormonal, physiologic, and interpersonal changes, and negative reinforcements from the popular media, many older women (and men) may feel asexual, or they may suppress any erotic interests, believing them to be inappropriate, and possibly even morally wrong. However, some investigations indicate a hormonal basis for decreased sexual interest. Hormonally untreated postmenopausal women were less responsive (using vaginal pulse amplitude as a measure) to erotic films than younger, menstruating females or older premenopausal women.[41]

Dennerstein,[16] on the basis of the report of Studd and Parsons[50] states that "nearly half of all patients presenting at a menopause clinic offer symptoms of sexual dysfunction among their three main complaints."[16] Dennerstein notes that perimenopausal women with such complaints appear to be placebo-responsive[10] and therefore discusses only those data from six double-blind studies.[15] In one study described by Dow and Hart,[18] use of hormone replacement therapy (either estradiol alone, or estradiol and testosterone) appeared related to a significant reduction in the level of psychologic and vasomotor complaints and an improvement in sexual interest, responsiveness, orgasmic capacity, and satisfaction. There was no improvement in marital dissatisfaction, which rarely is based on a single factor.[27, 28]

Since the findings of sexual interest and behavior in menopausal and postmenopausal women in a variety of studies are discrepant, it may be that there have been methodologic differences and omission of impacting factors, such as overall health status, genital changes, presence and/or health of spouse/partner, or level of sex education. A definitive decision regarding the sexual interest and behavior of menopausal and postmenopausal women will require taking individual histories, consulting and counseling with the couple, and management at a number of levels. Older women (and men) can become sexually liberated and seek to do so. Various programs and approaches continue to validate the potential for the enhancement of the sexual lives of older persons.[11, 51]

Other women explore stimulation by different means: self or partner masturbation, cunnilingus, and breast stimulation. They are more aware of the need of the middle-aged and older partner for prolonged direct stimulation of the penis and/or testes and are more willing to engage in the caressing and touching of another, a prerogative so long thought to be for "men only." In heterosexual relationships, some men who may have been interested in ceasing sexual activity with his mate (or any other woman) greet the menopause as an excuse not to perform sexually for a wife/partner who can no longer procreate. In that case, the menopausal woman is more than ever convinced of her new-found failings and may retreat into a period of mourning for her now dying sexual self.

RECENT RESEARCH

Current research invalidates the negative sexual stereotype of middle-aged and older American men and women. The Starr-Weiner report of 1981[49] surveyed 800 adults between the ages of 60 and 91 years who represented four regions of the U.S.; 65% of the sample population was female. The questions, developed from a pilot study, were open-ended and had been traditionally considered appropriate for young individuals only. The analysis of responses demonstrated that not only have people in the middle and later years responded to the so-called revolution in sexual behavior but that they continue to change with time. Some respondents belittled the marriage contract as a sanction for sexual relations, and others noted that the feeling and needs of two adults superceded the standards set by society. A large number reported that sex was better than ever. Many women identified orgasm as essential to the sexual experience and said it was stronger than in their youth. They enjoyed nudity with their partners, and their fantasized ideal lover was close to their own age. Both women and men recognized that pleasuring each other, rather than aiming for an orgasm, relieved them of the necessity to "perform" and freed them for the joy of interaction. The authors perceive the largest change to be among women. Most women recognize they have at least as much passion and sexuality as men do, and they now have newfound choices.

Brecher et al.[6] used a survey questionnaire to readers of *Consumer Reports* and their relatives and friends to investigate the sexual behavior of older adults. This nonrandom group of 4,246 persons between the ages of 50 and 93 years were, in fact, self selected, in better than average health, and above average in income and education, and they generally appeared to have a greater than average interest in "sex." They found a "substantial majority of respondents . . . make use of effective counter measures to the changing thresholds of sexual responsivity and any other factors involved with ill health and aging."[6] Some women (and men) engaged in oral and manual stimulation of breasts and genitals and anal stimulation; some used vaginal lubricants, vibrators, and/ or the technique of "stuffing" a partially erect penis into the vagina. Some experimented with various coital positions, different times of the day. Some preferred the comfort and warmth of fondling and cuddling. It was also reported that some made use of sexually explicit or pornographic materials and/or fantasy. A large proportion of respondents were sexually active, and the levels of enjoyment, variety, quantity, and quality of sexual activities were surprising even to those analyzing the data. Age alone was not enough to eliminate interest, libido, activity, and pleasure for most persons.

SUMMARY

Human sexual behavior is varied and culturally dependent; it has been learned and relearned many times in many places. A recurrent theme has been the "for youth only" attitude regarding sexuality.[52] Age-related changes in most other body systems are accepted, but any sign of change in the sexual system is dreaded, because society has dictated that rolelessness and sexlessness must follow.

Early in human history, the perceived purpose of female sexuality was to procreate and to fulfill male sexual needs—not to give women pleasure. Regarding her sexual behavior, woman was either glorified as innocent, pure, and incapable of sexual desire or aligned with the devil as evil, oversexed adultress.[8, 52] However, the menopausal and postmenopausal woman most often was neither exalted nor debased, but assigned to the mythical state of asexuality.

Investigations into human sexuality in the first half of this century established that the most useful reportable data were related to the narrow physical aspect of human sexuality: the number of sexual encounters, the incidence of orgasm during intercourse, and the frequency of masturbation and oral/genital sex in both heterosexual and homosexual relations.[29, 30, 35, 36, 43] The mechanical emphasis on technique and the importance of orgasm left little room for attention to the meaning of human, affectional interactions, with or without orgasm.

Recent research have confirmed that changing sex roles are stimulating an awakening of the middle-aged woman to her potential as wife, lover, mother, and worker. More assured in her own sexuality apart from procreation, she maintains interest and is limited only by the lack of opportunity and the residue of ignorant societal attitudes. Health professionals have become more informed about the needs of the whole person and about sexuality as part of that whole. It is hoped that this awareness will lead to greater support for the older woman who seeks sexual fulfillment.

CONCLUSION

Sexuality is a human attribute that changes with time but continues until death. Sexual behavior is learned behavior, and changing sex roles in today's society have already brought about new attitudes concerning sexual behavior, especially for women.

The "neuter" label for the middle-aged and older woman has not only been in error, but it has contributed to unnecessary emotional and physical starvation for some women. Widespread sexual myths and misconceptions, continuing even into this century, have negatively influenced members of the medical profession and the men and women in their care. It was not until sexuality was accepted as a legitimate subject for scientific inquiry that it began to be properly understood.[34]

Evidence is overwhelming that the need for intimate, affective relationships exists for all ages, and perhaps especially during the middle and later years. "A better understanding of menopause-related events by physicians will flow over into improved education programs in the general population and specifically, in better informed patients. Hopefully, this will also witness a positive change in attitude by society toward menopause and aging and with an ultimate decrease in the psycho-socio-cultural contribution to symptom formation."[54] Utian went further in reminding all who are involved with the health care of middle-aged women "to keep an open and questioning mind, to accept developments where proven, and to avoid dogma and prejudice."[54]

It is my hope that sexual research will go beyond quantitation to include the study of the quality and meaning of relationships among persons at all ages. It is time, scientifically and in the nature of human development, for helping professionals to seize the opportunity to treat the person, not the disease, to be committed to the promotion and maintenance of the functional health of the multiple dimensions of a human being, including the sexual, during all of the lifespan.

REFERENCES CITED
1. Alington-Mackinnon D, Troll LE: The adaptive function of the menopause: A devil's advocate position. *J Am Geriatr Soc* 1971; 29:349.
2. Asso D: *The Real Menstrual Cycle.* New York, John Wiley & Sons, 1983.
3. Bates G: On the nature of the hot flash. *Clin Obstet Gynecol* 1981; 24:231.
4. Bell RR: Sexuality and Sex Roles. Paper prepared for working conference to develop teaching materials on family and sex roles. Detroit, Mich, Nov. 1–12, 1975.
5. Bell AP, Weinberg MS: *Homosexualities: A Study of Diversity Among Men and Women.* New York, Simon & Schuster, 1978.
6. Brecher E, and the editors of *Consumer Reports* books: *Love, Sex and Aging.* Boston, Little, Brown & Co, 1984.
7. Uncertainties at a certain age. *Br Med J* 2(6029):199–200, 1976.
8. Bullough VL: *Sexual Variance in Society and History.* New York, John Wiley & Sons, 1976.
9. Cherry SH: *The Menopause Myth.* New York, Ballantine Books, 1976.
10. Coope J: Double blind crossover study of estrogen replacement therapy, in Campbell S (ed): *The Management of the Menopausal and Post-menopausal Years.* Lancaster, England, MTP Press Ltd, 1976, pp 159–168.
11. Corby N, Solnick RL: Psychosocial and physiological influences on sexuality in the older adult, in Birren JE, Sloane RB (eds): *Handbook of Mental Health and Aging.* Englewood Cliffs, New Jersey, Prentice-Hall, 1980, pp 893–921.

12. Cosper B, Fuller S, Tobinson G: Characteristics of post hospitalization recovery following hysterectomy. *J Obstet Gynecol Neonatal Nursing* 1978; 7:7.
13. Datan N, Rodeheaver D: Beyond generativity: Toward a sensuality of later life, in Weg R (ed): *Sexuality in the Later Years: Roles and Behavior.* New York, Academic Press, 1983, pp 279–288.
14. Delaney J, Lupton MJ, Toth E: Psychology and the menopausal menace, in Delaney J, Lupton MJ, Toth E (eds): *The Curse: A Cultural History of Menstruation.* New York, EP Dutton & Co, Inc, 1976, pp 186–191.
15. Dennerstein L, Burrows GD: A review of studies of the psychological symptoms found at the menopause. *Maturitas* 1978; 1:55–64.
16. Dennerstein L: Psychological and sexual effects, in Mishell DR Jr (ed): *Physiology and Treatment of the Menopause.* Chicago, Yearbook Medical Publishers, in press.
17. Detre T, Hayashi T, Archer DF: Management of the menopause. *Ann Intern Med* 1978; 88:373.
18. Dow MGT, Hart DM: Hormonal treatments of sexual unresponsiveness in postmenopausal women: A comparative study. *Br J Obstet Gynecol* 1983; 90:361–366.
19. Flint M: Cross-cultural factors that affect age of menopause, in Van Keep PA, Greenblatt RB, Albeaux-Fernet M (eds): *Consensus on Menopause Research.* Baltimore, University PK Press, 1976, pp 73–83.
20. Freud S: In Freud EL (ed): *The Letters of Sigmund Freud.* New York, Basic Books, 1960.
21. Frey KA: Middle-aged women's experience and perceptions of menopause. Women Health 1981; 6:25.
22. Gagnon JH, Henderson B: *Human Sexuality: An Age of Ambiguity.* Social Issues Series, No 1. Boston, Educational Associates, division of Little, Brown & Co, 1975.
23. Greenblatt RB: Estrogens in cancer change the way you treat postmenopausal patients. *Mod Med* 1977; 45:47.
24. Jehlen M: Archimedes and the paradox of feminist criticism. *Signs* 1981; 6:575.
25. Kassel V: Long-term care institutions, in Weg RB (ed): *Sexuality in the Later Years: Roles and Behavior.* New York, Academic Press, 1983, pp 167–184.
26. Kaufert PA: The perimenopausal woman and her use of health services. *Maturitas* 1980; 2:191.
27. Kaplan HS: *The New Sex Therapy.* New York, Brunner Mazel, 1974.
28. Kaplan HS: *The Illustrated Manual of Sex Therapy.* New York, Quadrangle, 1975.
29. Kinsey A, Pomeroy WB, Martin CI: *Sexual Behavior in the Human Male.* Philadelphia, WB Saunders, 1948.
30. Kinsey A, Pomeroy WB, Martin CI, et al: *Sexual Behavior in the Human Female.* Philadelphia, WB Saunders Co, 1953.
31. Kirkpatrick M: Women's sexual complaints. *Med Aspects Human Sexuality* 1976; 10:118.
32. Kistner RW: The menopause, in Caplan RM, Sweeney WJ (eds): *Advances in Obstetrics and Gynecology.* Baltimore, Williams & Wilkins Co, 1978, pp 551–565.
33. Laner MR: Growing older female: Heterosexual and homosexual. *J Homosex* 1979; 4:267.
34. Masters WH: The gynecological consideration of the sexual act (an editorial). *JAMA* 1983; 250:22.
35. Masters WH, Johnson VE: *Human Sexual Response.* Boston, Little, Brown & Co, 1966.
36. Masters WH, Johnson VE: *Human Sexual Inadequacy.* Boston, Little, Brown & Co, 1970.
37. Masters WH, Johnson VE: Sex and the aging process. *J Am Geriatr Soc* 1981; 29:385.
38. Masters WH, Johnson VE: Kolodny RC: *Human Sexuality.* Boston, Little, Brown & Co, 1982.
39. McArthur JW: The contemporary menopause. *Primary Care* 1981; 8:141.
40. McKinlay S, McKinlay J: Selected studies on the menopause. *J Biosoc Sci* 1973; 5:533.
41. Morrell MJ, Dixen JM, Carter CS, et al: The influence of age and cycling status on sexual arousability in women. *Am J Obstet Gynecol* 1984; 148:66–71.
42. Neugarten BL, Datan N: The middle years. *J Geriatr Psychiatry* 1976; 9:45.
43. Pfeiffer E, Davis GC: Determinants of sexual behavior in middle and old age. *J Am Geriatr Soc* 1972; 20:151.
44. Ricci A: *100 Years of Gynecology.* Philadelphia, Blakeston Co, 1947.
45. Rubin L: Sex and sexuality: Woman at midlife, in Kirkpatrick M (ed): *Women's Sexual*

Experiences—Exploration of the Dark Continent. New York, Plenun Publishing Corp, 1982, pp 61–82.

46. Scully D, Bart P: A funny thing happened on the way to the orifice: Women in gynecological textbooks. *Am J Sociol* 1973; 78:1045.
47. Sloane E: *Biology of Women.* New York, John Wiley & Sons, 1980.
48. Sontag S: The double standard of aging. *Sat Rev* 1972; 55:29.
49. Starr BD, Weiner MB: *The Starr-Weiner Report on Sex and Sexuality in the Mature Years.* New York, McGraw-Hill Book Co, 1981.
50. Studd JWW, Parsons A: Sexual dysfunction: The climacteric. *Br J Sex Med* 1977; Dec. 11–12.
51. Sviland MAP: Helping elderly couples become sexually liberated: Psychosocial issues. *The Counseling Psychologists* 1975; 5(1):67–72.
52. Tannahill R: *Sex in History.* New York, Stein & Day, 1980.
53. Utian WH: Definitive symptoms of post menopause-incorporating use of vaginal aprabasal cell index. *Front Horm Res* 1975; 3:74.
54. Utian WH: *Menopause in Modern Perspective.* New York, Appleton-Century-Crofts, 1980.
55. Van Keep PA: Psychosocial aspects of the climacteric, in Van Keep PA, Greenblatt RB, Albeaux-Fernet M (eds): *Consensus on Menopause Research.* Baltimore, University Park Press, 1976, pp 5–8.
56. Verwoerdt A, Pfeiffer E, Wang HS: Sexual behavior in senescence, in Palmore E (ed): *Normal Aging: Reports from Duke Longitudinal Study, 1955–1969.* Duke, NC, Duke University Press, 1970, pp 282–299.
57. Voda AM, Eliasson M: Menopause: The closure of menstrual life. *Women Health* 1983; 8:137.
58. Weg RB: Sexual inadequacy in the elderly, in Goldman R, Rockstein M (eds): *The Physiology and Pathology of Aging.* New York, Academic Press, 1975, pp 203–227.
59. Weg RB: Young/Beautiful or Banished. Paper delivered at the Women: Midstream Decision Conference. Miami University, Oxford, Ohio, June 20–22, 1976.
60. Weg RB: Normal aging changes in the reproductive system, in Burnside IM (ed): *Nursing and the Aged,* ed 2. New York, McGraw-Hill Book Co, 1981, pp 362–373.
61. Weg RB: Beyond babies and orgasm. *Educ Horizons* 1982; 60:161.
62. Weg RB: The physiological perspective, in Weg RB (ed): *Sexuality in the Later Years: Roles and Behavior.* New York, Academic Press, 1983, pp 4–80.
63. Weg RB: Intimacy in the later years, in Lesnoff-Caravaglia G (ed): *Images of the Older Person.* New York, Human Sciences Press, in press.
64. Weideger P: *Menstruation and Menopause.* New York, Alfred A Knopf, 1976.
65. West ND: Sex in geriatrics: Myth or miracle? *J Am Geriatr Soc* 1975; 23:551.
66. Woods NF: *Human Sexuality in Health and Illness.* St. Louis, CV Mosby Co, 1979.

PART II

Beneficial Effects of Pharmacologic Agents

CHAPTER **11**

Treatment of Hot Flushes

DAVID R. MELDRUM, M.D.

ESTROGEN REPLACEMENT

Mechanism of Action.—Hot flushes are the consequence of the effects of ovarian failure on hypothalamic neurotransmitter concentrations.[1] Estrogen is the principle component of the negative feedback control exerted by the normally functioning ovary. Its replacement has been recognized to be the most effective means of treatment of this disturbance and therefore serves as a standard against which all other treatments must be compared.

Effectiveness.—Table 11–1 shows the effects of ethinyl estradiol, 50 μg, on the subjective symptoms and objective changes measured under controlled conditions.[2] The objective recording of finger temperature and skin resistance has provided a quantifiable means of comparing the effects of various modes of therapy. It can be seen that this high dose of a long-acting preparation reduces the occurrence of both subjective and objective changes to almost nil.

Although high doses of estrogen completely abolish the symptom complex in almost all women, there are no dose-response studies using any of the available estrogen preparations to indicate the appropriate dose and schedule of administration. The practitioner must therefore rely on collective and personal experience to guide his management of this problem.

Mode of Therapy.—General experience indicates that for the most common estrogen preparation used, conjugated equine estrogens, a dose of 0.625–2.5 mg is necessary to relieve hot flushes completely in all women. These doses are generally higher than those required for normalization of vaginal cytology and calcium excretion.[3] The reasons for this discrepancy most likely stem from the differences of the treatment from normal ovarian function. First, the ovary secretes estrogen continuously, whereas a single daily

TABLE 11–1.

Effect of Ethinyl Estradiol* on Rate of Occurrence (per Hour) of Subjective Flushes and Physiologic Events in Four Women

FACTOR	BASELINE	WITH ESTROGENS	P VALUE
Subjective flushes	1.10 ± 0.2	0.07 ± 0.04	< .02
Finger temperature	1.20 ± 0.2	0.60 ± 0.10	< .02
Skin conductance	1.10 ± 0.2	0.03 ± 0.03	< .02
Core temperature	1.10 ± 0.02	0.03 ± 0.10	< .02
Finger temperature and skin conductance	1.03 ± 0.2	0	< .02
Finger temperature, skin conductance, and core temperature	1.00 ± 0.2	0	< .02

*50 μg q.d. for 30 days.

oral dose results in peaks and troughs throughout the day. Second, the ovary produces progesterone as well as estrogen during approximately half of the menstrual cycle. The two hormones have additive or perhaps even synergistic effects on the hypothalamus, manifested during the luteal phase of the normal menstrual cycle by a marked reduction in the frequency of luteinizing hormone (LH) pulses.

It is now recommended for most postmenopausal women to prescribe a progestin along with estrogen for at least ten days[4] for protection of the endometrium, and perhaps the breasts, from excessive estrogen stimulation. Although not proven, there is every reason to expect that this adjunctive therapy will also aid in the control of hot flushes at lower doses of estrogen. We currently recommend that treatment be started at 0.625 mg, together with a progestin, for 10–14 days out of the cycle and that the dose of estrogen be increased only if the symptoms are not controlled after an adequate trial (one to three months).

Estradiol pellets have been used in the past to provide continuous estrogen therapy, but this modality is no longer approved for use. We have investigated the use of percutaneous estrogen therapy by means of an estradiol-releasing skin patch.[5] Figure 11–1 shows the effect of a prototype patch on objectively recorded hot flushes. Even though

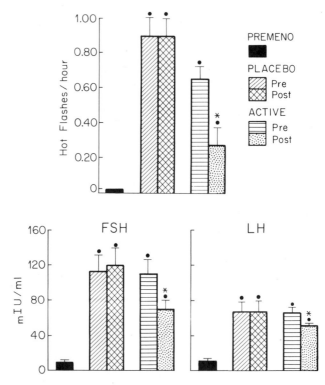

FIG 11–1.
Effects of transdermal estrogen treatment on the central nervous system. *Upper panel* shows the mean frequency of hot flushes in premenopausal control subjects and postmenopausal subjects before and after treatment with placebo or estradiol-containing (active) systems. *Lower panels* show the mean serum concentrations of FSH and LH in the same subjects. *Asterisk* denotes significant difference from baseline. *Solid circle* denotes significant difference from premenopausal control subjects.

the circulating estradiol level was elevated only to the early follicular phase range (70 pg/ml), there was a prominent reduction of hot flush episodes associated with significant reductions of the circulating levels of gonadotropins. A dose-response study is currently being completed. It is anticipated that levels of estradiol between 50 and 150 pg/ml, together with a progestin, will provide fully physiologic replacement with consistent relief of hot flushes.

Secondary Beneficial Effects of Therapy.—In a study by Campbell and Whitehead of women with severe hot flushes, estrogen treatment was accompanied by significant decreases in insomnia, anxiety, and irritability and by improvement of memory, compared with placebo.[6] The authors suggested that these improvements of other aspects of brain function may have been due to a "domino effect" by relief of hot flushes during sleep, improved quality of sleep, and prevention of the well-recognized adverse effects of a chronic sleep disturbance.

We have further investigated the relationship of hot flushes to sleep quality by the simultaneous recordings of finger temperature and skin resistance as objective indices of the hot flush and the use of the sleep polygraph to record the various stages of sleep.[7] Figure 11–2 shows the close temporal relationship of each hot flush to a waking episode (signified by an *asterisk*). In eight out of the nine subjects studied, it was possible to show a statistically significant relationship between the two events (in the remaining subject, the duration of sleep was very short). Figure 11–3 shows the sleep polygraph of a subject before and following treatment with 50 μg of ethinyl estradiol daily. Note the absence of hot flushes during treatment and the associated reduction of waking episodes and improvement of sleep quality. Other investigators have demonstrated that estrogen therapy decreases sleep latency and increases rapid eye movement sleep,[8] showing that this treatment is more physiologic than most sedatives or hypnotics used to treat insomnia.

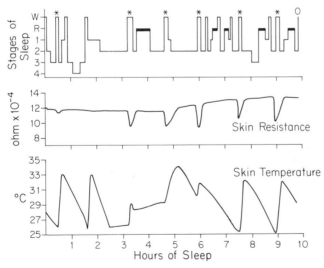

FIG 11–2.
Sleepgrams and recordings of the skin resistance and temperature in postmenopausal subject with severe hot flushes. Each *asterisk* marks occurrence of objectively measured hot flush. *Open circle* indicates arousal of patient by investigator at end of study.

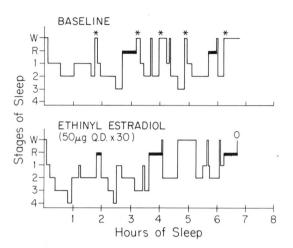

FIG 11–3.
Sleepgrams measured in symptomatic patient before and after 30 days' administration of ethinyl estradiol, 50 μg four times daily.

PROGESTIN THERAPY

Mechanism of Action.—Progestins such as medroxyprogesterone acetate have been shown to suppress the secretion of gonadotropins without altering the response of the pituitary to gonadotropin-releasing hormone,[9] thus suggesting a hypothalamic site of action. Therefore, progestins may also act to normalize the neurotransmitter changes resulting from ovarian failure. Since progestins alter the thermoregulatory set-point, it is also possible that they act in part directly on the thermoregulatory center. The hot flush represents a sudden downward resetting of this set-point. Thus progestins, by raising the set-point, may cause the thermoregulatory center to be more refractory to such stimuli.

Effectiveness.—The beneficial effect of progestins on hot flushes was first observed during the treatment of women with endometrial cancer with depomedroxyprogesterone acetate (depo-MPA). A subsequent double-blind study was carried out by Bullock et al. demonstrating relief of hot flushes in 90% of subjects by the injection of 150 mg monthly.[10] Abnormal bleeding was noted in 43% of those with intact uteri. Morrison and co-workers expanded on the observation by showing that beneficial effects were noted at monthly doses of 50–150 mg, although treatment failure were more common at the 50-mg dose.[11] No side effects other than bleeding (in two out of seven women with intact uteri) could be attributed to the drug, since they occurred with a similar frequency with placebo. Schiff et al. have examined the effects of 20 mg of MPA orally, using a double-blind cross-over study[12] (Fig 11–4). A 60%–74% reduction of hot flush episodes was observed, compared to a 26% reduction with placebo. Five out of the 12 women with intact uteri had vaginal bleeding. This group of investigators has also confirmed that 10 mg of MPA daily significantly reduced both subjective and objectively demonstrated hot flushes.[13] We have also studied megestrol acetate (MA) using objective recording[14] (Fig 11–5), and we noted a similar degree of effectiveness with 40–80 mg orally daily. These studies therefore indicated that 100–150 mg of depo-MPA intramuscularly administered monthly, or 10 mg MPA orally, or 40 mg of MA orally are highly effective in suppressing hot flushes. Since a fourth to half of those women

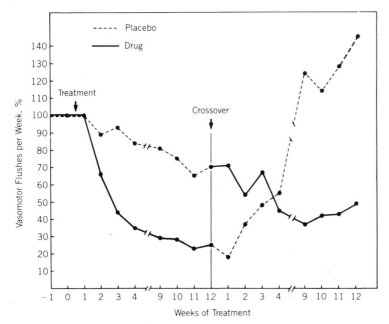

FIG 11–4.
Mean number of vasomotor flushes as a percentage change from pretreatment (week 1 to 0). Change of treatment regimen (crossover) occurred at 12 weeks. Weeks 5 to 8, unassociated with major variability, are not included.

with intact uteri had bleeding, this treatment would be primarily of benefit for women who have been previously hysterectomized, particularly those with contraindications to estrogen therapy. For women with breast or endometrial cancer, megestrol acetate or MPA may thus have beneficial effects on menopausal symptoms as well as their metastatic disease.

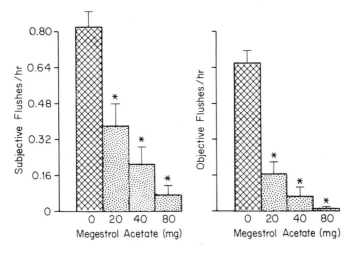

FIG 11–5.
The mean ($\pm$ SE) subjective and objective flushes per hour before and following the oral administration of the various doses of megestrol acetate. *Asterisk* denotes significant difference from baseline.

Mode of Therapy.—Although other progestins may also suppress hot flushes, the C-21 progestins, MPA and MA, would be preferred because of their lack of adverse effects on high-density lipoprotein (HDL) cholesterol.[15] If the treatment is begun by mouth, effectiveness and absence of side effects can be assured. Then the treatment can be given more economically, if necessary, by monthly injections of depo-MPA. It should be recognized that progestins are not approved in the United States for treatment of hot flushes.

Secondary Beneficial Effects of Therapy.—Both MPA and MA decrease calcium excretion[16] and therefore may protect against the development of osteoporosis. The necessary doses are 10–20 mg of MPA and 80 mg of MA. No studies are available of bone density during treatment with these agents. They should not be used as substitutes for proven treatments unless those medications are contraindicated. Medroxyprogesterone acetate appears to have better effects on both hot flushes and calcium secretion at lower doses than does MA.[16]

CLONIDINE

Mechanism of Action.—Clonidine is a centrally acting α-adrenergic agonist/antagonist. Several lines of investigation have suggested that the hot flush is triggered by the cyclic release of norepinephrine within the hypothalamus, which causes a periodic downward resetting of the thermoregulatory set-point.[1] Since norepinephrine acts by binding to α-adrenergic receptors, clonidine may act as an antagonist by inhibiting this binding. α-Methyldopa has also recently been found to have similar activity[17] through the central action of its metabolic product, methylnorepinephrine.

Effectiveness.—Clonidine has been examined for its effect on hot flushes in a number of adequately controlled studies, using subjective reporting of hot flushes, with conflicting results. We have performed a dose-response study (Fig 11–6) in normotensive

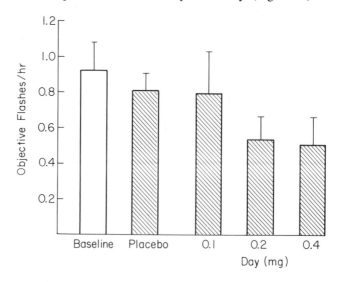

FIG 11–6.
Mean ± SEM of hot flushes (rate per hour) in six subjects at baseline, with placebo, and with 0.1, 0.2, and 0.4 mg of clonidine per day. Increasing dosage of clonidine was associated with a significant reduction of hot flushes as compared with baseline ($P < .005$) and with effects of placebo ($P < .05$).

women using objective documentation of hot flush episodes.[18] A significant treatment effect was observed at a dose of 0.1–0.2 mg b.i.d., although the treatment effect was clearly less than that seen with adequate doses of either estrogens or progestins. However, a high incidence of bothersome side effects was noted in these normotensive women, the most common of which was dizziness. Such side effects would be less likely to occur in hypertensive women, since the blood pressure would be unlikely to be lowered to below normal levels.

Mode of Therapy.—To limit side effects, clonidine should be started at 0.1 mg b.i.d., increasing to 0.2 mg b.i.d. if no side effects occur and the therapeutic effect is not adequate. It must be recognized that clonidine is not approved in the United States for treatment of hot flushes.

Secondary Beneficial Effects.—Women with hypertension have at least a relative contraindication for estrogen therapy, at least by the oral route. When percutaneous estradiol becomes available, it will be the preferred method for such women, since this route avoids the high hepatic concentration of estrogen and marked stimulation of renin substrate associated with oral absorption.[5] Currently, consideration should be made to incorporate clonidine into the regimen of treatment of hypertension, with the likelihood that relief of hot flushes will also occur.

BELLERGAL

Mechanism of Action.—This drug, which contains a combination of ergotamine tartrate, levorotatory alkaloids of belladonna, and phenobarbital, was introduced as an "autonomic stabilizer," since the manifestations of the hot flush are through the autonomic nervous system. Each of these agents could act at a central or peripheral level. It is not known which of the agents is responsible for its effectiveness.

Effectiveness.—Lebherz and French[19] carried out a double-blind study using subjective symptoms rated on a simple scoring system (0, none; 1, moderate; 2, severe). The mean score for hot flushes before treatment was 1.67, indicating that most patients had moderate to severe symptoms. After treatment, the score decreased to 0.66 with Bellergal and 1.30 with placebo. The reduction with active agent was highly significant. Significant reductions were also noted for nervousness, palpitation, nausea, insomnia, dizziness, and irritability. Some of these secondary benefits could have been due to secondary effects on hot flushes during sleep, relieving the resultant insomnia and the effects of a chronic sleep disturbance, or they may have been in part due to nonspecific effects of the phenobarbital component.

Mode of Therapy.—The drug is generally given b.i.d. Each tablet of Bellergal-S contains 40 mg of phenobarbital. The patient should therefore be cautioned about possible sedative effects, and the addictive potential of the drug should be considered.

The drug is contraindicated with peripheral or coronary vascular disease, hypertension, and glaucoma. Due to the multiple pharmacologic actions of the three ingredients, potential interactions with other drugs should be carefully considered.

ANDROGENS

Mechanism of Action.—We have definitively demonstrated, in a hypogonadal male with hot flushes, that androgen per se, independent of conversion to estrogen in the brain or other tissues, does suppress this disturbance.[20] Figure 11–7 shows objective recordings of the hot flushes before and after administration of testosterone, and during the admin-

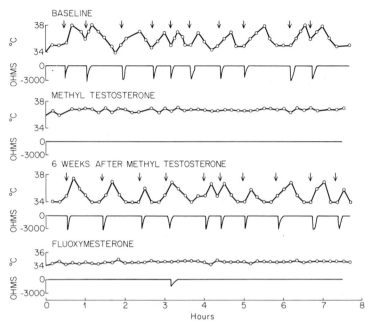

FIG 11–7.
Finger temperature (° C) and skin resistance (ohms) recordings in a man with testicular insufficiency before treatment, during and six weeks following methyl testosterone therapy, and during fluoxymesterone administration.

istration of fluoxymesterone, a nonaromatizable androgen. Other studies corroborate this direct action of androgen on the hypothalamus.

Effectiveness.—Clinically, administration of testosterone to provide normal male circulating levels is effective in abolishing this syndrome in castrated or hypogonadal males. It is not known whether androgen treatment of the female favorably affects hot flushes.

Mode of Therapy.—For the infrequent instances in which a testosterone pellet or a methyl testosterone conjugated equine estrogen tablet is prescribed to decrease breast tenderness associated with estrogen therapy or to increase libido in postmenopausal women, the androgen may contribute to suppression and control of hot flushes at a lower dose of estrogen.

Secondary Beneficial Effects.—It has been clinically observed that breast tenderness may resolve and libido may improve with the addition of testosterone to estrogen replacement therapy. Neither of these effects have been adequately studied to prove that they are specific therapeutic benefits of androgen treatment.

AGENTS FOUND NOT TO BE EFFECTIVE

A study by Erkkola et al.[21] showed that the number and intensity of hot flushes is significantly reduced with propranolol, a β-stimulating drug, and oxazepam, an anxiolytic. However, they did not control the study with placebo, and the reductions of hot flushes were identical to those demonstrated in many studies with placebo. A subsequent study by Coope and co-workers[22] demonstrated that the reductions caused by propranolol and placebo were almost identical. The lack of an effect of an anxiolytic beyond that observed with placebo suggests that sedatives have no specific effect on the hot flush.

SUMMARY

In summary, multiple pharmacologic agents have been found to be effective in treating the postmenopausal hot flush. Since each agent has its own unique contraindications and secondary benefits, the choice of therapy depends to a great degree on the presence of other medical disorders. In a healthy woman without contraindications to estrogen therapy, estrogen replacement remains the most specific and effective treatment of this disorder. When percutaneous or other continuous parenteral forms of estradiol become available, estrogen replacement will also be safe in most women with medical contraindications to oral estrogen therapy. Alternative treatments will always be necessary for women with estrogen-dependent neoplasms.

REFERENCES

1. Meldrum DR: Neuroendocrine aspects of the menopausal hot flash, in Givens JR (ed): *The Hypothalamus in Health and Disease.* Chicago, Year Book Medical Publishers, 1984, pp 229–243.
2. Tataryn IV, Lomax P, Meldrum DR, et al: Objective techniques for the assessment of postmenopausal hot flashes. *Obstet Gynecol* 1981; 57:340.
3. Geola FL, Frumar AM, Tataryn IV, et al: Biological effects of various doses of conjugated equine estrogens in postmenopausal women. *J Clin Endocrinol Metab* 1980; 51:620.
4. Judd HL, Cleary RE, Creasman WT, et al: Estrogen replacement therapy. *Obstet Gynecol* 1981; 58:267.
5. Laufer LR, DeFazio JL, Lu JKH, et al: Estrogen replacement therapy by transdermal estradiol administration. *Am J Obstet Gynecol* 1983; 146:533.
6. Campbell S, Whitehead M: Estrogen therapy and the post-menopausal syndrome. *Clin Obstet Gynecol* 1977; 4:31.
7. Erlik Y, Tataryn IV, Meldrum DR, et al: Association of waking episodes with menopausal hot flushes. *JAMA* 1981; 245:1741.
8. Schiff I, Regestein Q, Tulchinski D, et al: Effects of estrogens on sleep and psychological state of hypogonadal women. *JAMA* 1979; 242:2405.
9. Toppozada M, Parma C, Fotherly K: Effect of injectable contraceptives Depo-provera and norethisterone oenanthate on pituitary gonadotropin response to luteinizing hormone releasing hormone. *Fertil Steril* 1978; 30:545.
10. Bullock JL, Massey FM, Gambrell RD: Use of medroxyprogesterone acetate to prevent menopausal symptoms. *Obstet Gynecol* 1975; 46:165.
11. Morrison JC, Martin DC, Blair RA, et al: The use of medroxyprogesterone acetate for relief of climacteric symptoms. *Am J Obstet Gynecol* 1980; 138:99.
12. Schiff I, Tulchinsky D, Cramer D, et al: Oral medroxyprogesterone in the treatment of postmenopausal symptoms. *JAMA* 1980; 244:1443.
13. Albrecht BH, Schiff I, Tulchinsky D, et al: Objective evidence that placebo and oral medroxyprogesterone acetate therapy diminish menopausal vasomotor flushes. *Am J Obstet Gynecol* 1981; 139:631.
14. Erklik J, Meldrum DR, Lagasse LD, et al: Effect of megestrol acetate on flushing and bone metabolism in post-menopausal women. *Maturitas* 1981; 3:167.
15. Hirvonen E, Malkonene M, Manninen V: Effects of different progestogens on lipoproteins during postmenopausal replacement therapy. *N Engl J Med* 1981; 304:560.
16. Mandel FP, Davidson BJ, Erlik Y, et al: Effects of progestins on bone metabolism in postmenopausal women. *J Reprod Med* 1982; 27:511.
17. Hammond MG, Hatley L, Talbert LM: A double blind study to evaluate the effect of methyldopa on menopausal vasomotor flushes. *J Clin Endocrinol Metab* 1984; 58:1158.

18. Laufer LR, Erlik Y, Meldrum DR, et al: Effect of clonidine on hot flashes in postmenopausal women. *Obstet Gynecol* 1982; 60:483.
19. Lebherz TB, French LT: Nonhormonal treatment of the menopausal syndrome. A double-blind evaluation of an autonomic system stabilizer. *Obstet Gynecol* 1969; 33:795.
20. DeFazio J, Meldrum DR, Winer JH, et al: Direct action of androgen on hot flashes in the human male. *Maturitas* 1984; 6:8.
21. Erkkola R, Iisalo E, Punnonen R: The effect of propranolol and oxazepam on some vegetative menopausal symptoms. *Ann Clin Res* 1973; 5:208.
22. Coope J, Williams S, Patterson JS: A study of the effectiveness of propranolol in menopausal hot flushes. *Br J Obstet Gynaecol* 1978; 85:472.

CHAPTER **12**

Beneficial Effects of Pharmacologic Agents—Genitourinary

ARIEH BERGMAN, M.D.
PAUL F. BRENNER, M.D.

THE PHYSICAL CHANGES that occur in the vagina of the untreated postmenopausal woman produce a cascade of symptoms which initially may be local in nature but with time and without relief may result in a diverse spectrum of complaints and may even produce secondary symptoms in her partner. Local symptoms associated with vaginal atrophy include vaginal dryness, vaginal discharge, itching, burning, bleeding from the vagina, vaginismus, dyspareunia, uterine prolapse, a sensation of heaviness, pelvic pressure, or pelvic organs falling out of the vagina.[1] When these symptoms interfere with sexual performance, they can lead to a decrease in libido, anxiety, and a decrease in self-esteem, and eventually they may even affect the sexual performance of her male partner. Symptoms pertaining to vaginal atrophy are among those that postmenopausal women are most concerned about.

The rationale for estrogen therapy for postmenopausal women has been carefully scrutinized over the last decade. Again, the benefits and the risks have been carefully considered. At a minimum, there appears to be at least three important indications for the administration of estrogen therapy to postmenopausal women. The most important, from the standpoint of mortality and morbidity, is the prevention of osteoporosis. In terms of the number of persons affected, the relief of vasomotor symptoms may be needed by as many as 75% of all postmenopausal women. Third, and also very important, is the prevention or the reversal of the atrophy of the lower genitourinary system.

VAGINAL ABSORPTION OF SEX STEROIDS

Postmenopausal women take hormones by several different routes of administration, including oral, sublingual, vaginal, intramuscular, and transdermal. The most common route of administration of estrogen to postmenopausal patients is by oral ingestion. Medication administered per os is delivered to the intestinal tract, where it is absorbed and transferred via the enterohepatic circulation to the liver. Sex steroids are metabolized in the liver and may produce profound hepatic effects, depending on the steroidal configuration and the dose. Estrogens increase hepatic protein synthesis including clotting factors (fibrinogen, factor 7, factor 10), carrier proteins (ceruloplasmin, transferrin, thyroid-binding globulin, corticosteroid-binding globulin, and sex hormone-binding globulin) and angiotensinogen. The vaginal administration of estrogen is frequently used for postmenopausal women who have symptoms that are the result of atrophy of the vaginal mucosa or urethral mucosa. Prior to the availability of highly sensitive assays to measure small concentrations of estrogens in the peripheral circulation, the vaginal "topical" administration of estrogen was selected because of the misconception that any effect of the steroid would be limited to the site of application. The use of intravaginal estrogens was considered to have a local effect only and it was not thought to be a potential avenue for the absorption of sex steroids and their subsequent entrance into the peripheral circulation. The vaginal use of estrogen was incorrectly judged to be free of any systemic effects. It is now known that estrogens placed in the vagina are efficiently absorbed through the vaginal wall and appear in the circulation, where they may exhibit a variety of systemic actions. The pharmacodynamics of estrogen metabolism depends on the route of administration. There are significant differences between the oral and the vaginal routes.

Rigg and co-workers placed a single dose of micronized estradiol dissolved in normal saline in the posterior fornix of the vaginal vault of postmenopausal volunteers.[2] There was a significant increase in the 17β-estradiol levels in the peripheral circulation within the first five minutes after the intravaginal application of the micronized estradiol (Fig 12–1). This indicates that the absorption of estradiol through the vaginal mucosa is quite rapid. Peak responses were achieved two hours after the intravaginal administration of micronized estradiol and were sustained for several hours. The peak estradiol response was more than 100 times greater than the pretreatment estradiol concentration. The intravaginal administration of micronized estradiol also increased the levels of estrone

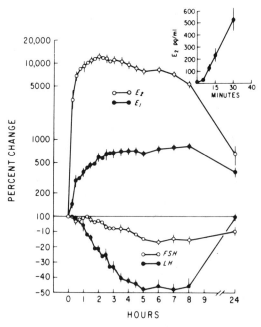

FIG 12–1.
Percent change (mean ± SEM) from basal levels in serum 17β-estradiol, estrone, FSH, and LH concentrations following the intravaginal administration of 1 mg micronized 17β-estradiol suspended in saline to eight estrogen-deficient women. The insert shows the rapidity of E_2 absorption during the first 30 minutes. (From Rigg LA, Milanes B, Villanueva B, et al: Efficacy of intravaginal and intranasal administration of micronized estradiol-17β. *J Clin Endocrinol Metab* 1977; 45:1261. Used by permission.)

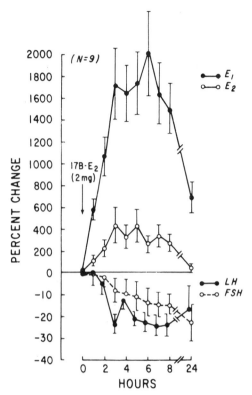

FIG 12–2.
Percent change (mean ± SEM) from basal levels in serum 17β-estradiol, estrone, FSH, and LH concentrations following ingestion of a single tablet containing 2 mg micronized 17β-estradiol. (From Yen SSC, Martin PL, Burnier AM, et al: Circulating estradiol, estrone, and gonadotropin levels following the administration of orally active 17β-estradiol on post-menopausal women. *J Clin Endocrinol Metab* 1975; 40:518. Used by permission.)

in the peripheral circulation, but the estrone response was smaller and slower than the estradiol response. The intravaginal application of micronized estradiol was demonstrated to have systemic activity when the gonadotropin levels were suppressed in these subjects.

These results are different than the circulating estrogen levels following the oral administration of a single dose of micronized estradiol. Estradiol is rapidly metabolized to estrone following the ingestion of micronized estradiol (Fig 12–2).[3] The conversion of estrogens is thought to occur in the mucosa of the small bowel. The intravaginal administration of micronized estradiol seems to preclude the conversion of estradiol to estrone, which occurs with the oral route of administration of the same drug. The serum estradiol levels are higher following the intravaginal administration of micronized estradiol than when it is given by mouth. A follow-up study by Rigg and co-workers indicated that both conjugated estrogens (Premarin) and micronized estradiol prepared as a vaginal cream are absorbed across the vaginal mucosa when administered intravaginally to estrogen-deficient postmenopausal volunteers.[4] The vaginal absorption of estrogen in a cream base is slower than when the steroid is suspended in saline. Therefore, the circulating estrogen levels achieved by the vaginal route of administration are dependent both on the dose and the vehicle in which the steroid is placed. Following the intravaginal administration of a single dose of conjugated estrogens, the estrone response exceeds that of estradiol and the concentrations of estrone are much higher than estradiol in the peripheral circulation (Fig 12–3). Following the intravaginal administration of a single dose of micronized estradiol in a cream base, the estradiol response is greater than that of estrone and serum estradiol levels are much higher than the estrone levels. A similar study design using single doses of 17β-estradiol and estrone in normal saline yielded the same results, indicating that both estrogens were efficiently absorbed across the vaginal wall into the systemic circulation and caused a decrease in circulating gonadotropin levels.[5] The daily intravaginal administration of conjugated estrogens or micronized estradiol in a cream base of 15 consecutive days did not have a cumulative effect on the serum concentrations of estrone or estradiol.[6] The estrogen levels on the 15th day of vaginal therapy were not significantly different from the levels determined 12 hours after the application on the first day.

Estrogens administered orally have a marked hepatic effect, which was postulated to be the result of the first-pass effect of the estrogens through the liver that occurs with this route of administration. If the hepatic metabolic alterations that result from the oral ingestion of estrogen are due to the immediate access of the estrogen to the liver via the

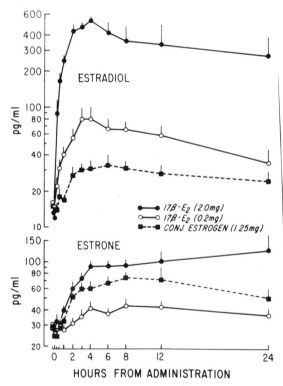

FIG 12–3.
Serum concentration (mean ± SEM) of 17β-estradiol and estrone prior to and after the intravaginal application of 2 mg and 0.2 mg 17β-estradiol cream and 1.25 mg conjugated estrogen cream in six estrogen-deficient women. (From Rigg LA, Hermann H. Yen SSC: Absorption of estrogens from vaginal creams. *N Engl J Med* 1978; 298:195. Reprinted by permission of the *New England Journal of Medicine.*

enterohepatic circulation, then the hepatic effects should be diminished or abolished by the vaginal application of estrogen preferentially in comparison to other systemic effects of exogenous estrogen. Mashchak and co-workers compared the bioavailability of 120 μg of ethinyl estradiol (EE) administered orally and 120 μg of EE in a polyethylene glycol base administered as a vaginal suppository.[7] The mean peak serum levels of EE were four times higher with the oral administration than with the vaginal route. Based on the bioavailability of estrogen administered orally being four times greater than the same dose of estrogen administered vaginally, these investigators performed a second study. Postmenopausal volunteers took orally administered EE for 25 consecutive days. After a six-week, medication-free interval, the same volunteers took EE vaginal suppositories for 25 consecutive days. In one group of the postmenopausal women, the daily oral dose was 5 μg EE and the daily vaginal dose was 20 μg. In a second group of postmenopausal women, the daily oral dose was 10 μg EE and the daily vaginal dose was 50 μg. Approximately four times more ethinyl estradiol administered orally than vaginally is necessary to suppress follicle-stimulating hormone (FSH), luteinizing hormone (LH), and low-density lipid cholesterol and to increase sex hormone-binding globulin, corticosteroid-binding globulin, and high-density lipid cholesterol. The potency ratio of the oral to vaginal administration of EE with respect to gonadotropin suppression (central nervous system effect) was the same as the ratio for carrier protein increase and lipid profile changes (hepatic effect). The vaginal administration of ethinyl estradiol does not appear to reduce selectively the hepatic metabolic alterations.

PREVENTION OF THE ATROPHY OF THE VAGINA

The prevention of the atrophy of the vaginal vault in a woman who has recently entered her postmenopausal years can be accomplished concomitantly with the administration of estrogen to relieve vasomotor flushes or with estrogen treatment to prevent osteoporosis. The dose of estrogen necessary to retard vaginal atrophy is usually less than that required to treat vasomotor symptoms or that which prevents the loss of bone mass. Additional estrogen therapy or estrogen given by another route of administration is not necessary. Either a continuous or a cyclic regimen of estrogen with or without gestagen supplementation is effective in preventing vaginal vault atrophy. There is evidence that a continuous daily dose of oral gestagen alone can be used to treat vasomotor symptoms. This therapy is not an acceptable alternative for the prevention of the atrophy of the vagina. The vagina is an estrogen-sensitive tissue and specifically requires estrogen to prevent atrophy.

The prevention of atrophy of the vaginal tissues for the postmenopausal woman who has no other indication for estrogen can be accomplished either by the oral route of administration or by the use of a vaginal cream.[8] The topical cream may have an advantage in also acting as a lubricant. The vagina offers a very efficient mechanism for the absorption of estrogen. The same metabolic alterations and systemic effects may be produced with the intravaginal administration of estrogen as with the oral ingestion of the steroid. The dose of estrogen needed to prevent vaginal atrophy is usually individual for each patient. The administration of estrogen every other day, or even less frequently, may be all that is necessary to prevent atrophic changes in the vagina.

In the postmenopausal years, the number of cytoplasmic estrogen receptors in the vaginal mucosa decreases. The estrogen receptors are never completely depleted and, in response to exogenous estrogen, the number of estrogen receptors in the vagina can return to concentrations normally found in the premenopausal years. The affinity of the vaginal estrogen receptor to bind with estrogen far exceeds the affinity of serum proteins to bind with estrogen. Therefore, the vagina responds to smaller doses of estrogen than those that are usually required to alter hepatic protein synthesis and produce metabolic alterations.

TREATMENT OF ATROPHY OF THE VAGINA

The optimal treatment to reverse the atrophic changes found in the unestrogenized postmenopausal vagina is estrogen. Estrogen therapy results in a shift in the maturation index to the right, an increase in the thickness of the vaginal mucosa, a decrease in the pH of the vagina, and a decrease in vaginal dryness.[9] While alternative therapy is available for the treatment of vasomotor symptoms, including gestagens derived from ace-toxy-progesterone, gestagens derived from 19-nortestosterone, and clonidine, there is no acceptable alternative to estrogen therapy for the atrophic changes in the vagina. More specifically, the therapy is low-dose estrogen, which can be administered orally or intravaginally, and the regimen can be individualized for each patient. Daily estrogen treatment of vaginal atrophy may be necessary for an interval of 2–12 weeks. Once the vaginal atrophy has been reversed, intermittent therapy two to three times a week is usually all that is necessary to maintain a symptom-free, well-estrogenized vaginal mucosa. The goal of the treatment is to provide each patient with the lowest dose of estrogen that satisfactorily relieves symptoms that have resulted from the atrophic changes in the vagina. The same absolute and relative contraindications that are applied to oral administration of estrogen should be used for the intravaginal administration of estrogen.[10] There are some individuals who do not absorb estrogen from the intestine very efficiently. These individuals are candidates for topical estrogen placed in the vagina.

Natural estrogens (conjugated equine estrogen, 0.3 and 0.625 mg; estrone sulfate, 0.3, 0.625, and 1.25 mg; micronized estradiol, 1.0 and 2.0 mg), synthetic estrogens (ethinylestradiol, 10 and 20 μg; quinestrol, 0.1 mg) and nonsteroidal estrogen (diethylstilbestrol, 0.1 and 0.5 mg) have all been used to treat vaginal atrophy.[11]

Campbell and Whitehead performed two double-blind, randomized, cross-over studies correlating the effect of estrogen therapy and menopausal symptoms.[12] The first was a short-term (four month) study for postmenopausal women with severe symptomatology, and the second was a long-term (12 month) study for postmenopausal women with a moderate degree of symptoms. Conjugated equine estrogen was administered orally 1.25 mg daily for three weeks, followed by a seven-day estrogen-free interval. This four-week course of treatment was given for a total of two cycles in the short-term study and a total of six cycles in the long-term study. During the placebo phases of the study, a placebo tablet was substituted for the estrogen. Changes in the 24-hour urinary excretion of total estrogen mirrored the responses of the maturation index. As estrogen excretion increased, the maturation index shifted to the right. In both studies the estrogen was significantly better than the placebo in relieving atrophic vaginitis.

Geola and co-workers studied 21 postmenopausal women before and after the oral administration of conjugated equine estrogen.[13] The doses studied ranged between 0.15 mg and 1.25 mg per day, and they were administered for a six-week treatment phase. Only the 1.25 mg daily dose altered the maturation index to that observed in premenopausal women. They concluded that, in order to achieve a physiologic estrogen effect on the vaginal mucosa, the daily administration of 1.25 mg of conjugated equine estrogen is necessary. Clinical experience indicates that a physiologic dose of estrogen is not necessary for a therapeutic response in cases of vaginal atrophy and that a 0.3 mg daily dose of conjugated equine estrogen produced a satisfactory therapeutic result for most women with vaginal mucosa atrophy.

In a follow-up study, Mandel and co-workers studied 20 postmenopausal women before and after the vaginal administration of conjugated equine estrogens.[14] The doses investigated ranged from 0.3 mg to 2.5 mg per day and were administered for a four-week treatment phase. The response in the maturation index to 0.3 mg of conjugated equine estrogen administered vaginally was equivalent to the response of 1.25 mg administered orally.

Callantine and co-investigators reported that 88% of patients treated with oral micronized estradiol had complete relief of their symptoms associated with genital atrophy.[15] Each subject was titrated to a dose of estrogen between 1 and 4 mg, which was administered cyclically in a regimen of 21 consecutive days of estrogen followed by a seven-day hormone-free interval.

Gordon and co-workers reported significant improvement in the vaginal symptoms of 54 postmenopausal women receiving 0.2 mg 17 β-estradiol in a 0.01% vaginal cream.[16] Fifty-four subjects completed one month of therapy and 51 subjects completed two months of therapy. In this study there was a significant decrease in the percent of parabasal cells in the maturation index by the fifteenth day of treatment. At the end of one month of treatment, 72% of subjects had no parabasal cells. Throughout the two months of observation, the percent of superficial cells steadily and significantly increased. Vaginal dryness, vaginal itching, atrophic vaginitis, and dyspareunia responded markedly to treatment. All symptoms responded to therapy within 15 days, and at the end of two months no subjects complained of vaginal dryness or dyspareunia.

Partial or complete prolapse of the uterus outside of the vaginal vault in the postmenopausal patient produces distressing if not intolerable symptomatology. This is generally considered an indication for surgery, even a vaginal hysterectomy, if the patient's general health permits her to undergo anesthesia and a surgical procedure. Frequently when there is a uterine procidentia, the cervix is ulcerated, and the vaginal mucosa may have bleeding sites and even ulcerations. Surgery can be greatly facilitated by taking the time to improve the tone, elasticity, and the thickness of the vaginal tissues. The uterus is replaced manually and retained within the vagina with the use of a pessary. Each evening the pessary is removed, cleansed, and then replaced in the vagina. Estrogen cream applied nightly around the pessary will facilitate the placement of the pessary and will markedly improve the appearance of the pelvic organs over a period of two to six weeks. The cervical ulcer heals, the vaginal mucosa thickens, and even the natural support of the uterus improves greatly. In the rare patient the support of the uterus responds so dramatically that surgery is no longer required.

The presence of a vaginal discharge in a postmenopausal women must be as thoroughly investigated as a discharge in a woman during her active reproductive years. For the postmenopausal woman with a vaginal discharge who is not receiving any exogenous source of estrogen, the underlying diagnosis will frequently be atrophic vaginitis. However, these women can also have candidiasis, trichomonas vaginitis, Gardnerella vaginalis vaginitis, gonorrhea, chlamydia trachomatis,[17] other sexually transmitted diseases, or cancer.[18] A thorough history, physical exam, pelvic exam, Pap smear, saline wet mount preparation, KOH wet mount preparation, and gonorrhea culture should be obtained. Where clinically indicated, aerobic and anaerobic cultures should be taken. A candidiasis vaginal infection in a postmenopausal woman not using estrogen therapy is an indication to screen the patient for diabetes mellitus. The glycogen content of the unestrogenized vaginal epithelial cell is low and usually not sufficient to support the candida organism in the nondiabetic woman.

TREATMENT OF POSTMENOPAUSAL STRESS URINARY INCONTINENCE

The peak incidence of stress urinary incontinence is in the postmenopausal years, when atrophy of estrogen sensitive tissues occurs.[19] The three principal pathophysiologic changes that lead to urinary incontinence are the attenuation of the urethral mucosa, loss of the intra-abdominal location of the proximal urethra, and loss of striated periurethral muscle tension following pelvic relaxation.

The urethra and trigone have a common embryonic origin with the distal vagina and contain a high concentration of estrogen receptors.[20–22] Thus, the urethra and trigone are considered estrogen-sensitive tissues. Estrogen treatment has a beneficial effect on each of the three factors that lead to urinary incontinence, that is, it thins the urethral mucosa, transmits abdominal pressure to the proximal urethra, and contracts the periurethral striated muscles.

Clinically, estrogen treatment improves and cures symptoms of urinary incontinence, as well as dysuria, urgency, and frequency secondary to atrophic urethritis.[23–25] In several studies it has been shown that a favorable clinical response (significant improvement or cure) can be achieved in approximately 50% of treated patients.[23, 25] In 33 patients with stress urinary incontinence whom we treated with estrogen for six weeks, subjective significant improvement or a cure occurred in 18 (55%) (Table 12–1).

The urethral mucosa is a primary target of estrogen treatment. In the premenopausal years the thickness of the urethral mucosa and the engorgement of blood vessels beneath the mucosa comprises 30% of the total urethral resistance.[26] Attenuation of the urethral mucosa in hypoestrogenic postmenopausal women correlates directly with a 30% decline in the urethral closure pressure[27] and with the appearance of stress urinary incontinence in these women. Since the urethral mucosa is an estrogen-responsive tissue containing estrogen receptors,[21, 22] it responds to estrogen treatment.

The urethral mucosa is covered proximally by transitional epithelium and distally by squamous epithelium. Daily estrogen treatment for at least six weeks matures the urethral squamous epithelium, with a shift of the urethral maturation index to the right, in a process similar to that seen in the vagina.[28–30] These cytologic alterations correlate clinically with a significant improvement of stress urinary incontinence. We treated a group of 11 patients with this condition with the daily application of 2 gm of conjugated

TABLE 12–1.

Evaluation in 33 Patients With Stress Urinary Incontinence Before and Following Six Weeks of Daily Application of 2 gm Premarin Vaginal Cream

PATIENTS' CONDITION	BEFORE TREATMENT	AFTER TREATMENT
Stress urinary incontinence	33 (100%)	15 (46%)
No stress urinary incontinence	0 (0%)	18 (54%)

equine estrogen vaginal cream for six weeks. Following estrogen treatment the urethral cytology of those patients who had a good clinical response showed a significant increase in intermediate and superficial squamous cells. The patients with a poor clinical response failed to demonstrate cytologic changes in their maturation index. These results suggest that a favorable estrogen response was achieved by positively affecting the "urethral mucosa" factor, causing proliferation and growth of the urethral mucosal cells (Table 12–2).

The second factor in the pathophysiology of stress urinary incontinence is poor abdominal pressure transmission to the proximal urethra. In a continent woman, the proximal third of the urethra is in the intra-abdominal pressure sphere, above the pelvic diaphragm (levator ani muscle and fascia). This anatomical factor results in an equal transmission of abdominal pressure to the bladder and to the proximal urethra at the time of a sudden valsalva. Thus, the pressure gradient between urethra and bladder (urethral closure pressure) is maintained even at times of stress, such as coughing or sneezing. In a postmenopausal, stress-incontinent woman, the pelvic diaphragm is relaxed, and support to bladder base is reduced. As a result, the poorly supported proximal urethra is no longer in the intra-abdominal pressure sphere. With every sudden valsalva maneuver (cough, sneeze), abdominal pressure is transmitted to the bladder and not to the urethra. The bladder pressure then exceeds the urethral pressure and results in the loss of urine. In a study using urodynamic testing in women with stress incontinence, the abdominal pressure transmission to the proximal urethra at the time of stress improved significantly following the administration of conjugated equine estrogen vaginal cream.[25] We reported that patients with stress incontinence who were treated for six weeks with daily application of 2 gm of conjugated equine estrogen vaginal cream improved their abdominal pressure transmission to the proximal urethra at the time of cough (Fig 12–4). These urodynamic findings correlate well with the improved clinical response to estrogen treatment. It is possible that the improved tension of the pelvic tissue results in a better support to the bladder base and proximal urethra. The improved support of the proximal urethra allows it to retain its intra-abdominal position, so that any increase in pressure at the time of stress is once again transmitted to the urethra as well as to the bladder.

The third factor in the maintenance of urinary continence is the contraction of the striated periurethral muscle fibers at the time of stress.[31] These muscle fibers need to be

TABLE 12–2.

Cytologic and Clinical Response in 13 Women Before and Six Weeks Following Estrogen Treatment for Stress Urinary Incontinence (SUI)

URETHRAL CYTOLOGY		GOOD CLINICAL RESPONSE NO SUI FOLLOWING TREATMENT (N = 7)	NO CLINICAL RESPONSE SUI BEFORE AND AFTER TREATMENT (N = 6)
Transitional Cells	Before	62	47
	After	17 P < .02	41 N.S.*
Squamous Intermediate Cells	Before	31	49
	After	72 P < .05	52 N.S.*
Squamous Superficial Cells	Before	7	5
	After	14 N.S.*	9 N.S.*

*N.S., no statistical significance by paired t test.

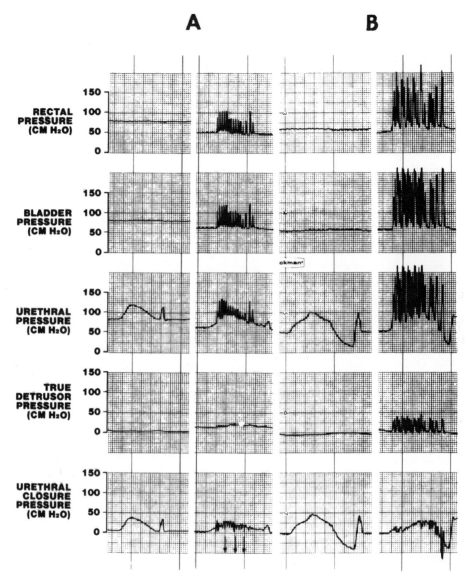

FIG 12–4.
Urethral pressure profile and urethral pressure cough profile before (A) and after (B) estrogen treatment. Note the increase in urethral closure pressure and functional length at rest. Note positive cough profile with pressure equalization between bladder and urethra before treatment (*arrows* point towards urine loss) and negative cough profile after treatment. (From Ostergard DR: *Gynecologic Urology and Urodynamics.* Baltimore, Williams & Wilkins Co, 1986. Used by permission.)

at an optimal tension in order to contract in response to stress. It is possible that the improved tissue tension following estrogen treatment has a positive effect, enabling a better muscle contraction. Furthermore, stress-reflectory periurethral muscular contraction is enhanced following estrogen therapy. α-Adrenergic receptors are present in the periurethral muscle. As a result of the α-adrenergic effect on the urethra, the urethral closure pressure is increased and the reflectory contraction of the periurethral muscle is improved at the time of stress.[32] A urethral pressure increase of 60% following α-sympathomimetic drug therapy has been reported.[33–35] An equivalent clinical response of 60% significant improvement or cure follows such treatment.[33, 35, 36] The reported effect of α-sympathomimetic drugs on the urethra in postmenopausal women is enhanced following priming with estrogens.

In order to produce a positive effect on the three factors that influence urinary continence (urethral mucosa thickness, intra-abdominal location of the proximal urethra, and periurethral muscle tension), estrogen must be given in an adequate dose and for a relatively long time. Therapy should start with a daily oral dose of 1.25 mg of conjugated equine estrogen (equivalent to 2 gm of conjugated equine estrogen vaginal cream). This dose should be continued for two to three months and then reduced to one half thereafter. Clinical improvement should not be expected before six weeks of treatment.

Estrogen therapy administered to postmenopausal women has a positive effect on the urethral mucosa, causing proliferation and thickening as well as an increase in tissue tone, thus promoting improved intra-abdominal pressure transmission to the urethra and a better contraction of periurethral muscle. It is not surprising that more than half of the postmenopausal patients with urinary incontinence respond favorably to estrogen treatment.

TREATMENT OF POSTMENOPAUSAL URGENCY INCONTINENCE AND URETHRAL SYNDROME

The term "urethral syndrome" refers to a symptom complex rather than a clearly defined clinical entity. Urethral syndrome is a disease of multiple causes, which include inflammation of the urethral glands, vitamin deficiency, and urethral stenosis in young patients and hypoestrogenism in postmenopausal patients.

The best working definition of urethral syndrome is the combination of the symptoms of urgency, frequency, dysuria, and suprapubic tenderness in the absence of urinary tract infection.

The true incidence of urethral syndrome is unknown, but it has been estimated that it occurs in 20% of all adult women and 15%–20% of all postmenopausal women.[37]

The etiology of urethral syndrome (senile urethritis) secondary to hypoestrogenism was first described by Cifuentes in 1947.[38] This author identified small white patches in the distal trigone, which on biopsy were found to be identical to the squamous vaginal epithelium. Youngblood et al.[28] studied urethral cells in postmenopausal women before and after estrogen treatment and found conversion of urethral epithelium from a hypoestrogenic to a mature, well-estrogenized state. The same author[39] demonstrated a marked clinical improvement in postmenopausal urethral syndrome in women receiving diethylstilbestrol urethral suppositories. Clinical improvement of urethral syndrome was directly correlated with the maturation of the urethral cytology to the well-estrogenized state.

Diagnosis of urethral syndrome (senile urethritis) is made essentially by excluding other conditions that cause urgency, frequency, dysuria, and suprapubic pain, and by demonstrating the pale-looking, atrophic urethra on urethroscopy. Urinary tract infection and the acute urethritis caused by gonorrhea and chlamydia should be excluded. A neurologic examination and cystometry should be performed to rule out bladder instability. Urethroscopy in these women usually demonstrates a pale, thin, friable urethral mucosa and trigone.

The treatment of urethral syndrome (atrophic urethritis) is estrogen replacement. The most convenient way is the intravaginal administration of estrogen cream. In a double-blind study, Youngblood et al.[39] obtained good results in 91% of postmenopausal women with senile urethral syndrome using urethral suppositories containing 0.01 mg of diethylstilbestrol. These suppositories are no longer available, and the vaginal cream is as effective as the urethral suppositories. The daily treatment with 2 gm (half an applicator) of conjugated equine estrogen vaginal cream (equivalent to 1.25 mg orally) for two to three weeks, reducing the dose to half thereafter, results in the relief of symptoms of the urethral syndrome in postmenopausal women.

Another entity causing urgency, frequency, nocturia, and urge incontinence in postmenopausal women is voiding difficulties and overflow incontinence. Normal voiding begins with voluntary urethral relaxation followed within two to five seconds by reflectory detrusor contractions.[40, 41] In order to achieve complete voiding without any residual volume, the urethra has to remain relaxed throughout voiding. Urethral contractions inhibit reflectory detrusor contractions, which results in incomplete voiding.[40, 42, 43] Numerous neurologic reflexes are involved in the initiation, maintenance, and cessation of voiding.[42–44]

Since voiding difficulties to postmenopausal women are attributed partly to the inability to relax the periurethral muscle secondary to impaired innervation, and partly to atrophic urethritis, a trial with estrogens should be the first therapeutic step. If voiding is still ineffective, urethral dilatation should be attempted next, since no effective treatment is known for central nervous system denervation. Using this regimen, Smith[45] successfully treated postmenopausal patients by daily application of 0.6 mg conjugated estrogens. This author observed that if symptoms persisted longer than a year, urethral dilatation was required in addition to estrogens in order to achieve satisfactory results.

Similar to estrogen treatment for stress urinary incontinence, hormonal treatment for atrophic urethritis and voiding difficulties is effective as long as the drug is administered, and thus should be continued indefinitely. Concomitant gestagen therapy is required in these cases, as in any condition where prolonged estrogen treatment is given to postmenopausal women.

REFERENCES

1. Dewhurst J: Postmenopausal bleeding from benign causes. *Clin Obstet Gynecol* 1983; 26:769.
2. Rigg LA, Milanes B, Villanueva B, et al: Efficacy of intravaginal and intranasal administration of micronized estradiol-17β. *J Clin Endocrinol Metab* 1977; 45:1261.
3. Yen SSC, Martin PL, Burnier AM, et al: Circulating estradiol, estrone, and gonadotropin levels following the administration of orally active 17β-estradiol on postmenopausal women. *J Clin Endocrinol Metab* 1975; 40:518.
4. Rigg LA, Hermann H, Yen SSC: Absorption of estrogens from vaginal creams. N Engl J Med 1978; 298:195.
5. Schiff I, Tulchinsky D, Ryan KJ: Vaginal absorption of estrone and 17β-estradiol. *Fertil Steril* 1977; 28:1063.
6. Martin PL, Yen SSC, Burnier AM, et al: Systemic absorption and sustained effects of vaginal estrogen creams. *JAMA* 1979; 242:2699.
7. Goebelsmann U, Mashchak CA, Mishell DR Jr: Comparison of hepatic impact of oral and vaginal administration of ethinyl estradiol. *Am J Obstet Gynecol* 1985; 151:868.
8. Hammond CB, Maxson WS: Current status of estrogen therapy for the menopause. *Fertil Steril* 1982; 37:5.
9. Semmens JP, Wagner G: Estrogen deprivation and vaginal function in postmenopausal women. *JAMA* 1982; 248:445.

10. Quigley MM, Hammond CB: Estrogen replacement therapy—Help or hazard? *N Engl J Med* 1979; 301:646.
11. Carr BR, MacDonald PC: Estrogen treatment of postmenopausal women. *Adv Intern Med* 1983; 28:491.
12. Campbell S, Whitehead M: Oestrogen therapy and the menopausal syndrome. *Clin Obstet Gynecol* 1977; 4:31.
13. Geola FL, Frumar AM, Tataryn IV, et al: Biological effects of various doses of conjugated equine estrogens in postmenopausal women. *J Clin Endocrinol Metab* 1980; 51:620.
14. Mandel FP, Geola FL, Meldrum DR, et al: Biological effects of various doses of vaginally administered conjugated equine estrogens in postmenopausal women. *J Clin Endocrin Metab* 1983; 57:133.
15. Callantine MR, Martin PL, Bolding OT, et al: Micronized 17β-estradiol for oral estrogen therapy in menopausal women. *Obstet Gynecol* 1975; 46:37.
16. Gordon WE, Hermann HW, Hunter DC: Safety and efficacy of micronized estradiol vaginal cream. *South Med J* 1979; 72:1252.
17. Golmeier D, Ridgway GL, Oriel JD: Chlamydia vulvovaginitis in a postmenopausal woman. *Lancet* 1981; 2:476.
18. Galask RP, Larsen B: Identifying and treating genital tract infections in postmenopausal women. *Geriatrics* 1981; 36:69.
19. Mattingly RP, Davis LE: Primary treatment of anatomic stress urinary incontinence. *Clin Obstet Gynecol* 1984; 27:445.
20. Batra S, Iosif S: Functional estrogen receptors in the female urethra. *Proc.* Second Joint Meeting of ICS and Urodynamic Society, Aachen, 1983, p 548.
21. Ingelman-Sundberg A, Rosen J, Gustafsson SA, et al: Cytosol estrogen receptors in the urogenital tissues in stress-incontinent women. *Acta Obstet Gynecol Scand* 1981; 60:585.
22. Iosif S, Batra S, Ek A, et al: Estrogen receptors in the human female lower urinary tract. *Am J Obstet Gynecol* 1981; 141:817.
23. Reed T: The effect of estrogens and gestagens on the urethral pressure profile in urinary continent and stress incontinent women. *Acta Obstet Gynecol Scand* 1980; 59:265.
24. Caine M, Roy S: The role of female hormones in stress incontinence. *Proc.* 16th Congress of International Society of Urology, Amsterdam, 1973.
25. Hilton P, Stanton SL: The use of intravaginal estrogen cream in genuine stress incontinence. *Br J Obstet Gynecol* 1983; 90:940.
26. Roy S, Ziegler M, Caine M: The vascular component in the production of intraurethral pressure. *J Urol* 1972; 108:93.
27. Reed T: Urethral pressure profile in continent women from childhood to old age. *Acta Obstet Gynecol Scand* 1980; 59:331.
28. Youngblood VH, Tombrin EM, Williams JO, et al: Exfoliative cytology of the senile female urethra. *J Urol* 1958; 79:110.
29. Smith P: Age changes in the female urethra. *Br J Urol* 1972; 44:667.
30. Walter S, Wolf H, Barlebo H, et al: Urinary incontinence in postmenopausal women treated with estrogens. *Urol Int* 1978; 33:135.
31. Tanagho EA, Miller ER: Functional consideration of urethral sphincteric dynamics. *J Urol* 1973; 109:273.
32. Applebaum SM: Pharmacological agents in micturition disorders. *Urology* 1980; 16:555.
33. Castleden CM, George CF, Renwich AG, et al: Imipramin—A possible alternative to current therapy for urinary incontinence in the elderly. *J Urol* 1981; 125:318.
34. Montague DK, Stewart·BH: Urethral pressure profiles before and after Ornade administration in patients with stress urinary incontinence. *J Urol* 1979; 122:198.
35. Stewart BH, Lynn WH, Benowsky LHW, et al: Stress incontinence: Conservative therapy with sympatomimetic drugs. *J Urol* 1976; 115:558.
36. Diokno AC, Taub M: Ephedrin in treatment of urinary incontinence. *Urology* 1975; 5:624.
37. Scotti RJ, Ostergard DR: The urethral syndrome. *Clin Obstet Gynecol* 1984; 27:515.
38. Cifuentes L: Epithelium of vaginal type in the female trigone: The clinical problems of trigonitis. *J Urol* 1947; 57:1028.
39. Youngblood VH, Tomlin EM, Davis JB: Senile urethritis in women. *J Urol* 1957; 78:150.
40. Tanagho EA: The anatomy and physiology of micturition. *Clin Obstet Gynecol* 1978; 5:3.

41. Tanagho EA, Miller ER: Initiation of voiding. *Br J Urol* 1970; 42:175.

42. Bradley WE, Bockswold GL, Timm GW, et al: Neurology of micturition. *J Urol* 1976; 115:481.

43. Blaivas JG: The neurophysiology of micturition: A clinical study of 550 patients. *J Urol* 1982; 127:958.

44. Ostergard DR: The neurologic control of micturition and integral voiding reflexes. *Obstet Gynecol Survey* 1979; 34:417.

45. Smith P: Postmenopausal urinary symptoms and hormonal replacement therapy. *Br Med J* 1976; 2:941.

CHAPTER **13**

Prevention of Postmenopausal Osteoporosis

ROGERIO A. LOBO, M.D.

WOMEN HAVE A smaller skeletal bone mass than men, and they enter their menopausal years with less bone. This smaller bone mass decreases further with the aging process (osteopenia) and is coupled with an accelerated rate of bone loss which is thought to result from estrogen deficiency. Overall, since bone loss after the menopause proceeds at about 1%–2% per year,[1] this may be expected to result in about a 50% reduction in bone mass in white women by age 80. The end result of this process is postmenopausal osteoporosis, a devastating disease.

The impact of this process of bone loss is staggering. Twenty-five percent of women older than 60 years gave radiographic evidence of vertebral crush fractures.[2] In 1979, 125,000 women in the U.S. sustained proximal femur fractures, and 13% died as a direct consequence of this event.[3, 4] In the United Kingdom, women with femoral neck fractures constitute the third largest group of nonpsychiatric hospitalized patients and have a mortality rate 20 times that expected for age.[5, 6, 7] During the 1980s in the U.S., the estimated cost for proximal femur fractures will exceed $3 billion annually.

Although some women lose bone at an accelerated rate compared to others,[8] estrogen deficiency stands as the most significant factor influencing the decline in bone mass. Immediately after oophorectomy, an accelerated decline in bone mass occurs and may achieve a rate of 3.9% per year for the first six years. This is followed, thereafter, by the normal rate of decline of about 1% per year.[9, 10] In women older than 50 who are still menstruating, the decline in bone mass is not as great as in amenorrheic age-matched patients.[11]

Although estrogen deficiency is the major factor responsible for bone loss in menopausal women, not all women are subject to the same risk. At least three factors are known to attenuate postmenopausal bone loss. These are race, obesity, and nutrition.

Figure 13–1 depicts the femur fracture incidence in several populations. While it is highest in the U.S. and Europe, it is lowest among dark-skinned races. It is generally believed that black women are less vulnerable to fractures from postmenopausal osteoporosis because their initial bone mass is greater than that of white women.[12]

Obese women also are less likely to have symptoms from postmenopausal osteoporosis because they, too, have a greater bone mass.[13] This may be due to the greater stress placed on the axial skeleton because of increased body weight, but it may also be due to the reduced calcium excretion resulting from higher levels of circulating total and unbound estrogen (Fig 13–2).[14]

A high-protein diet may result in increased urinary calcium excretion because of the additional acid load.[15] A high-phosphate diet also results in increased calcium excretion.

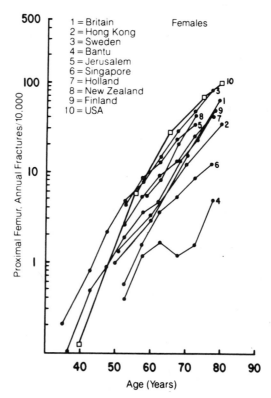

FIG 13–1.
Annual fracture rate of proximal femur from different populations. (From Gallagher JC: *Osteoporosis and Fractures.* Ayerst Laboratories, January, 1984. Used by permission.)

Nevertheless, the most important dietary factor in postmenopausal osteoporosis is calcium intake. Intestinal absorption of calcium decreases with age[16] and is even more pronounced in osteoporotic women.[17] In order to keep up with losses, postmenopausal women require an intake of 1,500 mg of elemental calcium daily. This requirement is clearly not met by the average U.S. diet. The importance of dietary calcium in the prevention of postmenopausal osteoporosis was confirmed by a study comparing two regions of Yugoslavia, one with a high and the other with a low dietary calcium intake. With a higher calcium intake (1,000 mg/day) there was greater bone mass and a lower fracture rate in this population compared to the one with a reduced calcium intake[17] (Fig 13–3).

There are other risk factors for osteoporosis in postmenopausal women. These include immobilization, smoking, alcohol excess, and hyperprolactinemia. The way in which certain factors in a woman's lifestyle may affect her bone mass is beyond the scope of this discussion. Whereas it has been suggested that rapid bone losers have lower serum progesterone levels than "slow" bone losers,[18] we have not found any correlation between serum progesterone levels and the degree of calcium loss in postmenopausal women.[19] However, recent data have implicated hyperprolactinemia as a significant risk factor for osteoporosis.[20, 21] This occurrence is associated with hypoestrogenism but may be an independent variable as well.

It· is still unclear as to why estrogen deficiency, by premature oophorectomy or spon-

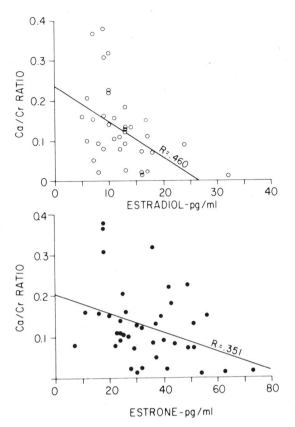

FIG 13–2.
Correlation of the Ca:Cr ratio with E_2 ($P < .005$) and E_1 ($P < .05$) levels. (From Frumar Am, Meldrum DR, Geola F, et al: Relationship of fasting urinary calcium to circulating estrogen and body weight in postmenopausal women. *J Clin Endocrinol Metab* 1980; 50:70. Used by permission.)

taneous menopause, results in accelerated bone loss. A recollection of some of the dominant theories on this controversy will help our understanding of how estrogen prevents postmenopausal osteoporosis. The effect of estrogen on bone turnover is thought to be through an indirect mechanism, because no estrogen receptors have been demonstrated on bone.[22, 23] The major theory suggests that estrogen sets a certain degree of sensitivity to bone of the resorbing effects of parathyroid hormone (PTH). Estrogen deficiency, therefore, results in an increased sensitivity of PTH at the level of bone, whereas at other organs, such as the intestine and kidney, the sensitivity remains unaltered. This results in increased bone resorption for the mobilization of calcium without substantial increased conservation of calcium by the kidney or intestine. If this theory were correct, there would be minimal changes in plasma PTH, which indeed is the case.

Somewhat related to this theory is the view that calcium malabsorption is the primary defect. In order to increase serum calcium levels, PTH levels in the circulation rise, resulting in more bone resorption. Since PTH levels are generally not elevated,[24, 25, 26] it is unlikely that this cascade of events plays the dominant role in postmenopausal osteoporosis. Also related to this theory is the possibility that a primary renal defect in

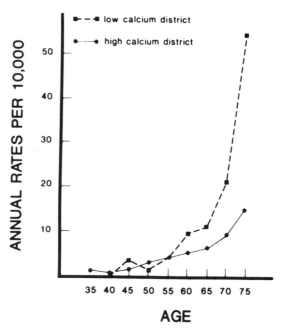

FIG 13–3.
Annual fracture rates in a low and a high calcium district in Yugoslavia. (Adapted from Gallagher JC, Riggs BL, Eisman J, et al: Intestinal calcium absorption and serum vitamin D metabolites in normal subjects and osteoporotic patients: Effect of age and dietary calcium. *J Clin Invest* 1979; 64:729.)

the formation of 1-25 dihydroxyvitamin D is operational. Here, there is evidence for[27] and against[28] a defect in the formation of 1-25 $(OH)_2$ vitamin D. Nevertheless, there are data supporting the increased formation of 1-25 $(OH)_2$ vitamin D with estrogen substitution therapy.[29] Whether this is mediated directly through renal 1 α hydroxylase, as in birds, or via PTH, is unsettled. One of the major problems in the interpretation of studies related to PTH-calcium homeostasis is the use of different immunoassays for PTH. The biologic activity of PTH may be vastly different from what is measured by the various assays, which are specific for different C-, mid- and N-terminal portions of the PTH molecule. One study in which the biologic activity of PTH was quantified, using measurements of urinary cyclic AMP, suggested that the activity of PTH was increased by estrogen.[30]

The other major theory proposed to explain postmenopausal osteoporosis involves the secretion of calcitonin. Calcitonin, which is secreted by the thyroid, opposes the effects of PTH by decreasing osteoclast number and function. The theory that estrogen deficiency results in postmenopausal osteoporosis because of declining calcitonin levels has been suggested for the following reasons: (1) high estrogen states, such as pregnancy, lactation, and oral contraceptive use, result in increased levels of calcitonin;[31] (2) calcitonin levels are lower in women than in men;[32, 33] (3) calcitonin levels decrease further as women age[34] and in postmenopausal women undergoing oophorectomy;[35] and (4) administration of calcitonin significantly increases total body calcium in women with postmenopausal osteoporosis.[36]

Indeed, at least three studies[25, 37–38] have demonstrated that postmenopausal estrogen replacement increases calcitonin levels. However, two other studies have not demonstrated such a difference.[26, 39] In our own study[26] (Fig 13–4), there were no differences in calcitonin levels between pre- and postmenopausal women before or after oral estrogen ingestion. Curiously, in one of the studies showing an effect of estrogen on calcitonin,[25] the effect could not be demonstrated with oral conjugated equine estrogens (Premarin), as in our study, although the increase was significant with parenteral forms of estrogen replacement. This raises some question about the importance of calcitonin as orally administered conjugated equine estrogen clearly has been demonstrated to prevent bone resorption. Perhaps difficulties in the interpretation of these data exist because of inherent problems in the measurement of immunoreactive as opposed to biologically active calcitonin. Investigators who have measured the monomeric form of calcitonin have suggested that immunoassays have not reflected the true biologic activity of circulating calcitonin.[40]

THE DETECTION OF BONE LOSS

While an in depth discussion of the methodology utilized for the detection of bone loss is beyond the scope of this review, some discussion is required in order to evaluate the effectiveness of various treatment modalities and to provide criteria for diagnosing postmenopausal osteoporosis.

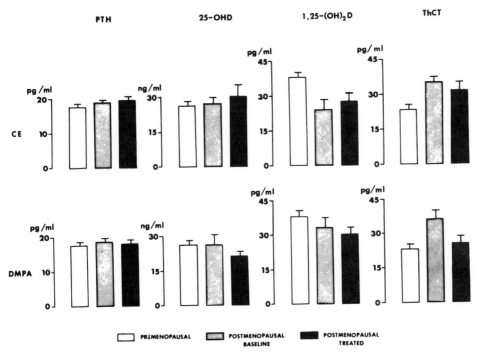

FIG 13–4.
Mean ± SE serum PTH, 25-OH-D, 1-25-(OH)$_2$D and CT in postmenopausal women before and after treatment with either 0.625 mg of conjugated estrogen or 150 mg of intramuscular depomedroxyprogesterone acetate and in 19 normal male and female subjects. (From Lobo RA, Roy S, Shoupe D, et al: Estrogen and progestin effects on urinary calcium and calciotropic hormones in surgically-induced postmenopausal women. *Horm Metab Res* 1985; 17:370. Used by permission.)

Several important points should be emphasized. First, although urinary calcium/creatinine and hydroxyproline/creatinine measurements are somewhat reflective of bone turnover, these techniques provide only crude approximations. As an example, although many different doses of estrogen will lower the urinary calcium/creatinine ratio to premenopausal levels,[19] and 0.3 and 0.625 mg of conjugated estrogen lowers this ratio to the same extent, only 0.625 mg of conjugated estrogen has been shown to prevent bone loss in all women.[41] A potentially new marker of bone loss is urinary α-carboxyglutamate (Gla) excretion, which has been shown to be increased in osteoporosis.[42] However, it is unlikely that this marker will replace the need for direct estimates of bone mass.

Secondly, the need arises to identify the patient at greatest risk for developing osteoporosis: the "fast bone loser." The biochemical techniques mentioned above cannot accomplish this identification. Repeated bone mass measurements may identify these individuals, but may take one to two years of observation. It has been suggested, however, that whole body retention of technetium-labelled diphosphonate may provide an index of bone turnover within one day.[43]

Thirdly, we need to consider the types of noninvasive bone mass determinations that will render the most information. Postmenopausal osteoporosis is largely a disease of trabecular bone rather than of peripheral or cortical bone. While the amount of cortical bone loss after oophorectomy may be 1%–3% per year, the loss in the axial skeleton (trabecular bone) may be as high as 15% in some patients. Most clinical studies up to now have focused on measurements of the peripheral skeleton, using techniques such as radiogrammetry and photon absorptiometry.[44, 45] Radiogrammetry usually measures cortical thickness and its area in x-ray studies of metacarpals. Single-photon absorptiometry measures the amount of cortical bone in the distal radius. However, as stated earlier, while these techniques may be quite accurate, they do not necessarily reflect the amount of mineral content of the axial skeleton.[46, 47] Vertebral bone mass has been measured by dual photon and neutron activation and computed tomographic (CT) techniques. While dual-photon beam studies measure both cortical and trabecular bone in the spine and hip, CT scans have the capability of measuring only trabecular bone mass in the spine.[48, 49] Currently, dual-photon beam absorptiometry[50] and CT scans are the preferred techniques for assessment of the axial skeleton. However, several investigators have combined either of these techniques with single-photon beam analysis to follow changes in cortical bone mass as well. The most sensitive method appears to be the use of the CT scan, which may detect changes in vertebral bone within six months,[51] because its precision has a reproducibility of 1%–3% with a single energy (80 kVp) technique. While the cost of a CT scan is currently $150, it may require only 10–15 minutes for an exam, and the radiation exposure is small (approximately 200 rem).

TREATMENT FOR THE PREVENTION OF PMO

Estrogen

It has been clearly established that estrogen prevents postmenopausal osteoporosis. However, several other therapies have been proposed and have been used singly or in combination with estrogen. Some of these are listed in Table 13–1.

Several prospective studies have unequivocally demonstrated that estrogen prevents bone loss in postmenopausal women when compared to placebo[52–56] (Fig 13–5). While

TABLE 13–1.

Various Proposed Treatments for the Prevention
of Postmenopausal Osteoporosis

Estrogen
Estrogen with progestins, with or without calcium
Progestins
Anabolic steroids
Calcium
Vitamin D
Fluoride
Thiazides
Calcitonin
Parathyroid hormone
Exercise

these studies have primarily demonstrated a retardation in loss of peripheral (cortical) bone, more recent studies confirmed a decrease in loss of spinal (trabecular) bone, a more significant observation[51, 57] (Fig 13–6). Several epidemiologic studies have also documented a reduced fracture rate in postmenopausal women treated with estrogen.[58–60]

Although these findings have been known for several years, only recently has the dose of estrogen required for a beneficial effect been established. While as little as 0.3 mg of conjugated estrogens will reduce calcium loss, using the fast urinary calcium/creatinine ratio, it has been established that 0.625 mg is the dose required to prevent

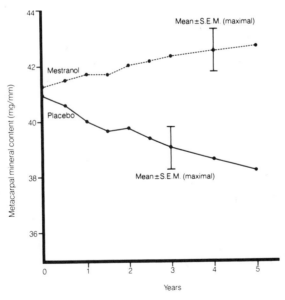

FIG 13–5.
Metacarpal content in women receiving mestranol (24 μg/day) or placebo. (From Lindsay R, Hart DM, Aitken JM, et al: Long-term prevention of postmenopausal osteoporosis by oestrogen: Evidence for an increased bone mass after delayed onset of oestrogen treatment. *Lancet* 1976; 1:1038. Used by permission.)

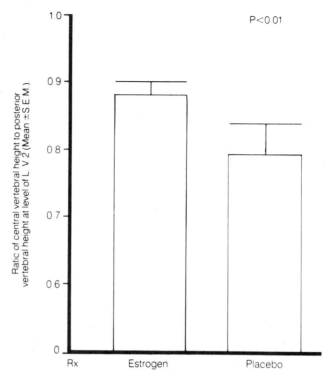

P<0.01

FIG 13–6.
Central vertebral height is preserved with estrogen compared to placebo. (Adapted from Lindsay R, Hart DM: *Osteoporosis: Pathogenesis and Treatment.* Haverstraw, New York, Regional Bone Center, Helen Hayes Hospital, p. 8. Used by permission.)

bone loss in all women.[41, 51] While 0.3 mg of conjugated estrogen, or its equivalent, may be sufficient to prevent bone loss in some women, the effect of estrogen upon bone cannot be predicted reliably. It has been suggested this lower dose may be sufficient if supplemented with 1,500 mg of calcium daily.[61] Indeed, because so many adjunctive measures, such as calcium, progestins and exercise, may be used for the treatment of postmenopausal women, it is conceivable that lower doses of estrogen may be recommended for all but those women at greatest risk for postmenopausal osteoporosis (Table 13–2).

Since the mechanism of action of estrogen on bone has not been determined, it has not been easy to compare the efficacy of various types of estrogen for the prevention of postmenopausal osteoporosis. It is known that estrogens have different potency ratios, depending on the response parameter that is used.[62]

This phenomenon may be particularly true for the effect of inhibition of bone resorption. While ethinyl estradiol is known to be more than 200 times as potent as the "natural" estrogens, an average of 25 mg was the dose shown by Lindsay et al. to prevent bone loss compared to placebo.[52] Nevertheless, 0.625 mg of conjugated estrogen will accomplish the same end. Even if 10 mg of ethinyl estradiol is sufficient, this dose would be equivalent to about 1–2 mg of conjugated estrogen, depending on the parameter used to compare estrogens.[62, 63] It appears, therefore, that a natural estrogen (conjugated equine estrogens) may prevent bone resorption to a greater extent than a

TABLE 13–2.

Common Risk Factors for Osteoporosis

Estrogen deficiency from any cause
Low calcium intake
Malabsorption of calcium
High phosphorus diet
High protein diet
Caucasian or oriental races
Lean body mass
Physical inactivity
Estrogen deficiency due to strenuous exercise
Hyperprolactinemia
Cigarette smoking
Alcoholism

synthetic estrogen would. However, a weaker natural estrogen, estriol, is much less potent, and large doses (more than 8 mg/day) are required to inhibit bone resorption.[64]

There has been considerable controversy about the effect of cessation of estrogen therapy. Earlier studies have suggested that withdrawal of estrogen results in an accelerated loss of bone.[65, 66] However, more recent studies[54, 67] have refuted this finding, agreeing with epidemiologic evidence that estrogen exposure is protective against bone loss.[58–60, 68] In a Danish study[54] the rate of loss of bone mass after switching from estrogen to placebo was similar to the loss after placebo treatment alone. However, therapy in this study, in contrast to others, consisted of estrogen with a progestin, together with calcium supplementation. It is suggested by these and other data (see below) that the addition of a progestin to estrogen may afford greater protection from bone loss.

Estrogen with Progestins

Three studies that have demonstrated a benefit of estrogen use in preventing resorption have been studies in which progestins have also been used.[54, 55, 57] Of particular interest in these three studies are data suggesting that bone mass may actually increase. In one of these studies (Fig 13–7),[55] if therapy was instituted within three years of the last menstrual period, bone mass increased. In another,[54] bone mass increased whenever the combination regimen was given (Fig 13–8). While in these studies calcium supplements were also used, the data strongly suggest that combination therapy has the ability to increase bone mass. In addition, it has been suggested that the combination of another progestin, norgestrel, to estradiol valerate, reduced bone turnover to a greater extent than the use of estrogen alone.[69]

While the mechanism of the synergy between estrogens and progestins on bone has not been determined, it has been suggested that their actions differ. It has recently been proposed, with some preliminary confirmatory data, that while estrogen prevents bone resorption, progestins increase its formation.[71] The combination of estrogen and progestin thus has been considered to be ideal treatment: resorption is inhibited and formation is stimulated. Nevertheless, it has not been determined what length or dose of progestin treatment is necessary for this function.

This different effect of progestins on bone may be related to a receptor-mediated process. Glucocorticoid receptors have been demonstrated on bone.[72] As progestins

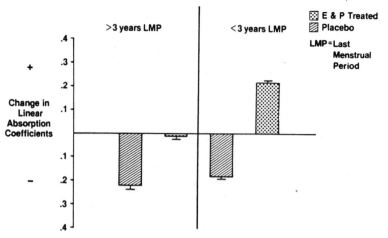

FIG 13–7.
Effect on estrogen/progestogen replacement on bone mass over a 10-year period. (Adapted from Upton GV: The perimenopause: Physiologic correlates and clinical management. *J Reprod Med* 1982; 27:15. Adapted from: Nachtigall LE, Nachtigall RH, Nachtigall RD, et al: Estrogen replacement therapy I: A 10-year prospective study in the relationship to osteoporosis. *Obstet Gynecol* 1979; 53:277.

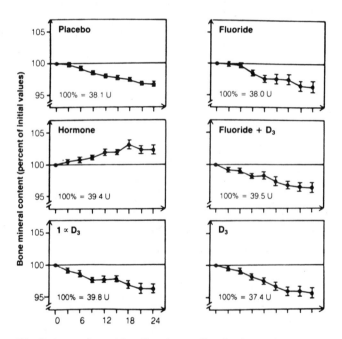

*All patients were given calcium either alone or with sodium fluoride, estrogen + progestogen, vitamin D with or without fluoride, or 1α-vitamin D.

FIG 13–8.
Changes in bone mineral levels with various supplement regimens. (From Christiansen C, Christiansen MS, Rodbro P: Effect of 1,25-dihydroxy-vitamin D in itself or combined with hormone treatment in preventing postmenopausal osteoporosis. *Eur J Clin Invest* 1981; 11:305. Used by permission.)

have the ability to displace glucocorticoids from their receptors, it is possible that progestin therapy may stimulate bone formation by blocking the inhibitory effects of glucocorticoids upon this process.

Progestins Alone

From the above discussion, it may be postulated that progestins have a beneficial effect on bone. While its use in conjunction with estrogen may result in bone formation, there is evidence that when used alone it also prevents resorption. Several studies have demonstrated this effect by indirect means with the use of medroxyprogesterone acetate, megestrol, and norethindrone.[73–76] While reduction in urinary calcium excretion has been consistently demonstrated with the use of progestins alone, only two studies[74, 76] have demonstrated a reduction in urinary hydroxyproline/creatinine ratios as well.

Although only some data exist, it must be realized that not all progestins exert the same beneficial effects. The type, dose, and duration of therapy appear to be critical in the prevention of postmenopausal osteoporosis. As an example, two similar 17-acetoxyprogestins (megestrol and medroxyprogesterone acetate) appear to be vastly different in bone resorption properties. The latter is about four times more potent than the former.[75]

Studies in postmenopausal women using depot injections of progestins have demonstrated that bone mass does not decrease.[73, 77] Our recent study[76] demonstrated that the reduction in fasting calcium/creatinine and hydroxyproline/creatinine ratios after trimonthly administration of 150 mg of depomedroxyprogesterone acetate were similar to the effects of 0.625 mg of conjugated estrogen administered daily (Fig 13–9).

A synthetic compound with progestin-like properties, 17α hydroxy 7 methyl 19 norpregn-5-(10)en-20-yn-3-one (ORG OD14), has been studied extensively in Europe and has been found to afford good protection from bone loss.[78] An oral dose of 2.5 mg daily has been beneficial in alleviating vasomotor symptoms in addition, without causing significant side effects.[79–83]

Anabolic Steroids

The withdrawal of androgen from men may result in osteoporosis. It is therefore entirely possible that androgens exert an effect in men similar to the effect of estrogens or progestins in women. When used in women, androgens may increase bone matrix and have been shown to increase total body calcium.[84, 85] In osteoporotic women with fractures, administration of methandrostenolone, 5 mg daily for six months, protected against further calcium loss.[83] However, it is unlikely that androgens will play a therapeutic role in postmenopausal osteoporosis, since androgenic side effects are likely to preclude continuous use.

For several years it had been suggested that stanozolol would play a role in the treatment of postmenopausal osteoporosis. While it has been documented that stanozolol increases total body calcium in patients who have established osteoporosis,[86] its role in the prevention of postmenopausal bone loss remains to be determined.

Calcium

Clearly, the U.S. recommended dietary intake of 800 mg of calcium per day is inadequate. In estrogen-deficient women, a negative calcium balance of approximately 40 mg/day occurs with this intake.

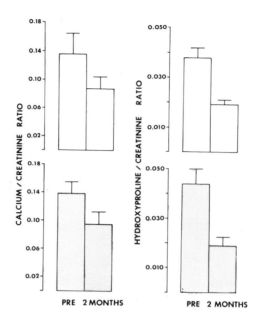

FIG 13–9.
Pretreatment calcium/creatinine and hydroxyproline/creatinine ratios ($\bar{x} \pm$ SE) and after two months of receiving either conjugated estrogens (*open bars*) or depo-medroxyprogesterone acetate (*closed bars*). (From Lobo RA, McCormick W, Singer F, et al: Depomedroxyprogesterone acetate compared with conjugated estrogens for the treatment of postmenopausal women. *Obstet Gynecol* 1984; 63:1. Reprinted with permission from the American College of Obstetricians and Gynecologists.)

Although the rate of calcium absorption may remain subnormal, total absorption will increase by substantially increasing oral intake. Theoretically at least, an increase in circulating calcium may inhibit PTH, which may in turn decrease the rate of bone resorption.

Although somewhat controversial, the consensus of opinion regarding the effects of calcium in postmenopausal patients is that calcium is beneficial as an adjunctive measure in preventing postmenopausal osteoporosis but can not replace the protective effects of estrogen therapy.[87–90] Nevertheless, the doubling of calcium intake in one population during lifetime exposure, from 500 to 1,000 mg daily, substantially reduced the risk of fractures (see Fig 13–3). This difference in fracture rate was greater the older the population became. Nevertheless, it appears that replacement of calcium alone in postmenopausal women is insufficient for preventing bone loss, while its combination with even suboptimal doses of estrogen may be beneficial.[61]

In one study, using single-photon beam absorption,[89] treatment with 0.625 mg of conjugated estrogen and 5 mg of methyl testosterone resulted in bone loss of 0.73% per year compared to a loss of 2.8% in control subjects. Women ingesting calcium only (2,600 mg of calcium carbonate daily) lost 1.8% per year. In another more recent study, women receiving 1,500 mg of calcium daily were compared to untreated women and women treated with 1,500 mg of calcium and 0.3 mg of conjugated estrogen daily.[61] Untreated women lost 8.5% of lumbar trabecular bone by CAT scan after one year. The loss in the calcium-only group was also substantial (6.2%). However, in the estrogen-plus-calcium group, only two subjects lost any bone and most women either did not lose or increased (0.6%) their bone mass (Fig 13–10).

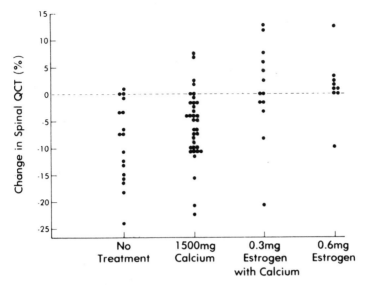

FIG 13–10.
Vertebral trabecular bone loss following menopause. The change in spinal quantitative computed tomography over 12 months is shown as a function of treatment. (From Genant HK, Cann CE, Ettinger B, et al: Quantitative computed tomography for spinal mineral assessment in osteoporosis. *Proceedings of the Copenhagen International Symposium on Osteoporosis.* p 69, 1984. Aalborg Stiftsbogtrykkeri. Used by permission.)

The current recommended dietary intake of calcium in postmenopausal women should be equivalent to 1,500 mg daily. This intake should be maintained whether or not the patient is receiving hormonal replacement. Table 13–3 lists the calcium content of food and other preparations.

TABLE 13-3.

Calcium-Containing Foods and Supplements

	QUANTITY	MG OF CALCIUM
Food		
Plain lowfat yogurt	1 cup	415
Sardines	3 oz	372
Whole milk	1 cup	291
Swiss cheese	1 oz	272
Cheddar cheese	1 oz	204
Ice cream	1/2 cup	88
Cottage cheese	1/2 cup	63
Supplements		
Tums antacid (calcium carbonate)	1 tablet	200
Caltrate 600 (calcium carbonate)	1 tablet	600
Os Cal (calcium carbonate)	1 tablet	500
Calcium lactate	1 tablet	100
Calcium gluconate	1 tablet	47, 62

Vitamin D

Although vitamin D theoretically should increase the calcium balance because 1-25(OH)$_2$ vitamin D increases calcium absorption, it has not been found to be a useful therapy in practice. In several studies, treatment with vitamin D or its metabolites has been found to be ineffective in preventing bone loss.[92, 93] During 1-25(OH)$_2$ vitamin D treatment, although Ca absorption increased, urinary calcium excretion also increased, causing a net negative effect on the process of bone resorption. Thus, although bone resorption may decrease, there appears to be a net negative effect.[93, 94] Long-term studies using vitamin D have indicated no effect on bone and, as a consequence, new fractures have occurred in osteoporotic patients.[93–95]

Fluoride

Fluoride therapy has been recommended for treatment of patients with established osteoporosis because of its stimulatory effects on osteoblast matrix synthesis.[96, 97] However, it does not appear to have a role in the prevention of osteoporosis. This occurs largely because there is a high percentage of serious side effects with fluoride treatment (40%) although only a minority of patients will not respond to therapy.[98] The significant side effects of fluorosis include hematemesis, anemia, neurologic problems, and joint pain. Figure 13–11 depicts the negative effect that fluoride can have with or without concomitant vitamin D therapy on bone mass in one study.[92]

Although the use of fluoride may be considered in patients with established osteoporosis, the bone formed is not normal bone. Since fluoride affects the cellular structure of bone, the resultant bone is abnormally crystalline and inelastic. Although a decreased

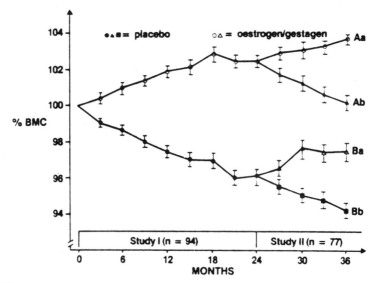

FIG 13–11.
Bone mineral content as a function of time and treatment. *A*, estrogen/progestogen; *B*, placebo; *a*, changeover to estrogen/progestin; *b*, changeover to placebo. (From Christiansen C, Christensen MS, Transbol I: Bone mass in postmenopausal women after withdrawal of oestrogen/gestagen replacement therapy. *Lancet* 1981; 1:459. Used by permission.)

fracture rate has been demonstrated with its use,[98] the increased bone mass with fluoride therapy does not add enough strength to bone to recommend its use for all osteoporotic patients. In combination with calcium and vitamin D, the fracture rate reported for fluoride in osteoporotic patients in one study was still in excess of 300 per thousand patient years.[99] The recommended dose is 25 mg of sodium fluoride twice daily.

Thiazides

Thiazides have been proposed for treatment of postmenopausal osteoporosis because renal calcium excretion is reduced. This effect is ascribed to a direct stimulation of calcium reabsorption from the distal tubule and an enhancement of proximal tubular reabsorption.[100, 101] However, thiazides also have the potential of accentuating PTH-dependent bone resorption.[102]

In a randomized study, thiazides were used as treatment in postmenopausal women. After a transient effect of six months during which bone density was sustained, the bone loss thereafter was similar to the control group.[103] Thiazides do not appear to have a role in the prevention of postmenopausal osteoporosis.

Calcitonin

Because of the observation that calcitonin levels are decreased in osteoporotic patients and because calcitonin is known to oppose PTH-dependent bone resorption, this therapy has been proposed to prevent postmenopausal osteoporosis. Despite some recent enthusiasm for this approach,[104, 105] the effects on bone resorption and formation have been viewed as being variable.[106]

Although calcitonin may prevent the PTH effects on bone resorption, when given alone it may stimulate PTH secretion, negating this inhibitory role. Furthermore, if bone resorption were to decrease with this therapy in conjunction with calcium, this should not lead to an increase in bone mass; since bone formation would decline commensurately.

More study will be needed on the role of calcitonin in postmenopausal osteoporosis before any use of calcitonin may be recommended for the prevention of osteoporosis.

Parathyroid Hormone

Although paradoxical, the use of PTH has been proposed to increase bone mass. Parathyroid hormone may activate osteoclasts and stimulate osteoblasts and new bone formation.[107] The life of osteoblasts is several times longer than that of osteoclasts.[108] Trabecular bone mass does increase in young rats treated with PTH.[109] Although encouraging results have been reported with use of 1-34 PTH in postmenopausal subjects,[110–114] the increase is primarily in trabecular bone, and cortical bone mass has been shown to be reduced.[114]

At present, PTH therapy requires the use of daily injections. While its use in established osteoporosis may be considered in some patients, there does not appear to be a place for PTH therapy in the prevention of postmenopausal osteoporosis.

Exercise

Although there are no definitive data linking exercise to a decreased fracture incidence, vigorous exercise has been thought to be of benefit. Preliminary information suggests that although perhaps only the exercised limb benefitted from exertion, exercise did increase total bone mass.[115] However, in osteoporotic patients, exercise has increased bone mineral content and total body calcium.[116, 117] More recent work has indicated that exercise does increase bone mass in athletes[118, 119] and that in postmenopausal women exercise may retard osteoporosis.[120–123] Although prospective long-term studies are still to be carried out, vigorous weight-bearing exercise, at least three times a week, should be recommended for all postmenopausal women. It is premature to decide whether exercise may be beneficial alone or as an adjunctive measure to proper nutrition and hormonal replacement in the prevention of postmenopausal osteoporosis. Nevertheless, its effect appears to be definitely positive at least as an adjunctive measure. Although it remains to be determined whether spinal bone will be preserved, any generalized increase in bone mass with exercise has to be viewed as positive. In addition, the potential improvement of cardiovascular status with exercise alone strengthens the argument for its recommendation.

ESTABLISHED OSTEOPOROSIS

All of the above treatments have been proposed for patients with established disease, either used alone or in various combinations. While the purpose of this chapter is to focus on the prevention of osteoporosis, several therapies may be mentioned again as candidates for the treatment of established osteoporosis. It appears that treatment of osteoporosis will require a combination of several agents. Candidates for this therapy include PTH, calcitonin, and fluoride, generally with calcium supplementation. Estrogen may also have some benefit because of its effect on depressing osteoclast function. Although not generally considered, progestins or androgens may also have an additive effect because of their stimulatory effect on bone formation.

One of the newest therapies that has been proposed is called coherence treatment.[108, 124] While multicellular bone units are usually out of phase with one another (activation and resorption effects), this treatment places units in phase, stimulating formation (Fig 13–12). In this treatment, a timed sequence of "activation-resorption and formation" is used to manipulate a large number of remodeling sites of bone. First an activating "pulse" of PTH is given for five days. This is followed by a drug to depress osteoclasts over a month, for example, calcium. During the ensuing two to three months when no drug is given, the stimulated osteoblasts would be allowed to form new bone. A reactivating cycle is then repeated. Various modifications of the basic scheme have been proposed and may be of benefit.[125] Nevertheless, this therapy is new, and much more work is necessary in order to recommend this regimen.

SUMMATION/ASSESSMENT

Quite clearly, our aim should be directed at the prevention rather than the treatment of osteoporosis. It appears that osteoporosis is largely a preventable disease and the risks and cost of treating most, if not all, peri- and postmenopausal women should be far less than the morbidity and mortality of, and the billions of dollars incurred from, osteoporotic fractures. Some of these cost issues for estrogen and progestin therapy have been reviewed elsewhere.[126]

Since the American diet is largely calcium-deficient, an important preventative measure would be to assure that all women enter the menopause with as much bone mass as possible. The average premenopausal patient has a negative calcium balance of about

Normal Sequence

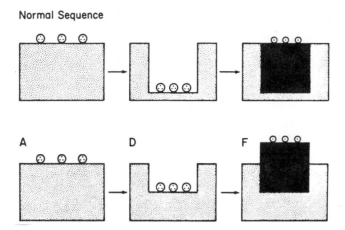

FIG 13–12.
Depiction of coherence treatment in an individual basic multicellular unit. Without ADFR sequence (*top*), the amount of bone destroyed (*top middle*) by osteoclasts is considered to be equal to the amount formed (*top right*) by osteoblasts. During the depression phase (*D*) of coherence treatment (*bottom middle*), less bone is destroyed by osteoclasts than without depression (*top middle*). Thus, the total amount of bone left is larger following ADFR sequence than without ADFR (compare *bottom right* with *top right*), assuming an equal amount of new bone formation (*shaded areas*). (From Pak CYC: Postmenopausal osteoporosis in the menopause, in Buchsbaum HJ (ed): *The Menopause*. New York, Springer-Verlag New York, 1983, p 35. Used by permission.)

20 mg/day.[127] Merely increasing dietary calcium in the pre- and perimenopausal years may significantly alter the fracture incidence in later years.

Since the other benefits of estrogen treatment of menopausal patients may be considerable as well (for example, the cardiovascular benefits, as discussed in Chapter 15), and as yet there is no sure way to determine the women at greatest risk for postmenopausal osteoporosis, it is my contention that all menopausal women, including women at low risk for developing postmenopausal osteoporosis (such as blacks and obese whites) should be treated with estrogen unless there is a major contraindication to such therapy. Unless there are strong personal objections by the patient, such treatment should be recommended even for the patient without vasomotor symptomatology. This therapy should be instituted within the first three years of the menopause and continued indefinitely or until other factors involving the benefit versus risk and cost issues emerge to guide us. If a woman has a contraindication for estrogen, progestins alone may be used with adjunctive measures such as increasing calcium intake and exercise.

More data are emerging to suggest that the benefits of estrogen in postmenopausal osteoporosis may be enhanced by the bone-forming properties of progestins. In this regard, we sorely lack data about the effects of various types of progestins and their duration of use in regard to prevention of osteoporosis as well as their effects, if any, on cardiovascular disease. The beneficial effects of estrogen on lipids and cardiovascular status may be attenuated or eliminated by the use of certain types and doses of progestins.[128] However, it is most plausible that by adding a low dose of progestin to a low dose of estrogen, and by supplemental calcium intake, the ideal preventative regimen would be achieved for postmenopausal women by balancing decreased resorption with increased bone formation. Nevertheless, the impact of such a regimen on cardiovascular disease will have to be analyzed independently. Further, the effect of the addition of progestins to estrogen therapy may have important implications in breast disease,[129, 130] an issue far from being settled. With the multiple, varied regimens of different doses of estrogens with progestins now being studied, used both cyclically as well as continually, we hope some of these issues will soon direct us further.

REFERENCES

1. Gordon GS, Vaughan C: Prevention of age related bone loss. *Proceedings Arnold O Beckman Conference on Clinical Chemistry* 1980; 3:1.
2. Heanly RP: Estrogens and postmenopausal osteoporosis. *Clin Obstet Gynecol* 1976; 19:791.
3. Judd HG, Cleary RE, Creasman WT, et al: Estrogen replacement therapy. *Obstet Gynecol* 1981; 58:267.
4. Carson SL: The perimenopause. *J Reprod Med* 1982, 27:27.
5. Stevenson JC, Whitehead MI: Postmenopausal osteoporosis. *Br Med J* 1982; 285:585.
6. Lewis AF: Fracture of neck of the femur: Changing incidence. *Br Med J* 1981; 283:1217.
7. Lane G, Whitehead MI, Stevenson JC: How to diagnose and treat osteoporosis after menopause. *Contemp Obstet Gynecol,* Jan 1983, p 38.
8. Lindsay R, Coutts JR, Hart DM: The effect of endogenous estrogen on plasma and urinary calcium and phosphate in oophorectomized women. *Clin Endocrinol* 1977; 6:87.
9. Lindsay R, Aitken JM, Anderson JB, et al: Long-term prevention of postmenopausal osteoporosis by oestrogen: Evidence for an increased bone mass after delayed onset of oestrogen treatment. *Lancet* 1976; 1:1038.
10. Horsman A, Simpson M, Kirby PA: Nonlinear bone loss in oophorectomized women. *Br J Radiol* 1977; 50:504.
11. Meema HE, Bunker MC, Meema S: Loss of compact bone due to menopause. *Obstet Gynecol* 1965; 26:333.
12. Smith DM, Nance WE, Kang KW: *J Clin Invest* 1973; 52:2800.
13. Dalen N, Hallberg D, Lamke B: *Acta Med Scand* 1975; 197:353.
14. Frumar AM, Meldrum DR, Geola F, et al: Relationship of fasting urinary calcium to circulating estrogen and body weight in postmenopausal women. *J Clin Endocrinol Metab* 1980; 50:70.
15. Licata AA. *J Gerontol* 1981; 36:14.
16. Ireland P., Fordham JS: Effect of dietary calcium and age on jejunal calcium absorption in humans studied by intestinal perfusion. *J Clin Invest* 1973; 52:2672.
17. Gallagher. *J Clin Invest* 1979; 64:729.
18. Johnston CC Jr, Norton JA Jr, Khairi RA, et al: Age-related bone loss, in Barzel NS (ed): *Osteoporosis.* New York, Grune & Stratton, 1978, vol 2, p 91.
19. Lobo RA, Brenner PF, Mishell DR Jr: Metabolic parameters and steroid levels in postmenopausal women receiving lower doses of natural estrogen replacement. *Obstet Gynecol* 1983; 62:94–98.
20. Klibanski A, Neer R, Beitius I, et al: Decreased bone density in hyperprolactinemia women. *N Engl J Med* 1981; 303:1511.
21. Schlechte JA, Sherman BM, Martin R: Bone density in amenorrheic women with and without hyperprolactinemia. *J Clin Endocrinol Metab* 1983; 56:1120–1123.
22. Nutik G, Cruess RL: Estrogen receptors in bone. An evaluation of the uptake of estrogen into bone cells. *Proc Exp Biol Med* 1974; 146:265.
23. Chen TL, Feldman D: Distinction between alpha-fetoprotein and intra-cellular estrogen receptors: Evidence against the presence of estradiol receptors in rat bone. *Endocrinology* 1978; 102:236.
24. Gallagher JC, Riggs BL, Eisman J: Intestinal calcium absorption and serum vitamin D metabolites in normal subjects and osteoporotic patients. *J Clin Invest* 1979; 64:729.
25. Stevenson JC, Abeyasekera G, Hillyard CJ, et al: Calcitonin and the calcium-regulating hormones in postmenopausal women: Effect of oestrogens. *Lancet* 1981; 1:693.
26. Lobo RA, Roy S, Shoupe D et al: Estrogen and progestin effects on urinary calcium and calcitrophic hormones in surgically-induced postmenopausal women. *Horm Metab Res* 1985; 17:369–392.

27. Slovik DM, Adams JS, Neer RM, et al: Deficient production of 1,25 dihydroxyvitamin D in elderly osteoporosis patients. *N Engl J Med* 1981; 305:372.

28. Riggs BL, Hamstra A, Deluca HF: Assessment of 25-hydroxyvitamin D 1 hydroxylase reserve in postmenopausal osteoporosis by administration of parathyroid extract. *J Clin Endocrinol Metab* 1981; 53:833.

29. Gallagher JC, Riggs BL, DeLuca HF: Effect of estrogen on calcium absorption and serum vitamin D metabolites in postmenopausal osteoporosis. *J Clin Endocrinol Metab* 1980; 51:1359.

30. Lindsay R, Sweeney A: Urinary cyclic—AMP in osteoporosis. *Scott Med J* 1976; 21:231.

31. Whitehead MI, Lane G, Young O, et al: Interrelations of calcium regulating hormones during normal pregnancy. *Br Med J* 1981; 283:10–12.

32. Heath H III, Sizemore GW: Plasma calcitonin in normal. *J Clin Invest* 1977; 60:1135–1140.

33. Hillyard CJ, Stevenson JC, MacIntyre I: Relative deficiency of plasma-calcitonin in normal women. *Lancet* 1978; 1:961–962.

34. Deftos LJ, Weisman MH, Williams G, et al: Influence of age and sex on plasma calcitonin in human beings. *N Engl J Med* 1980; 302:1351–1353.

35. Whitehead MI, Lane G, Morsman J, et al: Effect of castration on calcium-regulating hormones. *Maturitas* 1984; 6(2):207.

36. Chestnut CH III, Baylink DJ, Gruber HE, et al: Treatment of postmenopausal osteoporosis with salmon calcitonin: Preliminary results, in DeLuca HF, Frost HM, Jee WSS, et al (eds): *Osteoporosis: Recent Advances in Pathogenesis and Treatment.* Baltimore, University Park Press, 1981, pp 411–418.

37. Morimoto S, Tsuji M, Okada Y, et al: The effect of oestrogens on human calcitonin secretion after calcium infusion in elderly female subjects. *Clin Endocrinol* 1980; 13:135.

38. Stevenson JC, Abeyasekera G, Hillyard CJ, et al: Regulation of calcium-regulating hormones by exogenous sex steroids in early postmenopause. *Eur J Clin Invest* 1983; 13:481.

39. Leggate J, Farish E, Fletcher CD, et al: Calcitonin and postmenopausal osteoporosis. *Clin Endocrinol* 1984; 20:85–92.

40. Body JJ, Heath H: Estimates of circulating monomeric calcitonin: Physiologic studies in normal and thyroidectomized man. *J Clin Endocrinol Metab* 1983; 57:897.

41. Lindsay R, Hart DM, Clark DM: The minimum effective dose of estrogen for prevention of postmenopausal bone loss. *Obstet Gynecol* 1984; 63:759.

42. Gundbery CM, Lian JB, Gallup PM, et al: Urinary carboxyglutamic acid and serum osteocalcin as bone markers: Studies in osteoporosis and Paget's Disease. *J Clin Endocrinol Metab* 1983; 57:1221.

43. Fogelman I, Bessent RG, Cohen HN, et al: Skeletal uptake of diphosphonate: Method for prediction of post-menopausal osteoporosis. *Lancet* 1980; 2:667–670.

44. Garn SM: *The Earlier Gain and Later Loss of Cortical Bone, in Nutritional Perspective.* Springfield, Ill, Charles C Thomas, Publisher, 1970, p 146.

45. Cameron JR, Soreno J: Measurement of bone mineral in vivo: An improved method. *Science* 1963; 142:230–232.

46. Wilson CR: Prediction of femoral neck and spine bone mineral content from BMC of the radius of ulna and the relationship between bone strength and BMC, in Mazess R (ed): *International Conference on Bone Mineral Measurement,* Publication NIH-75-684, US Dept of Health, Education and Welfare, 1974, pp 51–59.

47. Dalen N, Jacobsen B: Bone mineral assay: Choice of measuring sites. *Invest Radiol* 1974; 9:174–185.

48. Orphanoudakis SC, Jensen PS, Rauschkolb EN, et al: Bone mineral analysis using single-energy computed tomography. *Invest Radiol* 1979; 14:122–130.

49. Ruegsegger P, Elsasser U, Anliker M, et al: Quantification of bone mineralization using computed tomography. *Radiology* 1976; 121:93–97.

50. Madsen M, Peppler W, Mazess RB: Vertebral and total body mineral content by dual photon absorptiometry, in Pors-Nielsen S, Hjorting-Hansen E (eds): *Calcified Tissues 1975.* Copenhagen, FAPL Publishing, 1976, pp 361–364.

51. Cann CE, Genant HK, Ettinger B, Gordon GS: Spinal mineral loss in oophorectomized women: Determination by quantitative computed tomography. *JAMA* 1980; 244:2056.

52. Lindsay R, Hart DM, Aitken JM, et al: Long term prevention of postmenopausal osteoporosis by estrogens. *Lancet* 1976; 1:1038–1041.

53. Atken JM, Hart DM, Lindsay R: Oestrogen replacement therapy for prevention of osteo-porosis after oophorectomy. *Br Med J* 1973; 3:515–518.
54. Christiansen C, Christensen MJ, Transbøl I: Bone mass in postmenopausal women after withdrawal of oestrogen/gestagen replacement therapy. *Lancet* 1981; 1:459–461.
55. Nachtigall LE, Nachtigall RH, Nachtigall RD, et al: Estrogen replacement therapy: A 10-year prospective study in the relationship to osteoporosis. *Obstet Gynecol* 1979; 53:277–281.
56. Reese W: A better way to screen for osteoporosis. *Contemp Obstet Gynecol* Nov 1983.
57. Lindsay R, Hart DM, Forrest C, et al: Prevention of spinal osteoporosis in oophorectomized women. *Lancet* 1980; 2:1151–1154.
58. Hutchinson TA, Polansky SM, Feinstein AP: Postmenopausal estrogens protect against frac-tures of hip and distal radius. *Lancet* 1979; 2:705–709.
59. Gordan GS, Pichi J, Roof BS: Antifracture efficacy of long term estrogens for osteoporosis. *Trans Assoc Am Physicians* 1973; 86:326–332.
60. Weiss NS, Ure CL, Ballard JH, et al: Decreased risk of fractures of the hip and lower forearm with postmenopausal use of estrogen. *N Engl J Med* 1980; 303:1195.
61. Ettinger B, Cann L, Genant K: Menopausal bone loss: Effects of conjugated oestrogen and/or high calcium diet. *Maturitas* 1984; 6(2):108 (#39).
62. Mashchak CA, Lobo RA, Dozono-Takano R, et al: Comparison of pharmacodynamic prop-erties of various estrogen formulations. *Am J Obstet Gynecol* 1982; 144:511.
63. Mandel FP, Geola FL, La JK, et al: Biologic effects of various doses of ethinyl estradiol in postmenopausal women. *Obstet Gynecol* 1982; 59:673.
64. Lindsay R, Hart DM, Maclean A, et al: Bone loss during estriol therapy in postmenopausal women. *Maturitas* 1979; 1:279.
65. Lindsay R, Hart DM, Maclean A, et al: Bone response to termination of oestrogen treat-ment. *Lancet* 1978; 1:1325–1327.
66. Horsman A, Nordin BEC, Crilly RG: Effect on bone of withdrawal of oestrogen therapy. *Lancet* 1979; 2:33.
67. Christiansen C, Christiansen M, McNair P, et al: Prevention of early postmenopausal bone loss: Controlled 2-year study in 315 normal females. *Eur J Clin Invest* 1980; 10:273–279.
68. Paganini-Hill A, Ross RK, Gerkins VR, et al: A case control study of menopausal estrogen therapy and hip fractures. *Am Intern Med* 1981; 95:28.
69. Crilly RG, Marshall DH, Nordin BEC: The effect of oestradiol valerate and cyclic oestradiol valerate/DL-norgestrel on calcium metabolism. *Postgrad Med J* 1978; 54:47.
70. Nachtigall LE, Nachtigall RH, Nachtigall RD, et al: Estrogen replacement therapy I: A 10-year prospective study in the relationship to osteoporosis. *Obstet Gynecol* 1979; 53:277.
71. Riis BJ, Nilas L, Christiansen C, et al: Effect of oestrogen: Progestogen treatment on bone turnover in early post-menopausal women. *Maturitas* 1984; 6:169.
72. Manolagas SC, Anderson DC: Detection of high-affinity glucocorticoid binding in rat bone. *J Endocrinol* 1978; 76:379.
73. Lindsay R, Hart DM, Purdie D, et al: Comparative effects of oestrogen and a progestogen on bone loss in postmenopausal women. *Clin Sci Mol Med* 1978; 54:193–195.
74. Mandel FP, Davidson BJ, Erlik Y, et al: Effects of progestins on bone metabolism in postmenopausal women. *J Reprod Med* 1982; 27(8):511.
75. Erlik Y, Meldrum DR, Lagasse LD, et al: Effect of megestrol acetate on flushing and bone metabolism in post-menopausal women. *Maturitas* 1981; 3:167.
76. Lobo RA, McCormick W, Singer F, et al: Depo-medroxyprogesterone acetate compared with conjugated estrogens for the treatment of postmenopausal women. *Obstet Gynecol* 1984; 63:1–5.
77. Dequeker J, Meryl der E de, Ferin J: The effect of long-term lynestrenol treatment on bone mass in cyclic women. *Contraception* 1972; 15:717.
78. Lindsay R, Hart DM, Kraszewski A: Prospective double-blind trial of a synthetic steroid (OD14) for preventing postmenopausal osteoporosis. *Br Med J* 1980; 1:1207–1209.
79. Fioretti EP, Grimaldi GB, Melis M, et al: Tibolone (ORG od 14) in the control of the climacteric. *Maturitas* 1984; 6(2):113, (#44).
80. Farish E, Fletcher CD, Hart DM, et al: ORG OD 14: Long term effects on serum lipopro-teins. *Maturitas* 1984; 6(2):110, (#41).

81. Cortes-Prieto J, Kicovic PM: Coagulation and fibrinolysis in post-menopausal women treated with org OD 14. *Maturitas* 1984; 6:99 (#28).
82. Aloysio de D, Fabiani AG, Mauloni M, et al: Use of ORG OD 14 for the treatment of climacteric complaints. *Maturitas* 1984; 6:83, (#6)
83. Tas L, Kicovic PM: Clinical profile of ORG OD 14. *Maturitas* 1984; 6:196 (#143)
84. Aloia JF, Kapoor A, Vaswani A, et al: Changes in body composition following therapy of osteoporosis with methandrostenolone. *Metabolism* 1981; 30:1076.
85. Chestnut CH III, Nelp NB, Baylink DJ, et al: Effect of methandrosteneolone on postmenopausal bone wasting as assessed by changes in total bone mineral mass. *Metabolism* 1977; 26:267.
86. Chestnut CH III, Ivey JL, Nelp WB, et al: Assessment of anabolic steroids and calcitonin in the treatment of osteoporosis, in Barzel US (ed): *Osteoporosis II*. New York, Grune & Stratton, 1979; pp 135–150.
87. Horsman A, Gallagher JC, Simpson M, et al: Prospective trial of oestrogen and calcium in postmenopausal women. *Br Med J* 1977; 11:789.
88. Nordin BEC, Horsman A, Crilly RG, et al: Treatment of spinal osteoporosis in postmenopausal women. *Br Med J* 1980; 281:451.
89. Recker PR, Saville PD, Heaney RP: Effect of estrogens and calcium carbonate on bone loss in postmenopausal women. *Ann Intern Med* 1977; 87:649.
90. Riggs BL, Seeman E, Hoidgson SP, et al: Effect of the fluoride calcium regimen on vertebral fracture occurrence in postmenopausal osteoporosis. *N Engl J Med* 1982; 306:446.
91. Matkovic V, Kostial K, Simonovic I, et al: Bone status and fracture rates in two regions of Yugoslavia. *Am J Clin Nutr* 1979; 32:540.
92. Christiansen C, Christensen MS, Rodbro P, et al: Effect of 1,25-hydroxyvitamin D in itself or combined with hormone treatment in preventing postmenopausal osteoporosis. *Eur J Clin Invest* 1981; 11:305.
93. Davies M, Maner EB, Adams PH: Vitamin D metabolism and the response to 1,25-D1 hydroxycholecalciferol in osteoporosis. *J Clin Endocrinol Metab* 1976; 42:1139.
94. Riggs BL, Jowsey J, Kelly POJ, et al: Effects of oral therapy with calcium and vitamin D in primary osteoporosis. *J Clin Endocrinol Metab* 1976; 42:1139.
95. Wandless I, Jarvis S, Evans JG, et al: Vitamin D_3 in osteoporosis. *Br Med J* 1980; 280:1326.
96. Jowsey J, Schenk RK, Reutter FW: Some results of the effect of fluoride on bone tissue in osteoporosis. *J Clin Endocrinol Metab* 1968; 28:869.
97. Rich C, Ensinck J: Effect of sodium fluoride on calcium metabolism of human beings. *Nature* 1961; 191:184.
98. Riggs BL, Seeman E, Hodgson SF, et al: Effect of the fluoride/calcium regimen on vertebral fracture occurrence in postmenopausal osteoporosis. *New Engl J Med* 1982; 306:446.
99. Riggs BL, Hodgson SF, Hoffman DL, et al: Treatment of primary osteoporosis with fluoride and calcium. *JAMA* 1980; 243:446–449.
100. Sutton RAL, Dirks JH: Renal handling of calcium: Overview, in Massry SG, Ritz E, (eds): Phosphate metabolism. *Adv Exp Med Biol* 1977; 81:15.
101. Porter RH, Cox BG, Heaney D, et al: Treatment of hypoparathyroid patients with chlorthalidone. *N Engl J Med* 1978; 298:577.
102. Parfitt AM: Chlorothiazide-induced hypercalcemia in juvenile osteoporosis and hyperparathyroidism. *N Engl J Med* 1969; 281:55.
103. Transbol I, Christensen MS, Jensen GF, et al: Thiazide for the postponement of postmenopausal bone loss. *Metabolism* 1982; 31:383.
104. Wallach S, Cohn SH, Atkins HL, et al: Effect of salmon calcitonin on skeletal mass in osteoporosis. *Curr Ther Res Clin Exper* 1977; 22:556.
105. Rasmussen H, Bordier P, Marie D, et al: Effect of combined therapy with phosphate and calcitonin on bone volume in osteoporosis. *Metab Bone Dis Relat Res* 1980; 2:107.
106. Jowsey J, Riggs BL, Goldsmith RS, et al: Effects of prolonged administration of porcine calcitonin in postmenopausal osteoporosis. *J Clin Endocrinol Metab* 1971; 33:752.
107. Ashton BA, Owen MR, Eagleson CC, et al: *Endocrinology of Calcium Regulating Hormones*. Amsterdam, Excerpta Medica, 1981.

108. Frost HM: Treatment of osteoporosis by manipulation of coherent bone cell populations. *Clin Orthop* 1979; 143:227.

109. Kalu DN, Pennock J, Doyle FH, et al: Parathyroid hormone and experimental osteosclerosis. *Lancet* 1970; 1:1363.

110. Reeve J, Williams D, Hesp R, et al: Anabolic effect of low doses of a fragment of human parathyroid hormone on the skeleton in postmenopausal osteoporosis. *Lancet* 1976; 1:1035.

111. Slovik DM, Neer RM, Poots JT: Short-term effects of synthetic human parathyroid hormone (1-34) administration on bone mineral metabolism in osteoporotic patients. *J Clin Invest* 1981; 68:1261.

112. Parsons JA, Meunier P, Podbesek R, et al: Pathological and therapeutic implications of the cellular and humoral response to parathyroin. *Biochem Soc Trans* 1981; 9:383.

113. Reeve J, Arlot M, et al: Calcium-47 kinetic measurements of bone turnover compared to bone histomorphometry in osteoporosis: The influence of human parathyroid fragment (hPTH1-34) therapy. *Metab Bone Dis Rel Res* 1981; 3:23.

114. Reeve J, Meunier P, Parsons JA, et al: Anabolic effect of human parathyroid hormone fragment on trabecular bone in involutional osteoporosis: A multicenter trial. *Br Med J* 1980; 2:1340.

115. Gordon GS, Haiden A, Vaughn C: *Medical Times* page no., vol. no.?, April 1971.

116. Kleerekoper M, Tolia K, Parfitt AM: Nutritional endocrine and demographic aspects of osteoporosis. *Orthop Clin North Am* 1981; 12:547–558.

117. Aloia JF, Cohn SH, Ostune JA, et al: Prevention of involutional bone loss by exercise. *Ann Intern Med* 1978; 89:356–358.

118. Dalen N, Olsson KE: Bone mineral content and physical activity. *Acta Orthop Scand* 1974; 45:170–174.

119. Nilsson B, Westin N: Bone density in athletes. *Clin Orthop* 1971; 77:179–182.

120. Brewer V, Meyer BM, Keele MS, et al: Role of exercise in prevention of involutional bone loss. *Med Sci Sports Exerc* 1983; 15:445.

121. Oyster N, Morton M, Linnell S: Physical activity and osteoporosis in postmenopausal women. *Med Sci Sports Exerc* 1984; 16:44.

122. Smith EL, Reddan W, Smith PE: Physical activity and calcium modalities for bone mineral increase in aged women. *Med Sci Sports Exerc* 1981; 13:50.

123. Montoye HJ, Smith EL, Farden DF, et al: Bone mineral in senior tennis players. *Scand J Sports Sci* 1980; 2:26–32.

124. Frost HM: Coherence treatment of osteoporosis. *Orthop Clin North Am* 1981; 12:649.

125. Rasmussen H, Bordier P, Marie P, et al: Effect of combined therapy with phosphate and calcitonin on bone volume in osteoporosis. *Metab Bone Dis Rel Res* 1980; 2:107–111.

126. Weinstein MC, Schiff I: Cost effectiveness of hormone replacement therapy in the menopause. *Obstet Gynecol Surv* 1983; 38:445.

127. Heaney RP, Recker RR, Saville PD: Menopausal changes in calcium balance performance. *J Lab Clin Med* 1978; 92:953–963.

128. Ottosson UB, Johansson BG, von Schoultz B: Subfractions of high-density lipoprotein cholesterol during estrogen replacement therapy: A comparison between progestogens and natural progesterone. *Am J Obstet Gynecol* 1985; 151:746–750.

129. Pike MC, Henderson BE, Krailo MD, et al: Breast cancer in young women and use of oral contraceptives: Possible modifying effect of formulation and age at use. *Lancet* 1983; 2(8349):556–558.

130. Gambrell RD, Maier RC, Sanders BI: Decreased incidence of breast cancer in postmenopausal estrogen-progestogen users. *Obstet Gynecol* 1983; 62:435.

CHAPTER 14

Effects of Pharmacologic Agents Used During Menopause: Impact on Lipids and Lipoproteins

TRUDY L. BUSH, Ph.D.
VALERY T. MILLER, M.D.

CORONARY HEART DISEASE (CHD) is the major cause of death among menopausal and postmenopausal women in the United States, accounting for more than 36% of all deaths in women. Clinical and epidemiologic evidence has clearly demonstrated that serum lipids and lipoproteins are powerful determinants of CHD in both women and men. A large proportion of perimenopausal and menopausal women use pharmacologic agents for the relief of menopausal symptoms and for other medical conditions. These drugs may significantly influence serum lipid and lipoprotein levels and thus potentially affect the risk of developing CHD. The purpose of this chapter is to examine the effects on lipid and lipoprotein levels of selected pharmacologic agents commonly used in the menopausal period.

LIPIDS, LIPOPROTEINS, AND CORONARY HEART DISEASE RISK

The major lipid of interest in the pathogenesis of CHD is serum cholesterol. Most (90 + %) of the cholesterol in serum is carried by two major lipoproteins: low-density-lipoprotein cholesterol (LDL-C) and high-density-lipoprotein cholesterol (HDL-C). Some cholesterol and most of triglycerides are carried by very-low-density lipoprotein cholesterol (VLDL-C).

Total Cholesterol.—Numerous reports have consistently shown that elevated total serum cholesterol levels are associated with an increased risk of CHD.[1-3] Even relatively small increases in absolute levels of serum cholesterol have been shown to influence the subsequent risk of disease. For example, observations from the Framingham Study show that an increase of 10 mg/dl of total cholesterol is associated with a 12% increase in the risk of disease.[4] Further, small reductions in total serum cholesterol levels have been shown to decrease the risk of CHD in men. Results from the Lipid Research Clinics Coronary Primary Prevention Trial have demonstrated that the risk of CHD declines 2% for each 1% reduction in serum cholesterol level.[5] The decline in CHD risk was seen when cholesterol levels were reduced by dietary means or by pharmacologic interventions.

Triglycerides.—While total cholesterol is an accepted etiologic factor in the development of CHD, the role of triglycerides in the pathogenesis of CHD is less clear. It has been suggested that elevated triglyceride levels increase the risk of CHD;[6, 7] however, to date, no independent effect of triglyceride level on CHD risk has been demonstrated.[8] The true association of triglyceride levels with CHD remains unknown. However, it is unlikely that modestly elevated triglyceride levels in the presence of normal cholesterol levels significantly contributes to the development of CHD.

Lipoproteins (HDL-C, LDL-C, and VLDL-C).—Two lipoprotein carriers of cholesterol, HDL-C and LDL-C, have been shown to be strong and consistent predictors of CHD.[8-11] High levels of HDL-C have been shown to be protective against the development of CHD, while high levels of LDL-C have been shown to increase the risk of CHD. Compared with total cholesterol, both HDL-C and LDL-C are more sensitive and specific indicators of CHD risk.[9] HDL-C is comprised of several subfractions defined by density. It is currently unknown which of the two major subfractions of total HDL-C (HDL_2 and HDL_3), is the more sensitive indicator of CHD risk. Unfortunately, little information is available on either the effect of VLDL-C level on the risk of CHD, or the effect of pharmacologic agents of VLDL-C levels.

AGENTS COMMONLY USED DURING MENOPAUSE

Pharmacologic agents used during the menopausal period for the relief of menopausal symptoms include: estrogens (given alone or cycled with progestins), progestins (prescribed alone or with estrogens), and the antihypertensive drug clonidine. Other agents commonly used by women during their menopausal years include antihypertensives and tranquilizers. With the growing awareness that osteoporosis is a significant health problem of postmenopausal women, drugs that prevent this condition are also being prescribed more frequently.

Magnitude and Patterns of Drug Usage.—There are few sources of information on the numbers and characteristics of menopausal women who may use prescription drugs. Some data are available from older surveys of selected populations[12-14] or from marketing information on various agents[15] or from physician surveys.[16] These data suggest that a very high proportion of women may be exposed, during some years of their lives, to agents prescribed from menopausal symptoms. Estimates from surveys completed in the 1970s suggest that between 8% and 50% of perimenopausal women at any one time were taking estrogens for menopausal symptoms.[12, 14]

Use of specific prescription agents for menopausal symptoms has varied considerably over the last 40 years.[17] Until the middle 1960s, most of the drugs used for relief of menopausal symptoms were synthetic estrogens, mainly ethinylestradiol and mestranol. Usually no additional agents were added to this regimen, i.e., unopposed estrogens were prescribed. In the middle to late 1960s, the synthetic estrogens were gradually replaced with natural estrogens, mainly Premarin (conjugated equine estrogens). During the late 1960s and early 1970s, these natural estrogens were more likely to be prescribed with no additional agents, although between 8% and 18% of prescriptions also included testosterone.[12, 14] Use of estrogens cycled with progestins at this time (before 1975) was rare.

Because of reports in the mid-1970s that showed that use of unopposed menopausal estrogens increased the risk of endometrial cancer, estrogen use in the U.S. declined during the late 1970s and early 1980s. Recent information suggests that estrogen use is again increasing.[15] However, unlike the previous decades, progestins are much more likely to be cycled with estrogens during the course of menopausal therapy.[16]

In addition to those agents used for the relief of menopausal symptoms, both antihypertensives and tranquilizers are frequently prescribed for women of menopausal age.

The high prevalence of hypertension in the United States and the popularity of the benzodiazepines for treatment of patients of all ages account for these exposures. As noted previously, pharmacologic agents, including estrogens, are being more frequently prescribed to menopausal women solely for the prevention of osteoporosis. It is likely that as both physicians and women become aware of the seriousness of this disorder, drug use for the prevention of osteoporosis will increase.

UNOPPOSED ORAL ESTROGEN THERAPY

There are numerous commercial estrogen preparations available for oral estrogen therapy. These formulations can be divided into two major groups: "natural" estrogens, or those whose chemical structure occur in nature, and "synthetic" agents, those whose structures must be synthesized.

The natural agents include 17β-estradiol, estriol, and estrone. The most frequently prescribed estrogen in the U.S. is Premarin, a mixture of conjugated equine estrogens (mainly estrone sulfate). Currently, Premarin accounts for about 70% of all replacement estrogen use in the U.S. Other frequently used natural formulations include estradiol succinate, piperazine estrone sulfate, and micronized 17β-estradiol.

The synthetic estrogens include ethinylestradiol, mestranol, quinestrol, and diethylstilbesterol (DES). Currently, these formulations are used most frequently for contraceptive purposes and are less often prescribed for menopausal therapy. Of the synthetic estrogens, ethinyl estradiol and mestranol are the most frequently used agents in menopausal therapy.

Oral Estrogens, Lipids, and Lipoproteins.—It has been recognized for over 30 years that oral estrogens are potent lipid- and lipoprotein-altering agents. The observation by Barr et al. in 1952 that estrogens increase alpha-lipoprotein (HDL-C) and decrease beta-lipoprotein (LDL-C) was the impetus for clinical trials of estrogen use in men.[18–20] Nearly all of the studies of estrogens and lipids and lipoproteins have demonstrated that estrogens consistently decrease total and LDL cholesterol, and increase HDL-C and triglycerides.[17] Questions still remain, however, regarding the precise effects of estrogens on lipids and lipoproteins. These questions remain because (1) the estrogen effect on lipids and lipoproteins may be significantly modified by type, dose, and route of administration; and (2) many of the published reports have methodologic problems, including small sample sizes and short durations of use and follow-up.

Natural Estrogens, Lipids, and Lipoproteins: Premarin.—A summary of selected studies of Premarin use and lipid and lipoprotein levels in menopausal women is presented in Table 14–1.[18–30] Generally speaking, total cholesterol and LDL-C levels are lower and HDL-C and triglyceride levels are higher after Premarin use, although these findings are not universally observed. The range of lipid and lipoprotein response reported in these studies is quite wide. For example, HDL-C levels are increased between 0% and 26%, and LDL-C levels are lowered between 4% and 19%.

The discrepancies in these values may be due to a variety of methodologic factors, including size of study population, duration of use within the study, and dose of Premarin. To account for these differences in studies, we have adjusted the results of each of the reports for sample size and duration of study. The results of this adjustment are graphically presented in Figure 14–1.

After adjustment for size and of duration of study, a dose-response effect of Premarin on lipids and lipoproteins is clearly seen (see Fig 14–1). With the low-dose (0.625 mg) formulation, total cholesterol levels are increased by approximately 1%, HDL-C levels

TABLE 14-1.
Effects of Oral Conjugated Equine Estrogens (Premarin) on Lipid and Lipoprotein Levels in Postmenopausal Women

REFERENCE	STUDY POPULATION	N	DURATION OF USE	DOSE/DAY	PERCENT CHANGE IN			
					TOTAL CHOLESTEROL	HDL CHOLESTEROL	LDL CHOLESTEROL	TRIGLYCERIDES
Notelovitz et al., 1983[21]	Oophorectomized women	35	3 mos	0.625 mg	+4%	+4%	-4%	+10%
Bolton et al., 1975[22]	Oophorectomized women, 32–46 yrs	17	3 mos	0.625 mg	-4%	—	—	+24%
Campagnoli et al., 1981[23]	Women > 45 yrs in menopause clinic	12	5 mos	0.625 mg	-1%	+26%	—	+2%
Bradley et al., 1978[24]	HMO population; users vs. nonusers	265	?	< 0.625 mg	—	+9%	—	—
Cauley et al., 1983[25]	Participants in bone loss study	48	?	0.1–1.0 mg	+1%	+24%	—	-3%
Bradley et al., 1978[24]	HMO population; users vs. nonusers	477	?	> 1.25 mg	—	+16%	—	—
Lind et al., 1979[26]	Women 49–54 yrs	6	12 mos	1.25 mg	-9%	—	—	+5%
Notelovitz et al., 1983[21]	Oophorectomized women	35	3 mos	1.25 mg	-1%	0%	-6%	+29%
Bolton et al., 1975[22]	Oophorectomized women, 32–46 yrs	17	3 mos	1.25 mg	-4%	—	—	+24%
McConathy et al., 1981[27]	Postmenopausal women	6	4 mos	1.25 mg	-2%	-1%	—	+24%
Paterson et al., 1980[28]	Menopause clinic patients	15	12 mos	1.25 mg	-6%	—	—	+17%
Robinson et al., 1965[29]	Hyperlipidemic women, 40–62 yrs	44	1 mo	1.25–2.50 mg	-7%	+7%	-11%	+51%
Wahl et al., 1983[30]	Population survey, users vs. nonusers	239	?	?	-5%	+13%	-19%	+24%

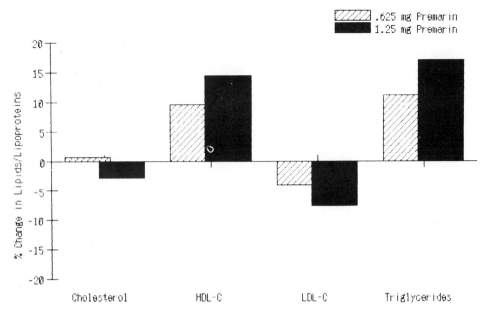

FIG 14–1.
Percent change in lipid/lipoproteins by dose of premarin.

by nearly 10%, and triglycerides by 11%. At this dose (0.625 mg) LDL-C is decreased by about 4%. (The small increase in total cholesterol at 0.625 mg is probably due to the relatively large increase in HDL-C.)

At the higher dose of Premarin (1.25 mg), total cholesterol and LDL-C are decreased 3% and 8% respectively, and HDL-C and triglycerides are increased 14% and 17% respectively. These findings indicate that favorable changes in regard to CHD risk in the lipoprotein profile can be demonstrated at all dose levels of Premarin.

Natural Estrogens, Lipids, and Lipoproteins (excluding Premarin).—A summary of selected studies of the effects of natural estrogens (excluding Premarin) on lipids and lipoproteins in menopausal women is presented in Table 14–2.[21, 23, 26, 28, 31–39] As with the data in Table 14–1, these results also vary widely. For example, total cholesterol is reported to be decreased 14%[35] and increased by 6%[33] at the same dose of the same agent. Again, differences in sample size and study duration may account for much of this discrepancy. Overall, it appears that HDL-C levels are consistently increased and LDL-C levels are consistently decreased with all natural estrogen formulations. Again, the range of lipid and lipoprotein response to natural estrogen is wide, with HDL-C levels increased between 1% to 34% and LDL-C decreased between 1% and 22%.

To compare the relative effects of type of conjugated estrogens on lipid and lipoprotein levels, the studies presented in Tables 14–1 and 14–2 were summarized after adjustment for sample size and duration of study. The adjusted percent changes in lipids and lipoproteins by type of conjugated estrogens are presented in Table 14–3. All of the natural estrogens evoked a favorable lipoprotein profile, i.e., increased HDL-C and decreased LDL-C levels.

Of these natural estrogens, estradiol valerate (2 mg/day) appears to have the most favorable impact on the lipoprotein profile, increasing HDL-C levels by approximately 15% and decreasing LDL-C levels by about 16%. Triglyceride levels are only slightly

TABLE 14–2.
Effects of Oral Conjugated Estrogens (Excluding Premarin) on Lipid and Lipoprotein Levels in Postmenopausal Women

REFERENCE	STUDY POPULATION	N	DURATION OF USE	TYPE OF ESTROGEN	DOSE/DAY	TOTAL CHOLESTEROL	HDL CHOLESTEROL	LDL CHOLESTEROL	TRIGLYCERIDES
							PERCENT CHANGE IN		
Wallentin et al., 1977[31]	Women with menopausal symptoms	19	6 mos	Estradiol valerate	2 mg	−3%	+12%	−7%	−6%
Silfverstolpe et al., 1982[32]	Women hysterectomized for cervical cancer	11	6 wks	Estradiol valerate	2 mg	—	+15%	−19%	—
Paterson et al., 1980[28]	Women attending menopause clinic	14	12 mos	Estradiol valerate	2 mg	−3%	—	—	+21%
Saunders et al., 1970[33]	Oophorectomized women, 30–50 yrs	10	1 mo	Estradiol valerate	2 mg	+6%	—	—	−8%
Lind et al., 1979[26]	Women 49–54 yrs	7	12 mos	Estradiol valerate	2 mg	−8%	—	—	+17%
Vilska et al., 1983[34]	Postmenopausal women, x̄ age = 55 yrs	53	6.4 yrs	Estradiol valerate	2 mg	+2%	+15%	—	−1%
Tikkanen et al., 1979[35]	Hyperlipidemic women	29	12 mos	Estradiol valerate	2 mg	−14%	+16%	−22%	+9%
Vilska et al., 1983[34]	Postmenopausal women, x̄ age = 53 yrs	42	6.4 yrs	Estradiol succinate	2 mg	0%	+8%	—	−1%
Saarikoski et al., 1981[36]	Postmenopausal women with symptoms	14	3 mos	Estradiol succinate	4 mg	−4%	+1%	—	−7%
Saarikoski et al., 1981[36]	Postmenopausal women with symptoms	7	6 mos	Estradiol succinate	8 mg	+1%	+30%	—	+20%
Saarikoski et al., 1981[36]	Postmenopausal women with symptoms	7	6 mos	Estradiol succinate	16 mg	+4%	+34%	—	+6%

Study	Group	n	Duration	Agent	Dose				
Notelovitz et al., 1983[21]	Oophorectomized women	35	3 mos	Micronized 17β-estradiol	1 mg	-1%	+10%	-7%	0%
Notelovitz et al., 1983[21]	Oophorectomized women	35	3 mos	Micronized 17β-estradiol	2 mg	+3%	+9%	-1%	+9%
Borglin et al., 1975[37]	Women treated for estrogen deficiency	105	6 mos	17β-estradiol + estriol	2 mg + 1 mg	-1%	—	—	-11%
Borglin et al., 1975[37]	Women treated for estrogen deficiency	127	6 mos	17β-estradiol + estriol	4 mg + 2 mg	-4%	—	—	-18%
Campagnoli et al., 1981[23]	Women > 45 years attending menopause clinic	10	5 mos	Estriol	2 mg	-1%	+17%	—	-15%
Issacs et al., 1977[38]	Menopausal women and women with gonadal dysgenesis	22	6 mos	Piperazine estrone sulfate	1.5-3.0 mg	-5%	+5%	-11%	+13%
Lind et al., 1979[26]	Women 49-54 yrs	7	12 mos	Piperazine estrone sulfate	1.50 mg	+1%	—	—	-2%
Lagrelius et al., 1981[39]	Perimenopausal women, 40-53 yrs	20	12 mos	Piperazine estrone sulfate	2.5 mg	-8%	+11%	—	+7%
Paterson et al., 1980[28]	Women attending menopause clinic	14	12 mos	Piperazine estrone sulfate	3 mg	-7%	—	—	+1%

TABLE 14–3.

Adjusted* Percent Change in Lipids and Lipoproteins by Type of Conjugated Estrogens

| | | CHANGE IN | | | |
TYPE OF ESTROGEN	NUMBER OF STUDIES	TOTAL CHOLESTEROL	HDL CHOLESTEROL	LDL CHOLESTEROL	TRIGLYCERIDES
Equine estrogens	10	−9%	+10%	−6%	+20%
Estradiol valerate	7	−4%	+15%	−16%	+4%
Estradiol succinate	2	0.0%	+12%	0.0%	+2%
Piperazine estrone sulfate	4	−6%	+8%	−11%	+7%

*Adjusted for sample size and duration of study

increased (4%) with this agent. Given its antiatherogenic potential, estradiol valerate, 2 mg/day, may be the agent of choice in menopausal therapy.

Synthetic Estrogens, Lipids, and Lipoproteins.—Although natural estrogens are the most commonly used formulations for menopausal therapy, the synthetic estrogens are occasionally prescribed for menopausal symptoms. A summary of the effects of synthetic estrogens on lipid and lipoprotein levels in postmenopausal women is presented in Table 14–4. [22, 24, 30–32, 40–43]

As seen in the summaries of earlier reported studies, there are wide variations in the results of these reports. Depending on the particular study, HDL-C is increased by 9% to 52%, and LDL-C is decreased by 2% to 27%. However, as with the natural estrogens, the synthetic agents tend to decrease total and LDL-C levels and to increase HDL-C and triglyceride levels.

Synthetic estrogens are known to be more potent than natural estrogens at equivalent doses,[44] and this higher potency is reflected in the magnitude of the changes induced in lipid and lipoprotein levels. The average change in the lipids and lipoproteins induced by natural estrogens compared with synthetic estrogens is presented graphically (after adjustment for size and duration of study) in Figure 14–2. Overall, the changes induced by the synthetic estrogens are two to three times greater than those induced by the natural estrogens.

The changes in the lipid and lipoprotein levels induced by the synthetic estrogens appear to be even more favorable than those induced by the natural agents (e.g., HDL-C increased 29% vs. 12%; LDL-C decreased 17% vs. 11%). However, despite this ostensibly more favorable lipoprotein profile, the synthetic estrogens are not recommended for general use in menopausal therapy for two reasons. First, synthetic estrogens, when compared to natural agents, markedly increase triglyceride levels (31% vs. 8%), and this alteration theoretically has the potential to be atherogenic. Second, the side effects for estrogen therapy (uterine bleeding, nausea, breast tenderness) have been shown to be more pronounced with the synthetic formulations.[45, 46]

Oral Estrogens and HDL-C Subfractions.—High-density-lipoprotein cholesterol is comprised of several subfractions defined by density. The two major subfractions of this protective lipoprotein are HDL_2 (d = 1.063 − 1.125) and HDL_3 (d = 1.125 − 1.210). It has been hypothesized that HDL_2 is the more "protective" subfraction,[11, 47] ostensibly because patients with CHD and men have lower HDL_2 levels than women and persons without disease.

Unfortunately, there are few studies that examine the effects of oral estrogen therapy

TABLE 14-4.
Effects of Oral Synthetic Estrogens on Lipids and Lipoproteins in Postmenopausal Women

REFERENCE	STUDY POPULATION	N	DURATION OF USE	TYPE OF ESTROGEN	DOSE/DAY	PERCENT CHANGE IN			
						TOTAL CHOLESTEROL	HDL CHOLESTEROL	LDL CHOLESTEROL	TRIGLYCERIDES
Marmorston et al., 1958[40]	Women with prior MI, 48–82 yrs	26	8 mos	Ethinyl estradiol	0.01 mg	−15%	—	—	—
Bolton et al., 1975[22]	Oophorectomized women, 32–46 yrs	17	3 mos	Ethinyl estradiol	0.02 mg	−8%	—	—	+59%
Silfverstolpe et al., 1982[32]	Women hysterectomized for cervical cancer 27–45 yrs	11	6 wks	Ethinyl estradiol	0.02 mg	—	+9%	−2%	—
Bradley et al., 1978[24]	Health plan participants; users vs. nonusers	32	?	Ethinyl estradiol	0.02 mg	—	+26%	—	—
Wallentin et al., 1977[31]	Women with menopausal symptoms; x̄ age = 52 yrs	20	6 mos	Ethinyl estradiol	0.05 mg	−11%	+33%	−27%	+22%
Bolton et al., 1975[22]	Oophorectomized women, 32–46 yrs	17	3 mos	Ethinyl estradiol	0.05 mg	−6%	—	—	+76%
Blumenfeld et al., 1983[41]	Women post-oophorectomy. 48–51 yrs	11	2 mos	Ethinyl estradiol	0.05 mg	+4%	+26%	−21%	—
Bradley et al., 1978[24]	Health plan participants, users vs. nonusers	26	?	Ethinyl estradiol	0.05 mg	—	+26%	—	—
Wahl et al., 1983[30]	Women 45–65 yrs. users compared to nonusers	8	?	Ethinyl estradiol	?	0%	+41%	−21%	+47%
Wahl et al., 1983[30]	Women 45–65 years. users compared to nonusers	7	?	DES	?	+3%	+52%	−18%	+16%
Hart et al., 1984[42]	Oophorectomized women; participants in bone study	40	10 yrs	Mestranol	0.026 mg	−1%	+28%	−13%	+31%
Aitken et al., 1971[43]	Hysterectomized and oophorectomized women; 37–58 years	20	12 mos	Mestranol	0.2–0.4 mg	−17%	—	—	+27%

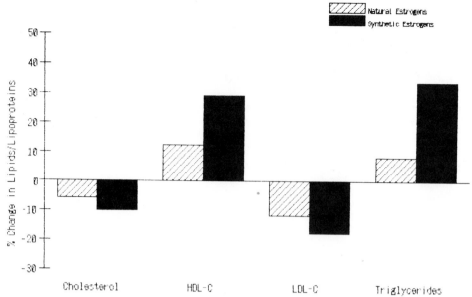

FIG 14–2.
Percent change in lipid/lipoproteins by type of estrogen.

on HDL-C subfractions. These studies, each of which used a different estrogen, are summarized in Table 14–5.[25, 41, 42, 47] In three of the four reports, the estrogen-induced increase in HDL-C is seen most clearly for the HDL$_2$ subfraction.[25, 42, 47] However, in the fourth study, it is the HDL$_3$ subfraction that is substantially increased by oral estrogen therapy.[41] Additional studies of the effects of oral estrogen therapy and HDL-C subfractions are needed.

Summary of Effects of Oral Estrogens on Lipids and Lipoproteins.—To date, the evidence that unopposed oral estrogen therapy modifies lipid and lipoprotein levels in a manner that should protect against the development of CHD (e.g., HDL-C levels increased and LDL-C levels lowered) is strong and consistent. It is also clear that the lipid and lipoprotein response is associated with both the dose of the estrogen used and the potency of the specific formulation, i.e., a more pronounced lipid/lipoprotein response is seen with higher doses and more potent agents. While the data are suggestive

TABLE 14–5.

Effects of Oral Estrogens on HDL Subfractions

STUDY	ESTROGEN/DOSE	N	REFERENCE GROUP	PERCENT CHANGE IN		
				HDL	HDL$_2$	HDL$_3$
Cauley, et al.[25]	Premarin 0.37 mg/day	48	Nonusers	+24%	+60%	+2%
Hart, et al.[42]	Mestranol 0.026 mg/day	21	Nonusers	+38%	+97%	+17%
Fahraeus et al.[47]	Estradiol 2–4 mg/day	19	Pretreatment	+19%	+21%	+14%
Blumenfeld, et al.[41]	Ethinyl estradiol 0.05 mg/day	11	Pretreatment	+30%	+29%	+76%

that estrogens selectively increase the HDL_2 subfraction of HDL-C, further work in this area is needed. Because of its nearly ideal lipid/lipoprotein altering properties, estradiol valerate, 2 mg/day, is suggested as the agent of choice in unopposed oral estrogen therapy in the menopause.

NON-ORAL ROUTES OF ESTROGEN THERAPY

Routes of estrogen administration other than oral are clinically effective for the relief of menopausal symptoms. In general, all routes of administration, whether in the form of vaginal creams, tablets, rings or solutions, in cutaneous gels or in subcutaneous pellets, have been found to raise serum estradiol levels to follicular phase levels of the normal cycle.[47–61] However, unlike oral estrogen, only subdermal pellets of estradiol significantly change lipoprotein values.[58, 59] The effects of nonoral estrogen on serum lipids and lipoproteins are presented in Table 14–6.[54–56, 58–61]

Vaginal Administration of Estrogens.—Estrogens can be administered via the vagina in the form of creams, tablets, saline solution, and rings. Systemic as well as local effects have been demonstrated with vaginal estrogen use and the effects are directly proportional to the dose and kind of estrogen, as well as the type of vehicle used. In several reports, use of 17β-estradiol in vaginal cream or tablets resulted in peaks of serum estradiol greater than 500 pg/dl.[49, 51] Unfortunately, in these reports, serum cholesterol and lipoproteins were not measured.

Mandel and colleagues, however, have compared the systemic effects (such as changes in hepatic proteins, FSH, and LH) of four doses of conjugated estrogens (0.3 mg, 0.625 mg, 1.25 mg, 2.5 mg) administered vaginally in a cream base.[61] Only the highest dose (2.5 mg, equivalent to 4 gm of estrogen cream) raised serum estrogen to early follicular phase levels. Levels of HDL-C, LDL-C, and VLDL-C remained unchanged. The authors concluded that the systemic effects of all doses of vaginal conjugated estrogen studied were substantially less than those of similar doses given orally.

Estrogens are withheld from women with histories of thrombophlebitis, severe hypertension, and certain familial hyperlipidemias, specifically those with hypertriglyceridemia.[62, 63] Low-dose vaginal estrogen (0.3 mg, equivalent to 0.5 gm of cream) is sufficient to treat the vaginal epithelium of menopausal women and does not have systemic effects.[61] It would appear that this dose may reasonably be given for the relief of vaginal symptoms in such patients.

Percutaneous Administration of Estrogen.—Estrogen (17β-estradiol) can be administered as an alcohol-water gel applied over the abdominal skin. Although follicular phase levels for serum estradiol are obtained with this route of administration, serum lipids and lipoproteins remain unchanged.[54–56] In two studies, serum estradiol levels were demonstrated to be similar to those seen with oral estrogen administration.[54, 56]

Estrogen Administered as Subdermal Pellets.—Pellets of 17β-estradiol inserted beneath the abdominal wall deliver physiologic doses of estrogen over a period of three to six months, depending on the initial dose of the pellet. In two studies, lipoprotein levels were significantly altered by estrogens administered via this route.[58, 59] Estrogen pellets of 25 mg and 100 mg increased HDL-C levels 48% and 32%, respectively. In contrast, a third study found only a modest increase (6%) in HDL-C levels in women using a 50-mg pellet.[60]

Of all of the nonoral routes of estrogen administration, only estrogens given via subdermal pellets were able to elicit lipoprotein responses, and these responses are far greater than the lipoprotein response to oral estrogen. The precise reasons for this effect

TABLE 14–6.
Effects of Nonoral Estrogen on Lipid and Lipoprotein Levels in Postmenopausal Women

REFERENCE	STUDY POPULATION	N	DURATION OF USE	DOSE/DAY	ROUTE	E LEVEL	PERCENT CHANGE IN LIPIDS			
							TOTAL-C	HDL-C	LDL-C	TRIGLYCERIDES
Mandel et al., 1983[61]	Natural menopause (no ages stated)	20	1 mo	0.3 mg	Vaginal cream	12 pg/ml	No change	No change	No change	No change
				0.625 mg		25 pg/ml	No change	No change	No change	No change
				1.25 mg		35 pg/ml	No change	No change	No change	No change
				2.5 mg		64 pg/ml	No change	No change	No change	No change
Fahraeus et al, 1982[54]	Natural and surgical, 42–58 yrs	17	6 mos	3.0 mg	Estradiol gel percutaneous	400 pmol/l	—	+4%	—	—
Basdevant et al, 1983[56]	Natural menopause, 44–60 yrs	20	2 mos	3.0 mg	Estradiol gel percutaneous	293 pmol/l	—	—	—	−14%
Elkik et al, 1982[55]	Natural menopause, 44–63 yrs	10	3 wks	3.0 mg	Estradiol gel percutaneous	—	—	—	—	−14%
Lobo et al, 1983[59]	Posthysterectomy, 29–50 yrs	22	3 mos	25.0 mg	Estradiol pellet	50–70 pg/ml	+2%	+48%	+3%	—
Farish et al, 1984[60]	Oophorectomized women 36–54 yrs	14	6 mos	50.0 mg	Estradiol implant	369 pmol/l	−3%	+7%	−6%	−8%
		14	4 mos	50.0 mg	Estradiol implant	339 pmol/l	−5%	+5%	−9%	−4%
Sharf et al, 1985[58]	Oophorectomized women 41–55 yrs.	8	14 wks	100.0 mg	Estradiol implant	306/pg/ml	−12%	+32%	−31%	−1%

remain unclear. Oral estrogens are absorbed by the intestines, and the concentration of estrogen in the portal system is four to five times higher than the concentration observed in the general circulation.[64] It has been hypothesized that the high level of portal estrogens stimulates the liver to produce the typical hepatic and gonadotropin effects (e.g., changes in levels of sex hormone-binding globulin, renin substrate, FSH, and LH) and to alter lipid and lipoprotein levels as well. It is not clear why estrogen pellets, but not vaginally or cutaneously administered estrogens, cause significant lipoprotein effects. Pellet estrogens are thought to be absorbed into the same lower abdominal circulation as are vaginally and cutaneously administered estrogens. Serum estradiol has been shown to reach high levels whether the administration was by percutaneous gel or subdermal pellet.[47, 56, 58] It is probable that peak or bolus concentrations in the portal system derived from pellet estrogen reach super-physiologic levels; these levels may be similar to those derived from oral estrogen.

UNOPPOSED ORAL PROGESTIN THERAPY

During the 1970s, estrogen therapy fell into disfavor among many physicians because of a combination of factors. First, studies of nonphysiologic doses of estrogens in men were shown to increase the risk of nonfatal CHD;[65–67] second, the estrogen content of oral contraceptives was implicated in thrombogenesis;[68, 69] and third, estrogens were shown to increase the risk of endometrial cancer in postmenopausal women.[70–71] The discovery that progestins could reverse estrogen-induced endometrial hyperplasia and decrease the risk of uterine cancer mandated that these agents be prescribed in women with intact uteri who needed estrogen therapy.

However, some practitioners became reluctant to prescribe any (opposed or unopposed) estrogen therapy for their patients. Because progestins have been shown to be relatively effective at reducing menopausal symptoms,[72–74] and are thought to have a positive effect on bone mass[75] as well as preventing endometrial hyperplasia and carcinomas,[76, 77] these agents have been proposed as effective menopausal agents for women in whom estrogen therapy is contraindicated.

Although there are a relative large number of progestins and progestin-like agents, only a few synthetic formulations are commonly used in the treatment of menopausal symptoms. Two of these compounds, norgestrel and norethisterone, are 19-nor steroids, and the third, medroxyprogesterone acetate or Provera, is a 17α hydroxyprogesterone derivative. The 19-nor steroids have pronounced androgenic and antiestrogenic effects, while medroxyprogesterone acetate is presumed to have little androgenic effect.[78]

Unopposed Oral Progestins and Lipids and Lipoproteins.—(The effect on lipids and lipoproteins of combined estrogen-progestin therapy are presented later.) Unfortunately, only a small number of studies have evaluated the effects of unopposed oral progestin on lipid and lipoprotein levels. Those studies are summarized in Table 14–7.[24, 79–81]

Both 19-nor derivatives (norgestrel and norethisterone) markedly decrease HDL-C levels (25%–31%) in postmenopausal women, and modestly increase LDL-C levels (6%–13%). These specific changes in lipoprotein patterns should be avoided since they are associated with an increased risk of CHD.

Spellacy and others would claim that the less androgenic medroxyprogesterone acetate is not associated with adverse lipid and lipoprotein changes.[79, 82, 83] This thesis is based on observations that total cholesterol is only slightly increased and triglycerides are modestly decreased with unopposed progestin therapy. Those reports did not examine

TABLE 14–7.

Adjusted* Percent Change in Lipoproteins by Unopposed Progestins

TYPE OF PROGESTIN	NUMBER OF STUDIES	PERCENT CHANGE IN HDL-C	LDL-C
Norethisterone[24, 79]	2	−31%	+13%
Norgestrel[79–81]	3	−25%	+6%
Medroxyprogesterone acetate[79–80]	2	−13%	—

*Adjusted for size and duration of study.

the subfractions of cholesterol; the modest changes in total cholesterol levels appear to be the result of simultaneous decreases in HDL-C and increases in LDL-C. When the lipoprotein fractions are specifically examined, HDL-C levels were decreased an average of 13% in women using oral medroxyprogesterone acetate alone.[79, 80] Unfortunately, LDL-C levels were not measured in these studies. (A closer reading of these reports reveals that most authors find no statistically significant adverse effect of medroxyprogesterone acetate on lipids and lipoproteins; however, due to very small sample sizes, all of the studies reviewed had less than a 5% chance of detecting a statistically significant decrease in HDL-C levels.) Since HDL-C is the most powerful predictor of CHD in middle-aged and older women, the impact of lowering HDL-C levels even 13% may be substantial.

Like estrogen, the effects of unopposed medroxyprogesterone acetate on lipids and lipoproteins may also be related to dose and route of administration. In one report, massive doses of medroxyprogesterone acetate (4,000 mg/month) given to women for treatment of uterine cancer induced a significant decrease in HDL-C levels.[84] (Post-menopausal women usually receive 100–140 mg/month). It is also unclear whether medroxyprogesterone acetate given intramuscularly adversely influences lipids and lipoproteins. One study has reported that HDL-C levels were significantly decreased after depo-medroxyprogesterone acetate therapy (150 mg every three months).[85] Another report using the same dosage found no change in HDL-C levels with this route of administration.[86] Again, further studies are needed to clarify the association between dose and route of unopposed medroxyprogesterone acetate use and lipid and lipoprotein levels.

Unopposed Progestins and HDL-C Subfractions.—One report in the literature evaluated the effects of norgestrel and medroxyprogesterone acetate on HDL_2 and HDL_3 subfractions.[81] In a sample of eight women, norgestrel lowered total HDL-C by 17%, HDL_2 by 30%, and HDL_3 by 7%. In comparison, use of medroxyprogesterone acetate decreased total HDL-C by 9%, HDL_2 by 8%, and HDL_3 by 10%.

From these studies it seems clear that unopposed oral 19 norprogestogens for the relief of menopausal symptoms should be avoided in most women. Use of unopposed medroxyprogesterone acetate for women with absolute contraindications for estrogen therapy may be acceptable if the lipoprotein profile is not adversely affected. Use of any unopposed progestin should be avoided in women who have very low (hypo-α) HDL-C levels prior to initiation of therapy.

COMBINED ESTROGEN AND PROGESTIN THERAPY

Current recommendations for menopausal therapy state that the lowest possible dose of estrogen be given for the first 25 days of the month, with the addition of a progestin to the regimen during the last 10 days of estrogen therapy.[87] Estrogens and progestins should be discontinued during the last five days of the month.

Currently, the addition of progestin to the estrogen therapy is solely for the protection of the endometrium. Therefore, women who have had a hysterectomy and thus are no longer at risk for uterine disease need not take a progestin. (Between 30% and 40% of menopausal women have had a prior hysterectomy).

A summary of the studies which have examined the impact on lipoproteins of various noncontraceptive estrogen/progestin formulations is presented in Table 14–8.[78, 79, 88–91] (Given that lipoproteins are more specific predictors of CHD, only those studies that reported estrogen/progestin effects on lipoproteins are addressed.) All of the studies reviewed here have very small sample sizes, and thus inferences made from these reports must be offered cautiously.

Although there is substantial variation in the results, it appears that even in the presence of estrogens, both norgestrel and norethisterone adversely affect HDL-C levels. For example, when estradiol valerate (2 mg/day) is given as an unopposed oral agent, HDL-C is increased by about 15%; however when norgestrel (0.25 mg–0.50 mg) is cycled with the estradiol valerate, the beneficial effect on HDL-C is not only negated but overwhelmed, as HDL is decreased an average of 10% from baseline. A similar effect on HDL-C is seen when norethisterone is cycled with estradiol valerate. That is, HDL-C is increased 15% over baseline with unopposed estradiol valerate and is decreased an average of 28% below baseline when norethisterone (10 mg) is added to the schedule. Even the addition of medroxyprogesterone acetate (10 mg) to a regimen of estradiol valerate negates any estrogen-induced beneficial change in HDL-C.

One study has reported that cycling 10 mg of medroxyprogesterone acetate with Premarin (conjugated equine estrogens) does not negate the estrogen-induced effects on HDL-C and LDL-C levels.[91] Unfortunately, these researchers did not specify when in the regimen lipid determinations were made. If samples were drawn during unopposed estrogen therapy, then the results would reflect estrogen effects only. In another study

TABLE 14–8.

Effects* of Noncontraceptive Cyclic Estrogen-Progestin Therapy on Lipoprotein Levels

AGENTS (ESTROGEN/PROGESTIN)	DOSE/DAY	REFERENCES	N†	PERCENT CHANGE FROM BASELINE	
				HDL	LDL
Estradiol valerate	2 mg	78,88	26	− 10%	
Norgestrel	0.25–0.50 mg				
Piperazine estrone sulfate	1.25 mg	89	9	− 8%	− 27%
Norgestrel	0.30 mg				
Estradiol valerate	2 mg	79,88	17	− 28%	+ 30%
Norethisterone	10 mg				
17β-estradiol	2 mg	90	9	− 14%	− 7%
Norethisterone	1 mg				
Estradiol valerate	2 mg	78,88	26	+ 1%	
Medroxyprogesterone	10 mg				
Premarin®	0.625–1.25 mg	91	20	+ 14%	− 16%
Medroxyprogesterone	10 mg				
Ethinylestradiol	0.3 mg	78	19	+ 16%	
Medroxyprogesterone	10 mg				

*Adjusted for size and duration of study
†Total number of women in study

in which lipid/lipoprotein determinations were done after completion of the progestin cycle, the addition of 10 mg medroxyprogesterone acetate to 2 mg of estradiol valerate negated (but did not overwhelm) the estrogen-induced effect on HDL-C.[79]

The ability of the progestin to negate and/or overwhelm any beneficial estrogen-induced changes in lipids and lipoproteins may be a function of the type and dose of estrogen used, as well as type of progestin. As noted above, Ottosson reported that an 8% increase in HDL-C induced by unopposed estradiol valerate was negated with a 10 mg/day dose of medroxyprogesterone acetate. However, when 30 μg of ethinylestradiol were cycled with the same dose of medroxyprogesterone acetate, only a slight decrease in HDL-C levels occurred.[79] Such doses of estrogen are appropriate for contraceptive purposes but are too potent for routine menopausal use.

In summary, medroxyprogesterone acetate (10 mg) cycled with estradiol valerate or other natural estrogens is appropriate for women with intact uteri and who are normolipidemic at baseline. However, such women cannot be expected to benefit from any estrogen-induced changes in lipoprotein profiles, since even this less-androgenic progestin has been shown to negate any beneficial estrogen·effect.

Given our current knowledge, there is no compelling reason to prescribe a progestin for women who, because of a prior hysterectomy, are without uteri. These women, who perhaps are at increased risk of CHD because of their surgery, may significantly benefit from a more favorable lipoprotein profile induced by unopposed estrogens. Finally, it has been suggested that women with significant hyperlipidemia may be treated for this disorder with unopposed natural estrogens.[92] In such cases, the addition of any progestin would interfere with estrogen-induced changes and would be contraindicated. Such women with intact uteri would need to be followed carefully for possible uterine disorders.

AGENTS USED TO TREAT OSTEOPOROSIS

Consideration of any drug for long-term use to prevent or treat osteoporosis should include the possible effects that drug may have on lipid and lipoprotein levels. The anabolic steroid stanozolol has been shown to increase bone mass in postmenopausal osteoporosis.[93] This steroid and two other related steroids, danazol and oxandrolone, have been shown to have adverse effects on lipoproteins.[93–95] For example, stanozolol has been shown to reduce total HDL-C by 53%, and HDL$_2$ by 85%.[94] Consequently, caution should be used in consideration of these drugs for long-term therapy, especially in younger menopausal women.

AGENTS USED TO TREAT HYPERTENSION

Diuretics.—Both chlorthalidone and the thiazide diuretics have been shown to increase significantly total serum cholesterol and LDL-C.[96–99] In one large study, chlorthalidone users had an average increase of 10 mg/dl of total cholesterol and an increase of 13 mg/dl of LDL-C.[96] In another report, both chlothalidone and hydrochlorothiazide were found to increase total cholesterol levels an average of 11 mg/dl.[97] These adverse effects of diuretic use were confirmed in a crossover, randomized, controlled trial.[98] However, in this same trial, it was reported that a cholesterol-lowering diet can largely prevent the diuretic-induced increase in total cholesterol and LDL-C levels. This latter result suggests that patients needing these specific antihypertensive agents should also be prescribed a cholesterol-lowering diet.

β-*blockers.*—β-blockers as well as diuretics are also considered as a first line of treatment for hypertension, and these agents have been shown to substantially alter serum lipid and lipoprotein levels.[100–106] Most studies demonstrate a uniform pattern of lipoprotein response induced by β-blockers, e.g., reduced HDL-C and increased VLDL-C.[104–105] These changes in lipid and lipoprotein levels may be substantial; for example, in one large cross-sectional study, HDL-C levels were 12 mg/dl lower in women using propranolol than in nonusers.[100]

Adverse lipoprotein responses have been reported with both nonselective (propranolol and exprenolol) and selective (atenolol and metaprolol) β-blockers.[106] It has been suggested that the increased levels of VLDL-C and decreased levels of HDL-C seen with all β-blockers is due to unopposed α-stimulation. Such stimulation may result in inhibition of adipose tissue lipase activity. This hypothesis is supported by the finding that an α-blocking antihypertensive, prazosin, reduces VLDL-C.[106]

Two other antihypertensive medications have been examined for their effects on lipids and lipoproteins. Aldomet is reported to have no effect on lipid levels, whereas hydralazine apparently lowers total cholesterol levels by about 11%.[107, 108] The effect of these two agents on lipoprotein levels has not been investigated.

To date, only one study has reported the combined effect of a diuretic and hormones on lipid and lipoprotein levels.[109] In this clinical trial, the thiazide diuretic (bendroflumethiazide) increased serum cholesterol levels, whereas the hormonal replacement therapy (a sequential estradiol-norethindrone regimen) decreased serum cholesterol. When the protocol included both the diuretic and hormones, serum cholesterol was slightly decreased. Blood pressures were significantly reduced with the thiazide (alone or in combination with the hormones); however, hormone therapy alone also induced a similar decrease in diastolic (but not systolic) pressures. Unfortunately, lipids and lipoproteins were not evaluated. This finding that estrogens may decrease blood pressure levels has also been reported in other studies.[110, 111]

It should not be inferred from these findings (e.g., that most antihypertensive medications have adverse effects on lipid and lipoprotein levels) that hypertension should not be treated. Rather, alternatives to drug therapy should be of special significance in minimally hypertensive menopausal women. In such cases, weight loss, exercise, and diminished alcohol intake may substantially lower blood pressure levels and should be the initial prescription. The patient should be fully counseled as to why these modalities are more preferable than drugs for blood pressure control.

For women who need drug therapy to control their blood pressures, a cholesterol-lowering diet should accompany the prescription for a diuretic or β-blocker. Given the results of the clinical trial reported above, it may be that the safest treatment for mild to moderate hypertension in menopausal women is indeed estrogen replacement (contrary to previous thought based on oral-contraceptive literature).

LIPID CHANGES DUE TO OTHER DRUGS

The benzodiazepine drugs are widely used by persons of all ages. Those most commonly used are diazepam, chlordiazepoxide, and flurazepam. A study from the Lipid Research Clinics Program Prevalence Study reported that men taking benzodiazepines, when compared to nonusers, had significantly higher mean triglyceride and VLDL-C levels and significantly lower mean HDL-C levels.[112] Women taking these drugs also had significantly higher triglyceride and VLDL-C levels and lower (but not significantly so) HDL-C levels. Because of the widespread use of these agents in the general population, the authors suggest that benzodiazepine use has the potential to affect cardiovascular risk negatively. Further research will be needed to clarify the importance of these findings.

Clonidine, a central α-adrenergic agonist initially prescribed for hypertension has been used successfully to treat menopausal flushing.[113] Unfortunately, the effect of clonidine on lipids and lipoproteins are unknown. As with most pharmacologic agents used in the menopausal years, studies of the impact of clonidine on lipid and lipoprotein levels are needed.

CONCLUSION

The purpose of this chapter was to review the effects of frequently used pharmacologic agents on lipid and lipoprotein levels in menopausal women. It was seen that hormones used to treat menopausal symptoms as well as agents used in the treatment of hypertension, osteoporosis, and anxiety can have significant beneficial or adverse impacts on lipid and lipoprotein levels. Given that coronary heart disease is the major killer of menopausal women and that lipids and lipoproteins are major determinants of CHD, physicians who treat menopausal women need to be aware of the lipid-altering properties of these agents.

REFERENCES

1. The Pooling Project Research Group: Relationship of blood pressure, serum cholesterol, smoking habit, relative weight and ECG abnormalities to incidence of major coronary events: Final report of the Pooling Project. *Am Heart Assoc Monograph* 1978; No. 60.
2. Keys A: Coronary heart disease in seven countries. *Circulation* 1970; 41(Suppl 1):1–211.
3. Kannel WB, Castelli WP, Gordon T, et al: Serum cholesterol, lipoproteins and the risk of coronary heart disease. *Ann Intern Med* 1971; 74:1–12.
4. McGee D: The probability of developing certain cardiovascular disease in eight years at specified values of some characteristics, in Kannel WB, Gordon T (eds): *The Framingham Study: An Epidemiological Investigation of Cardiovascular Disease.* US DHEW 1973; Pub No. 74–618: Section 27.
5. Lipid Research Clinics Program. The Lipid Research Clinics Coronary Primary Prevention Trial Results II. The relationship of reduction in incidence of coronary heart disease to cholesterol lowering. *JAMA* 1984; 251:365–74.
6. Beard RJ: Estrogens and the cardiovascular system, in Beard RJ (ed): *The Menopause: A Guide to Current Research and Practice.* Baltimore, University Park Press, 1976, pp 81–94.
7. Heyden S, Heiss G, Hames CG, et al: Fasting triglycerides as predictors of total and CHD mortality in Evans County, Georgia. *J Chronic Dis* 1980; 33:275–82.
8. Gordon T, Castelli WP, Hjortland MC, et al: High density lipoprotein as a protective factor against coronary heart disease: The Framingham Study. *Am J Med* 1977; 62:707–14.
9. Miller NE, Thelle DS, Forde OH, et al: The Thromso Heart Study. High-density lipoprotein and coronary heart disease: a prospective case-control study. *Lancet* 1977; 1:965–8.
10. Rhoads GG, Gulbrandsen CL, Kagan A: Serum lipoproteins and coronary heart disease in a population study of Hawaii Japanese men. *N Engl J Med* 1976; 294:293–8.
11. Ballantyne FC, Clark RS, Simpson HS, et al: High density and low density lipoprotein subfractions in survivors of myocardial infarction and in control subjects. *Metabolism* 1982; 31:433–7.
12. Rosenberg L, Shapiro S, Kaufman DW, et al: Patterns and determinants of conjugated estrogen use. *Am J Epidemiol* 1979; 109:676–86.
13. Markush RE, Turner SL: Epidemiology of exogenous estrogens. *HSMHA Health Rep* 1971; 86:74–86.
14. Stadel BV, Weiss N: Characteristics of menopausal women: A survey of King and Pierce Counties in Washington, 1973–74. *Am J Epidemiol* 1975; 102:209–16.

15. Kennedy DL, Baum C, Forbes MB: Noncontraceptive estrogens and progestins: Use patterns over time. *Obstet Gynecol* 1985; 65:441–6.
16. Pasley BH, Standfast SJ, Katz SH: Prescribing estrogen during menopause: Physician survey of practices in 1974 and 1981. *Public Health Rep* 1984; 99:424–9.
17. Bush TL, Barrett-Connor E: Noncontraceptive estrogens and cardiovascular disease. *Epidemiol Rev* 1985; 7:80–104.
18. Barr DP, Russ EM, Eder HA: Influence of estrogens on lipoproteins in atherosclerosis. *Trans Assoc Am Physicians* 1952; 65:102–13.
19. Oliver MF, Boyd GS: Influence of reduction of serum lipids on prognosis of coronary heart disease: a five year study using oestrogen. *Lancet* 1961; 2:499–505.
20. Coronary Drug Project Research Group. The Coronary Drug Project: Initial findings leading to modifications of its research protocol. *JAMA* 1970; 214:1303–13.
21. Notelovitz M, Gudat JC, Ware MD, et al: Lipids and lipoproteins in women after oophorectomy and the response to oestrogen therapy. *Br J Obstet Gynecol* 1983; 90:171–7.
22. Bolton CH, Ellwood M, Hartog M, et al: Comparison of the effects of ethinyl oestradiol and conjugated equine oestrogens in oophorectomized women. *Clin Endocrinol* 1975; 4:131–8.
23. Campagnoli C, Tousijn P, Belforte P, et al: Effects of conjugated equine oestrogens and oestriol on blood clotting, plasma lipids and endometrial proliferation in post-menopausal women. *Maturitas* 1981; 3:135–44.
24. Bradley DD, Wingerd J, Petitti DB, et al: Serum high-density-lipoprotein cholesterol in women using oral contraceptives, estrogens and progestins. *N Engl J Med* 1978; 299: 17–20.
25. Cauley JA, LePorte RE, Kuller LH, et al: Menopausal estrogen use, high density lipoprotein cholesterol subfractions and liver function. *Atherosclerosis* 1983; 49:31–9.
26. Lind T, Cameron EC, Hunter WM, et al: A prospective controlled trial of six forms of hormone replacement therapy given to postmenopausal women. *Br J Obstet Gynaecol* 1979; [Suppl]3:1–26.
27. McConathy WJ, Alaupovic P: The effect of oestrogens on the plasma lipoprotein system in premenopausal and postmenopausal women, in Greenhalgh RM (ed): *Hormones and Vascular Disease*. London, Pitman Medical, 1981, pp 319–30.
28. Paterson MEL, Sturdee DW, Moore B, et al: The effect of various regimens of hormone therapy on serum cholesterol and triglyceride concentrations in postmenopausal women. *Br J Obstet Gynecol* 1980; 87:552–60.
29. Robinson RW, Lebeau RJ: Effect of conjugated equine estrogens on serum lipids and the clotting mechanism. *J Atheroscler Res* 1965; 5:120–4.
30. Wahl P, Walden C, Knopp R, et al: Effect of estrogen/progestin potency on lipid/lipoprotein cholesterol. *N Engl J Med* 1983; 308:862–7.
31. Wallentin L, Larsson-Cohn V: Metabolic and hormonal effects of postmenopausal oestrogen replacement treatment. II. Plasma lipids. *Acta Endocrinol (Copenh)* 1977; 86:597–607.
32. Silfverstolpe G, Gustafson A, Samsioe G, et al: Lipid and carbohydrate metabolism studies in oophorectomized women: Effects produced by the addition of norethisterone acetate to two estrogen preparations. *Arch Gynecol* 1982; 231:279–87.
33. Saunders DM, Hunter JC, Shutt DA, et al: The effect of oestradiol valerate therapy on coagulation factors and lipid and oestrogen levels in oophorectomised women. Aust NZJ *Obstet Gynecol* 1978; 18:198–201.
34. Vilska S, Punnonen R, Rauramo L: Long-term post-menopausal hormone therapy and serum HDL-C, total cholesterol and triglycerides. *Maturitas* 1983; 5:97–104.
35. Tikkanen MJ, Kuusi T, Vartiainen E, et al: The treatment of post-menopausal hypercholesterolaemia with estradiol. *Acta Obstet Gynecol Scand* 1979; 88(Suppl):83–8.
36. Saarikoski S, Niemela A, Jokela H, et al: Effect of oestriol succinate on serum lipids. *Maturitas* 1981; 3:325–9.
37. Borglin NE, Staland B: Oral treatment of menopausal symptoms with natural oestrogens: Experiences with a new series of oestrogens and oestrogen-gestagen combinations. *Acta Obstet Gynecol Scand* 1975; 43(Suppl):1–11.
38. Isaacs AJ, Havard CWH: Effect of piperazine oestrone sulphate on serum lipids and lipoproteins in menopausal women. *Acta Endocrinol* 1977; 85:143–50.
39. Lagrelius A, Johnson P, Lunell N-O, et al: Treatment with oral estrone sulphate in the female climacteric. *Acta Obstet Gynecol Scand* 1981; 60:27–31.

40. Marmorston J, Magidson O, Lewis JJ, et al: Effect of small doses of estrogen on serum lipids in female patients with myocardial infarction. *N Engl J Med* 1958; 258:583–7.

41. Blumenfeld Z, Aviram M, Brook GJ, et al: Changes in lipoproteins and subfractions following oophorectomy and estrogen replacement in perimenopausal women. *Maturitas* 1983; 5:77–83.

42. Hart DM, Farish E, Fletcher CD, et al: Ten years post-menopause hormone replacement therapy—effect on lipoproteins. *Maturitas* 1984; 5:271–6.

43. Aitken JM, Lorimer AR, Hart DMc, et al: The effects of oophorectomy and long-term mestranol therapy on the serum lipids of middle-aged women. *Clin Sci* 1971; 41: 597–603.

44. Quirk JG Jr, Wendel GD Jr: Biologic effects of natural and synthetic estrogens, in Buchsbaum HJ (ed): *The Menopause*. New York, Springer-Verlag, 1983, pp 55–75.

45. Lebech PE: Effects and side-effects of estrogen therapy, in vanKeep PE, Greenblatt RB, Albeaux-Fernet M (eds): *Consensus on Menopause Research*. Baltimore, University Park Press, 1976, pp 44–56.

46. Lauritzen CH: The female climacteric syndrome: Significance, problems, treatment. *Acta Obstet Gynecol Scand* 1976; 51(Suppl):47–57.

47. Fahraeus L, Wallentin L: High density lipoprotein subfractions during oral and cutaneous administration of 17β-estradiol to menopausal women. *J Clin Endocrinol Metab* 1983; 56:797–801.

48. Martin PL, Yen SSC, Burnier AM, et al: Systemic absorption and sustained effects of vaginal estrogen creams. *JAMA* 1979; 242:2699–700.

49. Martin PL, Greaney MD, Burnier AM, et al: Estradiol, estrone and gonadotropin levels after use of vaginal estradiol. *Obstet Gynecol* 1984; 63:441–4.

50. Deutsch S, Ossowski R, Benjamin I: Comparison between degree of systemic absorption of vaginally and orally administered estrogen at different dose levels in postmenopausal women. *Am J Obstet Gynecol* 1981; 139:967–8.

51. Rigg LA, Herman H, Yen SSC: Absorption of estrogens from vaginal creams. *N Engl J Med* 1978; 198:195–7.

52. Ahren T, Victor HL, Vessby B, et al: Ovarian function, bleeding control and serum lipoproteins in women using contraceptive vaginal rings releasing five different progestins. *Contraception* 1983; 28:315–27.

53. Stumpf PG, Maruca J, Santen RS, et al: Development of a vaginal ring for achieving physiologic levels of 17β estradiol in hypoestrogenic women. *J Clin Endocrinol Metab* 1982; 54:208–10.

54. Fahraeus L, Larsson-Cohn U, Wallentin L: Lipoproteins during oral and cutaneous administration of estradiol-17β to menopausal women. *Acta Endocrinol* (Kbl) 1982; 101:597–602.

55. Elkik F, Gompel A, Mercier-Bodard C, et al: Effects of percutaneous estradiol and conjugated estrogens on the level of plasma proteins and triglycerides in postmenopausal women. *Am J Obstet Gynecol* 1982; 143:888–92.

56. Basdevant A, DeLignieres B, Guy-Grand B: Differential lipemic and hormonal responses to oral and parenteral 17 beta estradiol in postmenopausal women. *Am J Obstet Gynecol* 1983; 147:77–81.

57. Holst J, Cajander S, Carlstrom K, et al: A comparison of liver protein induction on postmenopausal women during oral and percutaneous estrogen replacement therapy. *Br J Obstet Gynecol* 1983; 90:355–60.

58. Sharf M, Oettinger M, Lanir A, et al: Lipid and lipoprotein levels following pure estradiol implantation in post menopausal women. *Gynecol Obstet Invest* 1985; 19:207–12.

59. Lobo RA, March CM, Goebelsmann UT, et al: Subdermal estradiol pellets following hysterectomy and oophorectomy. *Am J Obstet Gynecol* 1980; 138:714–9.

60. Farish E, Fletcher CD, Hart DM, et al: The effects of hormone implants on serum lipoproteins and steroid hormones in bilaterally oophorectomized women. *Acta Endocrinol* 1984; 106:116–20.

61. Mandel FP, Geola FL, Meldrum DR, et al: Biological effects of various doses of vaginally administered conjugated equine estrogens in postmenopausal women. *J Clin Endocrinol Metab* 1983; 57:133–9.

62. Glueck CJ, Scheel D, Fishbach J, et al: Estrogen-induced pancreatitis in patients with previously covert familial type V hyperlipidemia. *Metabolism* 1972; 21:657–66.

63. Thom M, Dubiel M, Kakkar VV, et al: The effects of different regimens of estrogen on the clotting and fibrinolytic system of the postmenopausal woman. *Front Horm Res* 1978; 5:192–8.
64. Pasetto N, Piccione EM, Pasetto F, et al: Treatment of patients at risk. Crossover study between natural estrogens, in Pasetto N, Paoletti R, Ambrus JL (eds): *The Menopause and Postmenopause*. Lancaster, England, MTP Press Ltd, 1980, pp 141–50.
65. Coronary Drug Project Research Group: The Coronary Drug Project: Initial findings leading to modifications of its research protocol. *JAMA* 1970; 214:1303–13.
66. Blackard CE, Doe RP, Mellinger GT, et al: Incidence of cardiovascular disease and death in patients receiving diethylstilbestrol for carcinoma of the prostate. *Cancer* 1970; 26: 249–56.
67. The Veterans Administration Co-operative Urological Research Group: Treatment and survival of patients with cancer of the prostate. *Surg Gynecol Obstet* 1967; 124:1011–17.
68. Inman WH, Vessey MP, Westerholm B, et al: Thromboembolic disease and the steroidal content of oral contraceptives: A report to the Committee on Safety of Drugs. *Br Med J* 1970; 2:203–9.
69. Sartwell PE: Oral contraceptives and thromboembolism: A further report. *Am J Epidemiol* 1971; 94:192–201.
70. Ziel HK, Finkle WD: Increased risk of endometrial carcinoma among users of conjugated estrogens. *N Engl J Med* 1975; 293:1167–70.
71. Smith DC, Prentice R, Thompson DJ, et al: Association of exogenous estrogen and endometrial carcinoma. *N Engl J Med* 1975; 293:1164–7.
72. Bullock JL, Massey FM, Cambrell RD Jr: Use of medroxyprogesterone acetate to prevent menopausal symptoms. *Obstet Gynecol* 1975; 46:165–9.
73. Paterson MEL: A randomized double-blind cross-over trial into the effects of norethisterone on climacteric symptoms. *Br J Obstet Gynaecol* 1982; 89:496–501.
74. Lobo RA, McCormick W, Singer F, et al: Depo-medroxyprogesterone acetate compared with conjugated estrogens for the treatment of postmenopausal women. *Obstet Gynecol* 1984; 63:1–4.
75. Mandel FR, Davidson BS, Erlik Y, et al: Effect of progestins on bone metabolism in postmenopausal women. *J Reprod Med* 1982; 27:511–6.
76. Gambrell RD: Estrogens, progestogens, and endometrial cancer. *J Reprod Med* 1977; 18:301–6.
77. Wentz WB: Progestin therapy in endometrial hyperplasia. *Gynecol Oncol* 1974; 2:362–7.
78. Ottosson UB: Oral progesterone and estrogen/progestogen therapy. *Acta Obstet Gynecol Scand* 1984; [Suppl] 127:5–37.
79. Silfverstolpe G, Gustafson A, Samsioe G, et al: Lipid metabolic studies in oophorectomized women: Effects on serum lipids and lipoproteins of three synthetic progestogens. *Maturitas* 1982; 4:103–11.
80. Tikkanen MJ, Nikkila EA, Kuusi T, et al: Different effects of two progestins on plasma high density lipoprotein (HDL$_2$) and postheparin plasma hepatic lipase activity. *Atherosclerosis* 1981; 40:365–9.
81. Kuusi T, Tikkanen MJ, Nikkila EA, et al: Progestagens and high-density lipoproteins. *Lancet* 1984; 2:1163.
82. Spellacy WN, Newton RE, Buhi WC, et al: Lipid and carbohydrate metabolic studies after one year of megestrol treatment. *Fertil Steril* 1976; 27:157–61.
83. Spellacy WN, Buhi WC, Birk SA: The effects of norgestrel on carbohydrate and lipid metabolism over one year. *Am J Obstet Gynecol* 1976; 125:984–6.
84. Crona N, Enk L, Samsioe G, et al: High-dose depo-medroxyprogesterone acetate—effects on lipid and lipoprotein metabolism. *Eur J Obstet Gynecol Reprod Biol* 1983; 16:97–104.
85. Kremer J, deBruijn HWA, Hindriks FR: Serum high-density lipoprotein cholesterol levels in women using a contraceptive injection of depo-medroxyprogesterone acetate. *Contraception* 1980; 22:359–65.
86. Barnes RB, Roy S, Lobo RA: Comparison of lipid and androgen levels after conjugated estrogen or depo-medroxyprogesterone acetate treatment in menopausal women. *Obstet Gynecol* 1985; 66:216–9.
87. Gambrell RD Jr: The menopause: Benefits and risks of estrogen-progesterone replacement therapy. *Fertil Steril* 1982; 37:457–74.

88. Hirvonen E, Malkonen M, Manninen V: Effects of different progestogens on lipoproteins during postmenopause replacement therapy. *N Engl J Med* 1981; 304:560–3.

89. Wren B, Garrett D: The effect of low-dose piperazine oestrone sulphate and low-dose levonorgestrel on blood lipid levels in postmenopausal women. *Maturitas* 1985; 7:141–6.

90. Mattsson LA, Samsioe G: Estrogen-progestogen replacement in climacteric women, particularly as regards a new type of continuous regimen. *Acta Obstet Gynecol Scand* 1985; 130(Suppl):53–8.

91. Notelovitz M, Gudat JC, Ware MD, et al: Oestrogen-progestin therapy and the lipid balance of post-menopausal women. *Maturitas* 1982; 4:301–8.

92. Tikkanen MJ, Nikkila EA: Natural oestrogen as an effective treatment for type II hyperlipoproteinaemia in postmenopausal women. *Lancet* 1978; 2:490–1.

93. Chestnut CH, Baylink DJ, Nelp WB: Stanozolol therapy in postmenopausal osteoporosis. Preliminary results. *Clin Res* 1979; 26:363A.

94. Taggert HMcA, Applebaum-Bowden D, Haffner S, et al: Reduction in high density lipoproteins by anabolic-steroid (stanozolol) therapy for postmenopausal osteoporosis. *Metabolism* 1982; 31:1147–50.

95. Allen JK, Frazer IS: Cholesterol, high density lipoproteins, and danazol. *J Clin Endocrinol Metab* 1981; 53:149–53.

96. Goldman AI, Steele BW, Schnaper HW, et al: Serum lipoprotein levels during chlorthalidone therapy. *JAMA* 1980; 244:1691–5.

97. Ames RP, Hill P: Elevation of serum lipid levels during diuretic therapy of hypertension. *Am J Med* 1976; 61:748–57.

98. Grimm RH, Leon AS, Hunninghake DB, et al: Effects of thiazide diuretics on plasma lipids and lipoproteins in mildly hypertensive patients. *Ann Intern Med* 1981; 94:7–11.

99. Rosenthal T, Holtzman E, Segal P: The effect of chlorthalidone on serum lipids and lipoproteins. *Atherosclerosis* 1980; 36:111–5.

100. Wallace RB, Hunninghake DB, Reiland S: Alterations of plasma high-density lipoprotein cholesterol levels associated with consumption of selected medications. *Circulation* 1980; 62(Suppl IV):77–84.

101. Arnesen E, Thelle D, Forde OH, et al: Serum lipids and glucose concentrations in subjects using antihypertensive drugs. Finnmark 1977. *J Epidemiol Comm Health* 1983; 37:141–4.

102. Rossnererand WL: Atenolol and metoprolol: Comparisons of effects on blood pressure and serum lipoproteins, and side effects. *Eur J Clin Pharmacol* 1983; 24:573–7.

103. Laren P, Helgeland A, Holme I, et al: Effect of propranolol and prazosin on blood lipids. The Oslo Study. *Lancet* 1980; 2:4–6.

104. Rossner S: Serum lipoproteins and ischemic vascular disease: On the interpretation of serum lipid versus serum lipoprotein concentrations. *J Cardiovasc Pharmacol* 1982; 4(Suppl 2):S201–5.

105. Johnson BF: The emerging problem of plasma lipid changes during antihypertensive therapy. *J Cardiovasc Pharmacol* 1982; (Suppl 3):S213–21.

106. Day JL, Metcalfe J, Simpson CN: Andrenergic mechanism in control of plasma lipid concentrations. *Br Med J* 1984; 2:1145–8.

107. Libman LF, Dormandy TL, Arrowsmith DE, et al: Blood lipids and the treatment of essential hypertension with methyldopa and bendrofluazide. *Postgrad Med J* 1974; 50:671–4.

108. Perry HM Jr, Mills EJ: The effect of oral hydralazine in circulating human cholesterol. *Am J Med Sci* 1962; 243:564–73.

109. Christiansen C, Christiansen MS, Hagen C, et al: Effects of natural estrogen/progestagen and thiazide on coronary risk factors in normal postmenopausal women. *Acta Obstet Gynecol Scand* 1981; 60:407–12.

110. Wren BG, Routledge AD: The effect of type and dose of estrogen on the blood pressure of postmenopausal women. *Maturitas* 1983; 5:135–42.

111. Pfeffer RI, Kurosaki TT, Charlton SK: Estrogen use and blood pressure in later life. *Am J Epidemiol* 1979; 110:469–78.

112. Hunninghake DB, Wallace RB, Reiland S, et al: Alterations of plasma lipid and lipoprotein levels associated with benzodiazepine use. The LRC Program Prevalence Study. *Atherosclerosis* 1981; 40:159.

113. Hammar M, Berg G: Clonidine in the treatment of menopausal flushing. A review of clinical studies. *Acta Obstet Gynecol Scand* 1985; 132(Suppl):29–31.

CHAPTER 15

Estrogen Use and Cardiovascular Disease

RONALD K. ROSS, M.D.
ANNLIA PAGANINI-HILL, Ph.D.
THOMAS M. MACK, M.D.
BRIAN E. HENDERSON, M.D.

ISCHEMIC HEART DISEASE is the number one cause of death in the United States.[1] However, it represents not a single disease entity but a complex of clinical syndromes, each of which has multiple known determinants. It is, therefore, a difficult subject for etiologic research. The possible role of estrogen in modifying the occurrence of ischemic heart disease has long been controversial. Despite decades of debate, we remain so ignorant about the role of estrogen in the etiology of ischemic heart disease that in recent reviews of the risks and benefits of estrogen replacement therapy ischemic heart disease has been cited as a hazard of such therapy,[2] as a benefit,[3] or the issue has simply been ignored.[4] While there is experimental evidence which can be interpreted as supporting both viewpoints, the epidemiologic literature overwhelmingly supports a beneficial effect, although the magnitude of the associated protection is undetermined.

Cardiovascular disease mortality has declined nearly 30% in the past 20 years.[1] The cause of this decline has been attributed both to improved medical care and changes in lifestyle,[5] although there is some evidence that the latter has been more important.[6] It is probable that multiple factors are actually involved, since the decline has occurred to a comparable degree in men and women and also in whites and nonwhites (Fig 15–1). It is highly doubtful that either lifestyle changes or access to more sophisticated diagnostic and treatment techniques have changed to a comparable degree among all four groups during this time period. Nonetheless, a marked decline in cardiovascular disease mortality in women is consistent with the increased prevalence of estrogen usage since 1960. Since men have shown a similar decrease in mortality, other factors associated with risk of coronary heart disease must have declined to a greater degree in men than in women. The prevalence of cigarette smoking, an important risk factor for coronary heart disease, decreased 26% in men but only 8% in women between the mid-1960s and mid-1970s. On the other hand, the proportion of adult women who were hypercholesterolemic decreased more during the same period than did the proportion of men.[1] The prevalence of other risk factors for coronary heart disease such as obesity, physical activity, and the ratio of low to high density lipoprotein cholesterol levels has almost certainly decreased as well, but the percent changes in men compared to women are not well documented.

In this review, we first discuss the relationship between estrogens and some of the well-established risk factors for ischemic heart disease. We then review the epidemio-

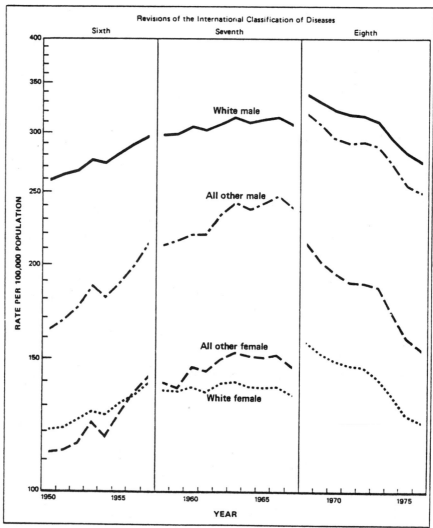

FIG 15–1.
Age adjusted mortality rates for ischemic heart disease by race and sex (United States, 1950–1976). (From the National Heart, Lung and Blood Institute Report by the Working Group of Heart Disease Epidemiology, NIH Publ No 79-1667, USDHEW, 1978.)

logic studies which have addressed the question of the association of estrogen use and heart disease directly. We also discuss related studies that provide indirect evidence of the possible influence of estrogen replacement therapy on the risk of cardiovascular disease. We end this review by estimating the impact of estrogen use on cardiovascular disease in the context of the other risks and benefits of such therapy.

ESTROGENS AND ISCHEMIC HEART DISEASE RISK FACTORS

The relationships of estrogens and ischemic heart disease risk factors are summarized in Table 15–1 and are individually discussed below.

TABLE 15–1.

Summary of the Relationships of Estrogen and
Ischemic Heart Disease Risk Factors

RISK FACTOR	ESTROGEN EFFECT
Lipid levels	↑ HDL cholesterol
	↓ LDL cholesterol
	↑ Triglyclerides
Hemostasis	↓ Antithrombin activity
Carbohydrate metabolism	↑ Fasting blood glucose
Blood pressure	↑ Renin substrate
Cigarette smoking	Early menopause
	↓ Urinary estrogens
Weight	↑ Circulating estrogens

Lipid Levels

The effects of exogenous hormones on lipid levels and lipid metabolism are extensively reviewed elsewhere in this volume. Early work in this area was concerned mainly
with oral contraceptives, in an effort to explain the increased risk of stroke, myocardial
infarction and other vascular diseases concurrent with such therapy. Oral contraceptives
increase serum triglycerides and cholesterol, the latter due primarily to higher concentrations of low-density lipoprotein (LDL) cholesterol.[7] These lipid changes are immediate and rapidly reversible with discontinuation of use.

The most extensive study of the effect of exogenous female hormones on lipoprotein
cholesterol was conducted by the Lipid Research Clinics Program.[8] They compared
lipoprotein cholesterol levels in 64 menstruating women under age 45 who did not use
oral contraceptives with levels in 374 menstruating women of similar age who were
taking one of seven oral contraceptive formulations. In addition, they compared lipoprotein cholesterol levels in 370 nonmenstruating women older than 45 with those in 254
nonmenstruating women of similar age who were taking estrogen replacement therapy.
All lipoprotein lipid levels were adjusted for age, weight, cigarette smoking, and alcohol
use. In the younger women, serum cholesterol and triglyceride levels were substantially
elevated in all the oral contraceptive users, regardless of the formulation (Table 15–2).
Low-density lipoprotein (LDL) cholesterol tended to be higher in oral contraceptive
users, especially in women using pills with a high progestin potency based on the delay
of menses test. High-density lipoprotein (HDL) cholesterol was not consistently affected
in oral contraceptive users. Very low-density lipoprotein (VLDL) cholesterol levels were
also substantially increased in oral contraceptive users. The highest median VLDL cholesterol level was observed in women using Ovulen, a pill with both a high estrogen
and a high progestin potency.

In older women, users of conjugated estrogens also had changes in their lipid profiles.
The median serum triglyceride level was increased 26%, and serum cholesterol was
decreased 4% in estrogen users, results which were both statistically significant. Larger
changes were observed in the lipoprotein cholesterol fractions than in the total cholesterol level. The median HDL cholesterol level was 10% higher and the VLDL cholesterol level was 23% higher in estrogen users than in nonusers, while the median LDL
cholesterol level was reduced by 11%. Others have found even larger decreases in LDL
cholesterol and even larger increases in HDL cholesterol in postmenopausal women
treated with estrogen replacement.[9]

TABLE 15–2.

Median Levels of Lipids and Lipoproteins in Users of Oral Contraceptives and Estrogens*

| TYPE OF EXOGENOUS FEMALE HORMONE | N | CHOLESTEROL | | | | TRIGLYCERIDE |
		TOTAL	HDL	LDL	VLDL	
Oral Contraceptives (20–44 years)						
Nonusers	642	176	54	109	11	72
Ortho-Novum	146	193†	58†	118	15†	113†
Norlestrin	41	195†	54	124†	14	111†
Ovral	76	195†	43†	135†	15†	101†
Ovulen	64	194†	54	124†	18†	141†
Estrogen Replacement (45–65 years)						
Nonusers	370	226	61	147	13	100
Equine estrogen	239	218†	67†	131†	16	126†

*From Wahl P, Walden C, Knopp R: Effect of estrogen/progestin potency on lipid lipoprotein cholesterol. *N Engl J Med* 1983; 308:862. Used by permission.
†Significantly different from nonusers at 0.05 level.

Hemostasis

Women taking estrogen replacement therapy have been shown to have hypercoagulability, an effect related primarily to decreased antithrombin activity.[10, 11] However, these changes in blood coagulability are not as pronounced as those associated with oral contraceptive use and are probably no greater than in premenopausal women taking no exogenous hormones.[12] There is some evidence that the natural conjugated estrogens used by the majority of menopausal estrogen users may be less thrombogenic than some of the synthetic estrogens, such as mestranol, that are widely used in oral contraceptives.[13]

Although combination oral contraceptives in premenopausal women clearly depress antithrombin activity, one study of combination estrogen and progestogen therapy in postmenopausal women did not find this effect.[14] In this study, in which naturally menopausal women received conjugated estrogens (0.625 or 1.25 mg for 21 of 28 days) and medroxyprogesterone acetate (10 mg for 7 of 28 days) for 18 months, hormone therapy had no effect on prothrombin time, activated partial thromboplastin time, or the amount or activity of fibrinogen. Plasminogen activity was actually enhanced by hormonal therapy.

In contrast to the situation with oral contraceptives, there is no apparent increase in venous thromboembolism in women taking estrogens as replacement therapy.[15]

Carbohydrate Metabolism

Most studies of carbohydrate metabolism in women taking combination oral contraceptives find elevated blood glucose and plasma insulin levels, especially during glucose tolerance testing.[16] However, the observed changes are generally small and seem to depend on the progestin more than the estrogen component of the pill.[17] Pills containing norgestrel seem to have the greatest effect, whereas carbohydrate metabolism seems to be largely unaffected in women using pills containing norethindrone.[18, 19]

One of the larger studies of the effect of estrogens alone on carbohydrate metabolism was conducted by Spellacy et al.[19] In that study, 171 hysterectomized women were randomly assigned to receive 1.25 mg Premarin, 0.08 mg mestranol, or 0.05 or 0.5 mg ethinyl estradiol for six months. Women were tested with a three-hour, 100-gm oral glucose tolerance test. The only statistically significant changes were a rise in fasting glucose for the Premarin group and a decrease in two-hour insulin for the mestranol group; but even for these, the absolute changes were small (4.6% and 11.7%, respectively). The significance of these findings in terms of cardiovascular disease risk is unstudied. However, in the absence of overt diabetes, hyperglycemia is a relatively weak predictor of risk.[20] In addition, large cross-sectional studies of postmenopausal women have generally found lower, not higher, fasting glucose levels in hormone users compared to nonusers.[21]

Blood Pressure

Young women using combination oral contraceptives are at increased risk of developing a reversible elevation in blood pressure.[22-24] The relative risk for hypertension in oral contraceptive users compared to nonusers is about 1.5.[23, 24] The hormonal component responsible for and the mechanism that explains this increased risk are not entirely clear. Several physiologic alterations induced by oral contraceptives that are consistent with an increase in blood pressure (increased renin substrate, increased cardiac output, increased plasma volume) are estrogen dose-dependent, yet development of hypertension does not appear to correlate well with estrogen dosage.[25] The most profound change related to blood pressure induced by oral contraceptives is a three- to fivefold increase in plasma renin substrate.[26] However, this may not be the mechanism to explain the increased risk of hypertension in oral contraceptive users, since the quantitative increase in renin substrate is similar in women who become hypertensive while taking oral contraceptives as in those who remain normotensive.[27]

Although most attention has focused on the estrogen component as the probable etiologic agent for oral contraceptive-induced hypertension, at least one large prospective study of oral contraceptive use found that the risk of hypertension increased with increased progestin dosage.[28]

Surprisingly few studies have been reported on the effects of estrogen use on blood pressure in postmenopausal women. Cross-sectional data from the Stanford Three-Community Study suggest that estrogen users have higher blood pressure than nonusers, even after adjusting for age and weight.[29] Data from other large cross-sectional studies, however, show slightly lower blood pressures among hormone users compared to nonusers.[21, 30] More consistent with these latter observations, noncontraceptive estrogen use does not appear to alter the risk of stroke.[31, 32]

Other Risk Factors

Each of the risk factors for ischemic heart disease discussed above may be altered by use of exogenous hormones. Two other risk factors, cigarette smoking and weight, appear to alter estrogen secretion and metabolism and may, therefore, potentially confound studies of the association of estrogen use and heart disease.

The epidemiologic literature strongly suggests that smokers have an earlier menopause than nonsmokers and that the age at menopause of ex-smokers is closer to those who have never smoked than to current smokers. The difference in the median menopausal age of smokers compared to nonsmokers is about 1.5 years.[33-36] MacMahon and colleagues have also demonstrated lower urinary estrogen levels in premenopausal smoking women compared to nonsmokers.[37] Consistent with this observation, smokers are at high risk of osteoporosis, a disease linked with estrogen deficiency in postmenopausal women.[38, 39] There is also some evidence that smokers are at low risk of endometrial cancer,[40, 41] a disease of estrogen excess, although not all studies have found this relationship.[42] Neither the high risk of osteoporosis in smokers nor the possibly low risk of endometrial cancer can be entirely explained by the earlier menopause of smoking women.[39, 40]

There is a well established relationship between body weight and circulating estrogen levels in postmenopausal women.[43] The reason for this is that the principal source of endogenous estrogen in the postmenopausal period is via conversion, primarily in adipose tissue, of androstenedione to estrogen.[43] With increasing body weight, a larger percentage of androstenedione undergoes this conversion, and circulating estrogen levels are correspondingly higher.

Certain steroid hormones such as estradiol may exist in plasma either bound to sex hormone-binding globulin (SHBG), bound more loosely to albumin, or in a 'free,' totally unbound state. Based on a variety of data, it is believed that those steroids bound to SHBG are unable to pass through capillary endothelium and are consequently inactive biologically, while those unbound to proteins are completely available to tissues.[44, 45] Most experts consider that the fractions of these steroids that are bound to albumin can also be transported across capillary endothelium and are thus available to tissues, although there is some disagreement on this point. Levels of sex hormone-binding globulin are reduced in obesity.[46] Therefore, obese women not only have increased levels of circulating estrogens, but a larger proportion of estrogen is available to tissue.

EPIDEMIOLOGIC STUDIES OF ESTROGEN USE AND CORONARY HEART DISEASE

There have been eight epidemiologic case-control studies that have evaluated the relationship between noncontraceptive estrogen use and various forms of coronary heart disease (Table 15–3).[47-54] Rosenberg et al. reported the first case-control study of this association in 1976.[47] They interviewed 336 women with nonfatal myocardial infarction whose conditions were diagnosed in 25 hospitals worldwide, to compare their use of estrogen with that of 6,730 control women of corresponding age selected from the same hospitals. The unadjusted relative risk was 0.5, but this low risk was completely accounted for by differences between cases and controls in other coronary heart disease risk factors (adjusted RR: 0.97). However, there was a low prevalence (3%) of estrogen use among both cases and controls in this study, so that the 95% confidence interval around this adjusted relative risk was quite large (0.48–1.95), despite the large study population.

The second case-control study was reported two years later by Pfeffer et al.[48] This population-based study included 171 female residents of a Southern California retirement community who suffered an acute myocardial infarction over an 11-year period. Pharmacy records from the central pharmacy in the medical center serving the community served as a source of information on estrogen use. Controls were 454 other female residents of the community without a known history of acute myocardial infarction. Information on other coronary heart disease risk factors, such as blood pressure, glucose tolerance, body habitus, and smoking was ascertained through outpatient medical charts. In this study, the unadjusted relative risk was 0.9 for any estrogen use and 0.6 for current estrogen use, both relative to no use at all. These relative risks were not greatly

TABLE 15–3.

Case Control Studies of Estrogen Replacement Therapy and Coronary Heart Disease

INVESTIGATOR/YEAR	DATA SOURCE	ENDPOINT‡	CRUDE RELATIVE RISK EVER USE	CURRENT USE	"ADJUSTED" RELATIVE RISK EVER USE	CURRENT USE
Rosenberg et al., 1976	Interviews	Nonfatal MI	Not reported	0.5	Not reported	1.0
Pfeffer et al., 1978	Pharmacy records	Fatal or nonfatal MI	0.9	0.6	0.9	0.7
Jick et al., 1978	Interviews	Nonfatal MI	Not reported	4.2	Not reported	Not reported
Rosenberg et al., 1980*	Interviews	Nonfatal MI	0.7 1.5	0.5 0.9	Not reported	Not reported
Ross et al., 1981†	Medical records	Fatal IHD	0.4 0.6	Not reported	0.4 0.6	Not reported
Bain et al., 1981	Mailed survey	Nonfatal MI	0.9	0.7	0.8	0.7
Adam et al., 1981	Doctors	Fatal MI	0.6	0.8	0.6	0.8
Szklo et al., 1984	Interviews	Nonfatal MI	0.5	0.4	0.4	0.4

*Rosenberg et al. reported the data on women aged 30–44 years *(top)* separately from those on women aged 45–49 years. "Adjusted" relative risks for postmenopausal women only were not reported.
†Ross et al. used two control groups for comparison: living controls *(top)* and deceased controls.
‡MI, myocardial infarction; IHD, ischemic heart disease.

affected by adjusting for other coronary heart disease risk factors; but after these adjustments, they were not statistically significant.

We studied the association between estrogen use and fatal ischemic heart disease in the same community studied by Pfeffer et al.[49] The 133 female residents of this community who died of ischemic heart disease over a five-year period were compared to women of the same age who died during the same time but from causes thought to be unrelated to estrogen use and to women of the same age who were still living in the community at the time of death of the cases. Medical records were the source of information on estrogen use. Using either control group for comparison, estrogen use was associated with a substantial reduction in risk of dying from ischemic heart disease. The relative risk using living controls was 0.4 (95% confidence interval: 0.2–0.8) and using deceased controls was 0.6 (95% confidence interval: 0.3-1.0). Although information on other important coronary heart disease risk factors was not consistently recorded, protection was conveyed to a comparable degree in women whose medical records indicated that they had other coronary heart disease risk factors (including a history of cigarette smoking, obesity, stroke, hypertension, diabetes, angina, or a previous myocardial infarction) as in those women for whom there was no such evidence of other risks.

Bain and associates collected information about myocardial infarction, use of female hormones after menopause, and coronary risk factors from 121,964 registered nurses aged 30 to 55 years during a mail survey conducted in 1976.[50] The relative risk estimate for myocardial infarction for current use of estrogens in this population was 0.7 but increased to 0.9 for those who had ever used these hormones. Neither result was statistically significant, and neither risk estimate changed greatly after adjusting for other coronary heart disease risk factors. Because of the young age group studied, most reported estrogen use in this study was of short duration. One subgroup of women, those who had had a bilateral oophorectomy and who also used estrogen replacement, received more substantial protection (RR: 0.4), an effect that did achieve statistical significance.

Adam, Williams, and Vessey studied all women in England and Wales aged 50–59 years who died of an acute myocardial infarction during a one-month period (November, 1978).[51] They collected information on estrogen use from the general practitioners who cared for the patients prior to death and compared these women to two randomly selected age-matched controls from the practice lists of the same physicians. The relative risk for women who received hormone replacement therapy at any time was 0.6.

In a study conducted to examine the role of various sociocultural factors on myocardial infarction risk in white women, Szklo et al. found a relative risk of 0.5 for any past use of estrogen.[52] This study was conducted on 102 women aged 35–64 who had been admitted to five general hospitals in Maryland with a first episode of myocardial infarction in 1971–72. Information on their estrogen use, obtained from personal interviews, was compared to that of 169 controls individually matched to the cases (67 triplets, 35 pairs) by hospital, age, and date of admission. The observed relative risk was essentially unchanged after simultaneous adjustment for cardiovascular diseases, smoking, education, and type of menopause, and it was similar for those who had very recently used estrogen and those who had used it less recently.

The other two case-control studies to examine this association were restricted to women younger than 50 years. Jick et al. compared noncontraceptive estrogen use in 14 previously healthy women under age 46 with 21 previously healthy control women hospitalized for other reasons.[53] In this small study, in seven cases, compared to four controls, there was estrogen use at the time of admission (RR: 4.2). This association might have been confounded by the high prevalence (90%) of cigarette smoking among the cases.

Rosenberg et al., in a second study of 477 women aged 30–49 years with a myocardial infarction and 1,832 hospital control subjects, found a relative risk of 0.5 and 0.9 for current estrogen use for women aged 30–44 and 45–49, respectively, who had had either a natural or an artificial menopause by bilateral oophorectomy.[54] The comparable relative risk estimate for any use was 0.7 for women younger than age 45, but 1.5 for the older age group. They did not report the average duration of use for menopausal women separately, but for pre- and postmenopausal women combined, the average duration of use for current estrogen users was 33 months for cases and 41 months for controls. For past users, the average duration of use was 19 months for cases and 20 months for controls.

There have been fewer cohort than case-control studies of the association between coronary heart disease and use of estrogen replacement therapy (Table 15–4). The most credible cohort study was recently reported by Bush and her colleagues, using data from the Lipid Research Clinics (Table 15–5).[55] The association of estrogen use with all-cause mortality was examined in 2,269 white women aged 40–69 years who had been followed for an average of 5.6 years in the Lipid Research Clinics Program Follow-Up Study. The relative risk of death was 0.4 in estrogen users compared to nonusers. A substantially lower mortality rate was observed in estrogen users compared to nonusers, regardless of hysterectomy status, although the lowest relative risk (0.1) was observed in women who had had bilateral oophorectomy. The relative risk for fatal cardiovascular

TABLE 15–4.

Cohort Studies of Estrogen Replacement Therapy and Coronary Heart Disease

INVESTIGATOR/YEAR	STUDY POPULATION	DESCRIPTION OF COHORT	ENDPOINT*	RELATIVE RISK
Burch et al., 1974	Surgical Practice Nashville, Tenn.	737 hysterectomized women	CHD	0.4
Hammond et al., 1974	Duke Medical Center	610 hypoestrogenic inpatients and outpatients	CHD	0.3
Petitti et al., 1979	Walnut Creek, Cal. Kaiser Permanente	1675 white women	MI	1.2
Bush et al., 1983	Lipid Research Clinics, USA	2269 white women	Fatal CHD	0.3
Wilson et al., 1985	Framingham, Mass.	1234 postmenopausal residents	CHD	1.9
Stampfer et al., 1985	Nurses Health Study, USA	32, 317 postmenopausal women	CHD	0.5

*CHD, coronary heart disease; MI, myocardial infarction.

disease in estrogen users compared to nonusers was 0.3. Differences between estrogen users and nonusers in levels of high density lipoprotein cholesterol accounted for some but not all of these differences in death rates. Interpretation of the results of this study suffers somewhat because of the limited estrogen history available on cohort members.

In a follow-up survey of over 32,000 female nurses, Stamfper et al. reported comparable relative risk estimates.[79] The age-adjusted risk of coronary disease in women who had ever used estrogen was 0.5 and the risk in current users was 0.3, both relative to women who had never used those hormones. Risk was similar for fatal and nonfatal coronary disease.

In the Framingham study, there was a 90% increase in risk of coronary heart disease

TABLE 15–5.

Age-Adjusted All-Cause Mortality Rates per 1,000 per Year (and 95% Confidence Limits) by Hysterectomy Status and Estrogen Use*

HYSTERECTOMY STATUS	ESTROGEN USE	
	NONUSERS	USERS
Intact uterus	9.0 (6.5–12.0)	4.9 (1.8–10.7)
Hysterectomy	8.2 (3.3–16.8)	2.8 (0.3–10.0)
Oophorectomy	11.8 (5.9–21.2)	1.4 (0.0–7.6)
Total	9.3 (7.2–11.9)	3.4 (1.5–6.4)

*From Bush TL, Cowan LD, Barret-Connor E, et al: Estrogen use and all-cause mortality. *JAMA* 1983; 249:903–906. Copyright 1983 by the American Medical Association.

observed in estrogen users, despite a generally favorable cardiovascular disease risk profile in these women.[80] Differences in age at menopause between estrogen users and nonusers may explain part of this excess risk. It has been reported that at any given age, postmenopausal women in the Framingham cohort have nearly a threefold increase in risk of cardiovascular disease compared to women who are still menstruating. Since estrogen use is associated with early menopause, to observe a protective effect on cardiovascular disease risk, the protective effect must be of sufficient magnitude to overcome this underlying association if results are left unadjusted for age at menopause.

Hammond and colleagues identified women with a variety of estrogen deficiency syndromes whose conditions were diagnosed over a 30 year period, 1940 to 1969, at Duke University and who were still being seen in 1974.[57] While estrogen users in this group had a much lower risk of cardiovascular disease, the methodology of this study has been seriously questioned for a variety of reasons,[58] including the questionable comparability of the estrogen users and nonusers, bias introduced by losses to follow-up, and the possible lack of generalizability of the findings.

Burch, Byrd, and Vaughn studied the effects of long-term estrogen therapy on women from a single surgical practice who had been hysterectomized over a 20-year period.[59] Nine deaths from heart disease were observed compared to an expected 24. The methodology for calculating the expected number of deaths was not described.

The only other cohort study to address this issue was conducted by Petitti et al., using data from the Walnut Creek, California, Kaiser Permanente Program.[60] They reported a relative risk of 1.2 for myocardial infarction among current noncontraceptive estrogen users. Participants in this study were generally quite young and only 26 cases of myocardial infarction were observed during follow-up, nine among estrogen users.

RELATED EPIDEMIOLOGIC STUDIES

The Coronary Drug Project was a nationwide collaborative study sponsored by the National Heart and Lung Institute to test the efficacy and safety of several lipid-lipoprotein influencing drugs, for the long-term therapy of coronary heart disease in men aged 30–64 years with a proven previous myocardial infarction.[61] By October 1969, 8,341 patients had been recruited by the 53 project centers and had been randomly assigned to one of six treatment groups, including two estrogen treatment groups. One of the treatment groups received conjugated estrogens, 5.0 mg/day, a second group received conjugated estrogens, 2.5 mg/day, while a third received lactose placebo. Within a year of the last patient enrollment, the 5.0 mg/day estrogen regimen was discontinued because of an excess number of nonfatal cardiovascular events compared to the placebo group.[61] In early 1973, the 2.5 mg/day estrogen group was also discontinued, since there was no evidence of therapeutic efficacy and a high incidence of side effects had led to poor adherence in this group.[62] Even this group, for which no adverse effects in terms of cardiovascular disease were observed, used an estrogen dose considerably higher than that used by the vast majority of postmenopausal women.

Prostate cancer is another condition for which high-dose estrogen treatment is sometimes indicated. Patients treated for prostate cancer with a 5.0 mg daily dose of the synthetic nonsteroidal estrogen diethylstilbestrol have an almost twofold increased risk of fatal and nonfatal cardiovascular disease.[63] Risk is particularly high in the first year of treatment.

In 1976, Phillips reported that young men with myocardial infarctions had significantly higher serum estradiol and estrone levels than age-matched healthy controls.[64] Other reports of raised circulating estrogen levels in young male survivors of myocardial infarction followed.[65, 66] Early studies of this association failed to adjust for weight, which is potentially an important confounder, since weight is related both to risk of myocardial infarction and to levels of circulating estrogens. However, a recent study suggested that increased weight in heart attack patients could explain little of this effect.[66]

Men with Klinefelter's syndrome have raised circulating estrogen levels, in the range of those reported in men with coronary artery disease.[67] The Medical Research Council Cytogenetics Registry in Edinburgh has been conducting a prospective mortality study of men with this disorder since 1959.[68] As of 1983, 17 deaths from coronary artery disease had been observed among members of this cohort, compared to the 19 expected based on national disease-specific mortality rates. The distribution of other coronary heart disease risk factors among men with Klinefelter's syndrome did not appear to differ from that of the general population. This finding suggests the possibility that the raised estrogen levels in survivors of myocardial infarction may have no etiologic significance.

The increased risk of vascular disease in women who use oral contraceptives is well documented. This high risk is observed over a wide range of vascular conditions, including venous thromboembolism, myocardial infarction, thrombotic stroke, hemorrhagic stroke, and subarachnoid hemorrhage.[69–72] Based on data from the Royal College of General Practitioners large cohort study, the risk of vascular disease overall is increased about fourfold in oral contraceptive users compared to nonusers.[73] The effect is especially strong in oral contraceptive users who smoke.[74, 75] However, recent reports from this study suggest that the risk of arterial disease is related to the progestin rather than the estrogen component of the pill.[76] The relative risk for any arterial disease in women using oral contraceptives containing 50 μg of ethinyl estradiol and various doses of norethindrone acetate (NEA) were 1.3 for 1 mg NEA, 2.0 for 3 mg NEA, and 2.5 for 5 mg NEA. Others have confirmed these results.[77]

Studies documenting an increased risk of coronary heart disease in women undergoing an early artificial or natural menopause strongly suggest that ovarian function influences risk.[56, 78]

ESTROGENS, HEART DISEASE, AND OTHER RISKS AND BENEFITS

Other known or possible risks and benefits of estrogen replacement therapy, such as endometrial cancer, breast cancer, osteoporosis, and cholecystitis, are covered in detail elsewhere in this volume and will not be reviewed here. Despite these other effects, if the risk of ischemic heart disease is influenced by postmenopausal estrogen use, as epidemiologic data suggest, in terms of mortality this would be the single most important factor in the cost-benefit equation, even if the relative change in risk is small.

One can crudely compute the effects on mortality through age 75 of high-dose (1.25 mg conjugated estrogen) and moderate-dose (0.625 mg conjugated estrogen) estrogen replacement therapy given at age 50 to 100,000 representative U.S. women. Assuming the best available measures of incidence and five-year survival for the relevant diseases (Table 15–6), and assuming the following relative risks for high- and moderate-dose estrogen replacement therapy, respectively: fractures (0.4, 0.4), gallbladder disease (2.0, 1.5), endometrial cancer (7.0, 2.0), breast cancer (1.5, 1.1), and ischemic heart

TABLE 15–6.

Conditions with Risk Changed by Estrogen Replacement Therapy,
Ages 50–75 Years

CONDITION	AVERAGE ANNUAL INCIDENCE RATE PER 100,000 WOMEN	CASE FATALITY RATE*	CUMULATIVE MORTALITY TO AGE 75 PER 100,000
Osteoporotic fractures	250	0.15	938
Gallbladder disease	100	0.001	3
Endometrial cancer	50	0.15	188
Breast cancer	250	0.30	1,875
Ischemic heart disease	700	0.60	10,500
Total			13,504

*Proportion of cases who die of their disease.

disease (1.0, 1.0), one would expect high-dose therapy to produce a net *increase* in deaths of about 6% and moderate-dose therapy to produce a net *decrease* in deaths of about 2% (Table 15–7).

If ischemic heart disease risk were reduced by as little as 20% (RR: 0.8), the net change in mortality would be a reduction of 10% for high-dose therapy and of nearly 18% for moderate-dose therapy. If the protection afforded by estrogen use were stronger (RR: 0.5), these reductions in mortality would be in excess of 33% and 41%, respectively.

All of these projections are crude and depend on a variety of assumptions. Nonetheless, these calculations suggest that even minor relative changes in risk of ischemic heart disease following estrogen use can have a major impact on the overall risk/benefit equation. Just as it is important for clinicians to consider the possible implications of estrogen therapy on the entirety of the risk/benefit equation, it is important that epidemiologists continue to refine these calculations through research aimed at measuring the effects of long-term low-dose versus high-dose therapy on risk of ischemic heart disease, assessing the effects of combined estrogen-progestin therapy on risk, and clarifying the interactions between the effect' of estrogen replacement therapy and those of known risk predictors of ischemic heart disease.

TABLE 15–7.

Estimated Changes in Mortality Induced by High and Moderate Dose Estrogen
Replacement Therapy, Ages 50–75 Years

CONDITION	HIGH DOSE		LOW DOSE	
	RR	CUMULATIVE CHANGE IN MORTALITY PER 100,000	RR	CUMULATIVE CHANGE IN MORTALITY PER 100,000
Osteoporotic fractures	0.4	−563	0.4	−563
Gallbladder disease	2.0	+3	1.5	+2
Endometrial cancer	7.0	+378*	2.0	+63*
Breast cancer	1.5	+938	1.1	+187
Ischemic heart disease	1.0	0	1.0	0
Net change		+756		−311
Net percent change		+6%		−2%

*Case fatality rate for estrogen-induced endometrial cancer estimated at 0.05.

REFERENCES

1. *Healthy People: The Surgeon General's Report on Health Promotion and Disease Prevention 1979:* DHEW (PHS) Publication No. 79-55071, U.S. Government Printing Office, Washington, D.C., 1979.
2. Quigley MM, Hammond CB: Estrogen-replacement therapy—help or hazard? *N Engl J Med* 1979; 301:646.
3. Hammond CB, Maxson WS: Current status of estrogen therapy for the menopause. *Fertil Steril* 1982; 37:5.
4. Weinstein MC: Estrogen use in postmenopausal women—costs, risks and benefits. *N Engl J Med* 1980; 303:308.
5. Walker WJ: Changing United States lifestyle and declining vascular mortality: Cause or coincidence. *N Engl J Med* 1977; 287:163.
6. Stewart AW, Beaglehole R, Fraser GE, et al: Trends in survival after myocardial infarction in New Zealand, 1974–81. *Lancet* 1984; ii:444.
7. Wallace RB, Hoover J, Barrett-Conner E, et al: Altered plasma lipid and lipoprotein levels associated with oral contraceptive and estrogen use. *Lancet* 1979; ii:111.
8. Wahl P, Walden C, Knopp R: Effect of estrogen/progestin potency on lipid lipoprotein cholesterol. *N Engl J Med* 1983; 308:862.
9. Wallentin L, Larsson-Cohn U: Metabolic and hormonal effects of postmenopausal oestrogen replacement treatment. II. Plasma lipids. *Acta Endocrinol [Copenh]* 1977; 86:597.
10. Coope J, Thomson JM, Poller L: Effects of "natural oestrogen" replacement therapy on menopausal symptoms and blood clotting. *Br Med J* 1975; 4:139.
11. Stangel JJ, Innerfield I, Reyniak JV, et al: The effect of conjugated estrogens on coagulability in menopausal women. *Obstet Gynecol* 1977; 149:314.
12. von Kaulla E, Droegmueller W, von Kaulla KN: Conjugated estrogens and hypercoagulability. *Am J Obstet Gynecol* 1974; 122:688.
13. Bonnar J: Effects of synthetic and natural estrogens on the coagulation system in postmenopausal women, in Campbell S (ed): *Management of the Menopausal and Postmenopausal Years.* Lancaster, England, MTP Press Ltd, 1976, p 321.
14. Notelovitz M, Kitchens G, Ware M, et al: Combination estrogen and progestogen replacement therapy does not adversely affect coagulation. *Obstet Gynecol* 1983; 62:596.
15. Boston Collaborative Drug Surveillance Program: Surgically confirmed gallbladder disease, venous thromboembolism and breast tumors in relation to postmenopausal estrogen therapy. *N Engl J Med* 1974; 290:15.
16. Kalkhoff RK: Effects of oral contraceptive agents on carbohydrate metabolism. *J Steroid Biochem* 1975; 6:949.
17. Spellacy WN, Buhi WC, Birk SA: The effect of estrogen on carbohydrate metabolism: Glucose, insulin, and growth hormone studies on one hundred and seventy-one women ingesting Premarin, mestranol, and ethinyl estradiol for six months. *Am J Obstet Gynecol* 1972; 114:378.
18. Spellacy WN, Buhi WC, Birk SA: Effects of norethindrone on carbohydrate and lipid metabolism. *Obstet Gynecol* 1975; 46:560.
19. Spellacy WN, Buhi WC, Birk SA: The effects of norgestrol on carbohydrate and lipid metabolism over one year. *Am J Obstet Gynecol* 1976; 125:984.
20. Miller NE, Forde OH, Thelle DS, et al: The Tromso heart study: High-density lipoprotein and coronary heart disease. A prospective case-control study. *Lancet* 1977; 1:965.
21. Barrett-Conner E, Brown V, Turner J, et al: Heart disease risk factors and hormone use in postmenopausal women. *JAMA* 1979; 241:2167.
22. Crane MG, Harris JJ, Winsor W III: Hypertension, oral contraceptive agents, and conjugated estrogens. *Ann Intern Med* 1971; 74:13.
23. Fisch IR, Freedman SH, Myatt AV: Oral contraceptives, pregnancy, and blood pressure. *JAMA* 1972; 222:1507.
24. Greenblatt DJ, Koch-Weser J: Oral contraceptives and hypertension. A report from the Boston Collaborative Drug Surveillance Program. *Obstet Gynecol* 1974; 44:412.
25. Roberts JM: Oestrogens and hypertension. *Clin Endocrinol Metab* 1981; 10:489–512.
26. Crane MG, Harris JJ, Winsor W: Hypertension and oral contraceptives. *Br Med J* 1978; 11:1165.

27. Beckerhoff R, Leutscher JA, Beckerhoff I, et al: Effects of oral contraceptives on the renin-angiotensin system and on blood pressure of normal young women. *Johns Hopkins Med J* 1972; 132:80.

28. Royal College of General Practitioners: Effect on hypertension and benign breast disease of progestogen component in combined oral contraceptives. *Lancet* 1977; i:624.

29. Stern MP, Brown BW, Haskell WL, et al: Cardiovascular risk and use of estrogens or estrogen-progestogen combination. *JAMA* 1976; 235:811.

30. Pfeffer RI, Kurosaki TT, Charlton SK: Estrogen use and blood pressure in later life. *Am J Epidemiol* 1979; 110:469.

31. Pfeffer RI, Van Den Noort S: Estrogen use and stroke risk in postmenopausal women. *Am J Epidemiol* 1976; 103:445.

32. Rosenberg SH, Fausone V, Clark R: The role of estrogens as a risk factor for stroke in postmenopausal women. *West J Med* 1980; 133:292.

33. Kaufman DW, Slone D, Rosenberg L, et al: Cigarette smoking and age at natural menopause. *Am J Public Health* 1980; 70:420.

34. Lindquist U, Bengtsson C: Menopausal age in relation to smoking. *Acta Med Scand* 1979; 205:73.

35. Jick H, Porter J, Morrison AS: Relation between smoking and age of natural menopause. *Lancet* 1977; 1:1354.

36. Willett W, Stampfer MJ, Bain C, et al: Cigarette smoking, relative weight and menopause. *Am J Epidemiol* 1983; 117:651.

37. MacMahon B, Trichopoulos D, Cole P, et al: Cigarette smoking and urinary estrogens. *N Engl J Med* 1982; 307:1062.

38. Daniell HW: Osteoporosis of the slender smoker. *Arch Intern Med* 1976; 136:298.

39. Paganini-Hill A, Ross RK, Gerkins VR, et al: Menopausal estrogen therapy and hip fractures. *Ann Intern Med* 1981; 95:28.

40. Weiss NS, Farewell VT, Szekely DR, et al: Oestrogens and endometrial cancer: Effect of other risk factors on the association. *Maturitas* 1980; 2:185.

41. Williams RR, Horn JW: Association of cancer sites with tobacco and alcohol consumption and socioeconomic status of patients: Interview study from the Third National Cancer Survey. *J Natl Cancer Inst* 1977; 58:525.

42. Garfinkel L: Cancer mortality in non-smokers: Prospective study of the American Cancer Society. *J Natl Cancer Inst* 1980; 65:1169.

43. Siiteri PK, MacDonald PC: Role of extraglandular estrogen in human endocrinology, in *Handbook of Physiology*, sect 7, vol 2, Part 1. Washington, DC, American Physiological Society, 1973, p 615.

44. Anderson DC: Sex hormone binding globulin. *Clin Endocrinol* 1974; 3:69.

45. Vermeulen A: Transport and distributions of androgens at different ages, in Martini L, Motta M (eds): *Androgens and Antiandrogens*. New York, Raven Press, 1977.

46. Siiteri PK, Hammond GL, Nisker JA: Increased availability of serum estrogens in breast cancer: A new hypothesis, in Pike MC, Siiteri PK, Welsch CW (eds): *Hormones and Breast Cancer*, Banbury Report 8. New York, Cold Spring Harbor Laboratory, 1981, p 87.

47. Rosenberg L, Armstrong B, Jick H: Myocardial infarction and estrogen therapy in postmenopausal women. *N Engl J Med* 1976; 294:1256.

48. Pfeffer RI, Whipple GH, Kurosuki TT, et al: Coronary risk and estrogen use in postmenopausal women. *Am J Epidemiol* 1978; 107:479.

49. Ross RK, Paganini-Hill A, Mack TM, et al: Menopausal estrogen therapy and protection from death from ischemic heart disease. *Lancet* 1981; i:858.

50. Bain C, Willett W, Hennekens CH, et al: Use of postmenopausal hormones and risk of myocardial infarction. *Circulation* 1981; 64:42.

51. Adam S, Williams V, Vessey MP: Cardiovascular disease and hormone replacement treatment: A pilot case-control study. *Br Med J* 1981; 282:1277.

52. Szklo M, Tonascia J, Gordis L, et al: Additional evidence supporting a protective effect of estrogen use on myocardial infarction risk. *Prev Med* 1984; 13:510–516.

53. Jick H, Dinan B, Rothman KJ: Noncontraceptive estrogens and nonfatal myocardial infarction. *JAMA* 1978; 239:1407.

54. Rosenberg L, Slone D, Shapiro S, et al: Noncontraceptive estrogens and myocardial infarction in young women. *JAMA* 1980; 244:339.

55. Bush TL, Cowan LD, Barrett-Conner E, et al: Estrogen use and all-cause mortality. *JAMA* 1983; 249:903–906.
56. Gordon T, Kannel WB, Hjortland MC, et al: Menopause and coronary heart disease: The Framingham study. *Ann Intern Med* 1978; 89:157.
57. Hammond CB, Jelovsek FR, Lee KL, et al: Effects of long-term estrogen replacement therapy. I. Metabolic effects. *Am J Obstet Gynecol* 1979; 133:525.
58. Vessey MP, Bungay FT: Benefits and risks of hormone therapy in the menopause, in Smith A (ed): *Recent Advances in Community Medicine.* New York, Churchill Livingstone, Inc, 1982, p 77.
59. Burch JC, Byrd BF, Vaughn WK: The effects of long-term estrogen on hysterectomized women. *Am J Obstet Gynecol* 1974; 118:778.
60. Petitti DB, Wingerd J, Pellegrin F, et al: Risk of vascular disease in women. Smoking, oral contraceptives, noncontraceptive estrogens and other factors. *JAMA* 1979; 242:1150.
61. The Coronary Drug Project: Initial findings leading to modifications of its research protocol. *JAMA* 1970; 214:1303.
62. The Coronary Drug Project: Findings leading to discontinuation of the 2.5 mg/day estrogen group. *JAMA* 1973; 226:652.
63. Blackard CE, Doe RP, Mellinger GT, et al: Incidence of cardiovascular disease and death in patients receiving diethylstilbestrol for carcinoma of the prostate. *Cancer* 1970; 26:249.
64. Phillips GB: Evidence for hyperestrogenemia as a risk factor for myocardial infarction in men. *Lancet* 1976; ii:14.
65. Entrican JH, Beach C, Carroll D, et al: Raised plasma oestradiol and oestrone levels in young survivors of myocardial infarction. *Lancet* 1978; ii:487.
66. Luria MH, Johnson MW, Pego R, et al: Relationship between sex hormones, myocardial infarction, and occlusive coronary disease. *Arch Intern Med* 1982; 142:42.
67. Forti G, Giusti G, Borghi A, et al: Klinefelter's syndrome: A study of its hormonal plasma pattern. *J Endocrinol Invest* 1982; 2:149.
68. Prince WH, Clayton JF: Oestrogens and coronary artery disease in men. *Lancet* 1983; 2:860.
69. Mann JI, Inman WHW: Oral contraceptives and death from myocardial infarction. *Br Med J* 1975; 2:245.
70. Vessey MP, Doll R: Investigation of relation between use of oral contraceptives and thromboembolic disease. *Br Med J* 1968; 2:199.
71. Collaborative Group for the Study of Stroke in Young Women: Oral contraception and increased risk of cerebral ischemia or thrombosis. *N Engl J Med* 1973; 288:871.
72. Petitti DB, Wingerd J: Use of oral contraceptives, cigarette smoking, and risk of subarachnoid hemorrhage. *Lancet* 1978; ii:234.
73. Royal College of General Practitioners' Oral Contraception Study: Further analysis of mortality in oral contraceptive users. *Lancet* 1981; i:541.
74. Mann JI, Vessey MP, Thorogood M, et al: Myocardial infarction in young women with special reference to oral contraceptive practice. *Br Med J* 1975; 2:241.
75. Jick H, Dinan B, Rothman KJ: Oral contraceptives and non-fatal myocardial infarction. *JAMA* 1978; 239:1403.
76. Kay CR: Progestogens and arterial disease—evidence from the Royal College of General Practitioners' Study. *Am J Obstet Gynecol* 1982; 142:762.
77. Meade TW, Greenberg G, Thompson SG: Progestogens and cardiovascular reactions associated with oral contraceptives and a comparison of the safety of 50- and 30-μg oestrogen preparations. *Br Med J* 1980; 280:1157.
78. Robinson RW, Higano N, Cohen WD: Increased incidence of coronary heart disease in women castrated prior to the menopause. *Arch Intern Med* 1959; 104:908.
79. Stampfer MJ, Willett WC, Colditz JA, et al: A prospective study of postmenopausal estrogen therapy and coronary heart disease. *N Engl J Med* 1985; 313:1044.
80. Wilson PWF, Garrison RJ, Custelli WP: Postmenopausal estrogen use, cigarette smoking, and cardiovascular morbidity in women over 50. *N Engl J Med* 1985; 313:1038.

CHAPTER 16

Psychologic and Sexual Effects

LORRAINE DENNERSTEIN, M.B., B.S., Ph.D., D.P.M., F.R.A.N.Z.C.P.

IN THE PERIMENOPAUSAL years there is an increase in many minor psychologic complaints, such as anxiety, mood lability, and difficulty in concentrating and making decisions. These changes are discussed more fully in Chapter 9. A longitudinal study[13] found that sexual interest, responsivity, and activity began to decline premenopausally and that this decline continued through the menopause. Morrell et al.,[20] in a psychophysiologic study, demonstrated that postmenopausal women (who were not receiving hormones) were significantly less responsive to erotic films as measured by vaginal pulse amplitude, than were either young regularly menstruating women or older premenopausal women. Semmens and Wagner[24] demonstrated a fall in vaginal pH and increases in transvaginal potential difference, quantity of vaginal fluid, and vaginal blood flow when oral conjugated estrogens were administered to 14 postmenopausal women. Among patients attending a menopause clinic, psychologic and sexual complaints are frequent. Studd and Parsons[27] report that nearly half of all patients presenting at a menopause clinical offer symptoms of sexual dysfunction among their three main complaints. This chapter will explore approaches to management of such problems, with special consideration of the role of exogenous hormones.

Evidence of the specific effects of steroid hormones on mood and sexual response derives largely from clinical trials. There have been considerable methodologic difficulties experienced in such studies. These have included the problems of defining and measuring the variables to be studied. The psychologic symptoms studied include many vague and ill-defined terms. In many of the studies reported, it is not clear whether investigator and patient have a clear and similar understanding of terms that can have different connotations when their popular meaning is compared to their clinical meaning. The use of varying measures of symptomatology may have produced some disparity. Psychometric tests have been used infrequently. When rating scales have been used, many workers have failed to provide information as to their sensitivity, validity, and reliability. Few researchers have adequately investigated the different components of female sexuality, which must include female interest or drive, and the physical and psychologic experience of sexual response during arousal, penetration, and orgasm, as well as the frequency of all sexual activities, whether they be autosexual, such as dreams or fantasies, or those involving others. In clinical trials, the menopausal status of subjects must be described, with evidence derived from hormone assays; there must be a sufficient number in the sample; measurements of variables must be valid and sensitive to change; the length of therapy must be sufficient to judge results; the crossover design must allow for interpatient variability in response and assessment of change; and bias must be reduced by double-blind techniques.

CLINICAL TRIALS

Since women with perimenopausal complaints have been shown to be highly responsive to placebo,[2] only those studies that were double-blind will be discussed here.

A review of six earlier double-blind studies[7] found that all except one study reported that, compared with placebo, there was a decrease in psychologic complaints such as irritability, fatigue, insomnia, anxiety, and depression when estrogen was given alone or in combination with a progestin. The one study that failed to find any difference between estrogen and placebo used a cross-over design, but only one month of therapy occurred before the cross-over. In this study,[16] treatment with placebo always followed a course of estrogen therapy. Since the effects of estrogen may persist for some time after they have been discontinued, the true effects of placebo may not have been accurately measured. Coppen et al.[3] also failed to find significant differences between a group treated with placebo and a group receiving estrogen (piperazine estrone sulphate 3 mg daily for 12 months). The estrogen group did show significantly lowered Beck Depression Inventory scores compared with their own baseline. Whitehead[31] attributed the negative findings of this study to a marked difference in pre-entry scores between groups. A cross-over may have overcome the problems of inter- and intrapatient variability. Fedor-Freybergh,[15] using an ordinal scale, found a significant beneficial effect of estrogen on libido, sexual activity, satisfaction, experience of pleasure, sexual fantasies, and capacity for orgasm.

The two largest double-blind, placebo-controlled, cross-over studies that have been published both report improvements with estrogen therapy over placebo for a variety of psychologic and sexual symptoms. Campbell and Whitehead[1] compared two months therapy of 1.25 mg conjugated estrogens (daily) with placebo in a short-term cross-over involving 64 patients with severe symptoms. Estrogen was found to be significantly more effective than placebo in alleviating 12 symptoms (hot flushes, insomnia, vaginal dryness, irritability, poor memory, anxiety, worry about age, headaches, worry about self, urinary frequency, optimism, good spirits) and produced increased coital satisfaction. There was no change in masturbation, orgasmic, or coital frequencies. In order to determine whether this improvement reflected relief of hot flushes, an analysis was made of the 20 patients who had not reported hot flushes. Vaginal dryness, poor memory, anxiety, and worry about age and self continued to be significantly improved by estrogens, indicating a direct positive effect of estrogen on mental status. It was not clear whether these 20 women were endocrinologically as postmenopausal as the other women in the study or if a large component of their symptoms reflected psychologic or sociologic causes that would be unlikely to respond to estrogens. In a longer-term study of 61 patients with less severe symptoms, estrogen and placebo were each given for six months. Five physical and psychologic symptoms were significantly relieved by conjugated estrogen compared with placebo (hot flushes, vaginal dryness, insomnia, urinary frequency, poor memory). Once again, it is unclear in which ways, if any, the sample of 61 differed from the 64 patients with more severe symptoms. The measure used in this study was an analogue scale.

In the other large double-blind, placebo-controlled cross-over study, Dennerstein et al.[10, 11] found that no changes were detected with analogue scales, whereas significant changes were evident on ordinal scales and in orgasmic and coital frequency rates recorded daily. This study differed from earlier studies in the following ways: First, all 49 women were of a definable endocrine status in that they had all received hysterectomy with bilateral oophorectomy, the results of which were confirmed with hormonal assays.[8] The operations were performed for benign diseases. Second, there was a detailed study of the mental status and sexual behavior of the women prior to admission to the study. Women with diagnosable psychiatric disorders or with significant interpersonal conflict were excluded, since it was thought that such problems may overwhelm any hormonal influence. Only women with stable, heterosexually active relationships were included, since one of the aims of the study was to measure the effects of hormones on sexual functioning. Most of these women denied any autosexual activity such as sexual dreams or masturbation but were prepared to discuss their sexual interest. Third, this study set out to measure the effects separately of an estrogen and a progestin and compare these with placebo. The study used a cross-over design so that each woman received three months each of the following medications, the order of which was randomly allocated: ethinyl estradiol, 50 μg/day; levonorgestrel, 250 μg/day; "Nordiol," the combination of these two compounds; and placebo. Drug-taking was continuous, there being no drug-free periods between medication. If women were unable to tolerate the side effects in any drug phase, they were changed to the next drug in the sequence. Ethinyl estradiol given alone was found to have the most beneficial effect on psychologic status as measured by Hamilton scores and ordinal ratings of general well-being, depression, fatigue, anxiety, irritability and insomnia. The combination, "Nordiol," was next in beneficial effect, with norgestrel scoring slightly better than placebo. Virtually all women in this study suffered from hot flushes, and the hormonal therapies have been shown to alleviate these significantly.[9] In order to determine whether the beneficial effects of estrogen were secondary to hot flush relief, an analysis of covariance of Hamilton scores was carried out. Although it appeared that at least some of the effects on mood were related to the effects on hot flushes, a significant effect of the hormones on the Hamilton scores remained, suggesting a direct beneficial psychotropic effect of estrogen.

This study also found that ethinyl estradiol had a beneficial effect on female sexual desire, enjoyment, and vaginal lubrication (all measured by ordinal scales) and on orgasmic frequency (recorded daily) (Figs 16–1, 16–2, and 16–3) (Dennerstein et al., 1980). There was a trend toward norgestrel being more inhibitory. The combination pill was less beneficial than estrogen alone. Finally, when the relationship between headaches and the administration of hormones was examined, it was found that an increase in headaches occurred when therapy was changed from estrogen-containing compounds to the nonestrogens (norgestrel or placebo).[12]

In a later double-blind, cross-over study, Paterson[22] studied 23 postmenopausal hysterectomized women. The women received three months each of either graded sequential mestranol and noresthisterone or placebo. Symptoms were measured by ordinal questionnaires. Active therapy resulted in a significant reduction in hot flushes and night sweats. There was a slight improvement in insomnia, and an increase in energy and confidence, but no alteration in depression, anxiety, memory, tension, libido, or vaginal dryness. These findings in part confirm those of the previous study[10] that when a progestin was added to estrogen, beneficial effects on mood and sexual functioning were reduced. These results were also confirmed in a recent study by Hammerback et al.[18] They studied 22 symptomatic postmenopausal women who were given either estrogen only (estradiol creme percutaneously for three weeks out of four) or with the addition of a progestin (lynestrenol 5 mg/day) in the last 11 days of the cycle. It was found that when the progestin was added to medication there was a significant cyclicity in mood

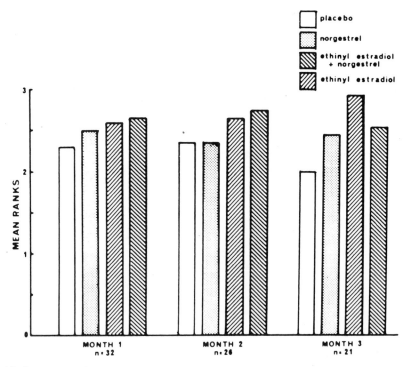

FIG 16–1.
Hormone therapy and sexual desire. (From Dennerstein et al: *Obstet Gynecol* 1980; 56:316. Used by permission.)

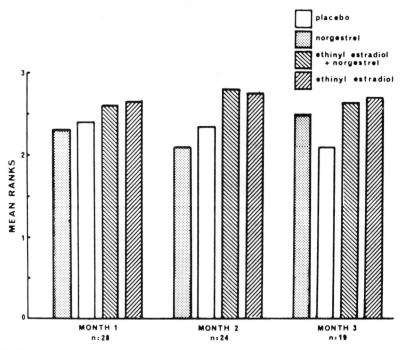

FIG 16–2.
Hormone therapy and sexual enjoyment. (From Dennerstein, et al: *Obstet Gynecol* 1980; 56:316. Used by permission).

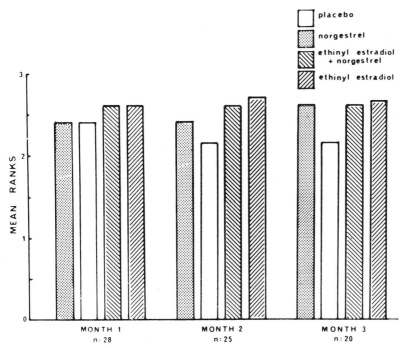

MEAN RANKS

placebo
norgestrel
ethinyl estradiol + norgestrel
ethinyl estradiol

MONTH 1
n: 28

MONTH 2
n: 25

MONTH 3
n: 20

FIG 16–3.
Hormone therapy and vaginal lubrication. (From Dennerstein, et al: *Obstet Gynecol* 1980; 56:316. Used by permission.).

and physical signs (such as breast tenderness and feelings of swelling) with a maximum symptom score during the final days of progestin treatment. Those receiving only estrogen did now show any deterioration of mood or physical signs during the treatment. Sexual feeling was the only unchanged parameter in this study.

There have been few double-blind studies of the role of androgens as part of hormone replacement therapy. Uncontrolled studies[28, 29] suggest significant sexual improvement in patients who had complained of loss of libido after receiving a combined hormone implant of 50 mg of estradiol and 100 mg of testosterone. Studd et al.[29] had found little improvement when women with loss of libido without primary coital discomfort were treated with oral conjugated equine estrogen therapy. Dow and Hart[14] studied 40 postmenopausal women referred for hormone replacement therapy, all of whom had reported a significant concern about a decline in sexual interest. These women were randomly allocated to one of two hormone implant treatment groups: either estradiol (50 mg) alone or estradiol (50 mg) and testosterone (100 mg). Comparison between the two groups revealed no significant differences on any measure. Both treatments were associated with a significant reduction in the severity of psychologic, somatic, and vasomotor symptoms and with a significant improvement in sexual interest, responsiveness, satisfaction, and orgasmic capacity, and a lessening of dyspareunia. These results indicated no advantages of testosterone administration over estradiol alone for sexually unresponsive postmenopausal women. The only variable that was not improved by the hormone treatment was marital dissatisfaction. This study did not include a placebo-control group, and the sample was mixed endocrinologically, in that some women had undergone hysterectomy and bilateral oophorectomy.

A recent study by Sherwin and Gelfand[25] attempted to overcome these flaws. These

researchers studied women who had been hysterectomized and bilaterally oophorectomized for benign causes. In a double-blind, cross-over design, 38 women were administered by intramuscular injection monthly for three months with the following substances: estrogen, testosterone, estrogen and testosterone combined, or placebo. There
was a control group of 10 women who were hysterectomized but not oophorectomized.
Three emotions—anxiety, depression, and hostility—were measured, using the multi-
ple-adjective affect checklist. It was found that the oophorectomized women who received any of the hormonal preparations were significantly less depressed than the placebo group. The women treated with androgens alone had significantly higher hostility
scores than all other groups. There were no effects on anxiety across time in any of the
groups studied. Sherwin et al.[25] also found that exogenous androgen significantly enhanced the intensity of sexual desire and arousal in the oophorectomized women. There
was no effect on coital frequency, suggesting that the major impact of androgen in
women is on sexual motivation rather than activity per se.

To summarize, most double-blind studies have found that estrogens have beneficial
effects on psychologic and sexual functioning. The addition of a progestin leads to less
favorable results. When the effects of addition of an androgen were studied, no additional benefits on either depression or sexual responsiveness were found over those
observed with the use of estrogen alone. The use of testosterone injections alone were
associated with an increase in hostility.

FACTORS INFLUENCING RESPONSE TO HORMONE THERAPY

Few studies have examined the factors that may influence patients' responses to hormone therapy. The importance of such factors was demonstrated recently in a study by
Hahn et al.[17] Forty postmenopausal women were studied. Twenty-two patients with an
intact uterus were given conjugated estrogen with 2.5 mg of norethindrone for the last
ten days of the cycle. All but three discontinued therapy over an 18-month period. The
22 patients who had been hysterectomized were treated with conjugated estrogens only.
None of these women discontinued therapy. The claimed reason for the discontinuation
of therapy was the monthly withdrawal bleeding. However, there is no indication as to
whether it was the bleeding per se, or perhaps associated symptomatology, such as the
premenstrual-like syndrome described by Hammerback et al.[18] with their cyclical regime, which led to noncompliance.

Factors involved in determining the acceptability of progestins were recently reviewed.[32] Personality variables, dosage and type of progestins used, and individual patient vulnerability may be important in determining the response to treatment.
Personality Variables.—Collins et al.[33] studied 17 symptomatic postmenopausal
women. They found a significant correlation in reduction of psychosomatic symptoms
(palpitations, dizziness, numbness, tingling of the skin, headache) and personality variables purporting to measure anxiety proneness, distance preference, and psychasthenia.
No significant correlations were found between personality variables and the reduction
of vasomotor, sleep-related, or psychologic symptoms. There was a high, positive, and
significant correlation between feminine interest scores and treatment of the following
symptoms: hot flushes, tingling of the skin, and tiredness. These results must be interpreted with caution, since it is possible that some of the symptoms and personality
variables may be measuring the same underlying dimension. Further studies are needed,
but it is possible that women who value traditional feminine interests will respond more

favorably to hormone therapy. Anxiety-prone, detached women may have a greater reduction of psychosomatic symptoms than other women.

Dosage.—De Lignieres and Vincens[5] noted that the same therapeutic regime induced different individual plasma levels of steroids. They studied symptomatic climacteric women and administered estradiol percutaneously and progesterone orally. Those women who had the lowest plasma estradiol levels before and after treatment were also likely to suffer moderate depressive symptoms. Only when a moderate increase in estradiol level occurred did the estradiol treatment lead to pleasant feelings of well-being. An excessive increase caused women to complain of unpleasant side effects of irritability and aggressiveness. Progesterone (micronized) had very few psychologic effects, if estradiol levels were low or slightly increased. When plasma estradiol was high, a moderate elevation of plasma progesterone induced a pleasant tranquilizing effect. A massive elevation of plasma progesterone levels immediately induced an inadequate hypnotic effect, sometimes with dizziness.

Whitehead (1983) reported that when dl norgestrel, 500 µg/day, was added to estrogen medication, about 10% of patients experienced a premenstrual tension-like syndrome with mastalgia during the progestin phase of treatment. Reducing the dosage to 150 µg daily reduced the frequency and intensity of these complaints.

Type of Progestin Used.—The 19 nortestosterone derivatives, which include norethisterone and dl norgestrel, possess androgenic activities that may be responsible for their adverse effects on plasma lipid and lipoprotein concentrations. It is possible that nonprogesterone activity may be involved in psychologic side effects. Progestins closer to the chemical structure of progesterone include dydrogesterone and medroxyprogesterone acetate; these have minimal androgenic activities and may warrant further investigation. Synthetic progestins may have different effects on the central nervous system than does progesterone itself, since the active metabolites of each of these substances may vary in proportion and amount. An oral, micronized preparation of progesterone is now available which produces adequate plasma and tissue levels of progesterone. This substance deserves further evaluation to assess whether it will antagonize the harmful effects of estrogen (as in the study of De Lignieres and Vincens[5]) and have less detrimental psychologic side effects than those reported by investigators such as Hammerback et al.,[18] who used 19 norsteroids.

Patient Individual Vulnerability.—Previous studies by the author have demonstrated significant interpatient variability in response to hormones.[10] The experience of patients attending a menstrual/menopause clinic suggests there may be a group of women who are more sensitive to the effects of hormones and in whom hormones may provoke symptoms. A history of the following may indicate risk factors of such hormonal sensitivity: mood symptoms while taking the oral contraceptive pill, postpartum depression, and premenstrual syndrome. The existence of such individual differences was suggested by the work of Cullberg,[4] who carried out a large comparison study of the oral contraceptive pill at different dosages of progestogen (norgestrel). He found that the only group in whom psychologic complaints developed while taking the pill were women with a previous history of premenstrual syndrome who reacted badly to the combination pill with the lowest amount of norgestrel. In another study, suggesting sensitivity to hormone provoked symptoms, Tonge[30] studied 100 consecutive deliveries prospectively. He reported that women who had developed postpartum depression were significantly more likely to have suffered from premenstrual complaints before pregnancy.

A further indication of individual sensitivity to hormones was indicated by patients attending a premenstrual tension clinic.[13] Of the first 80 patients, 77 had taken the oral contraceptive pill. Ninety-two percent of those women who suffered from a true premenstrual syndrome had ceased taking the pill because of side effects. When pregnancy had occurred, there was a history of postpartum depression in 67.74%. In 30.64%, depression had followed more than one pregnancy.

MANAGEMENT

The clinician is concerned not with what proportion of the climacteric population experiences symptoms, but rather with the individual woman who comes to the doctor seeking relief for her complaints. She may be pre-, peri-, or postmenopausal or have experienced hysterectomy with or without oophorectomy. Recent studies suggest that the percentages of women seeking help in each of these groups increases from approximately 33% for the premenopausal woman to 75% for the woman who has undergone hysterectomy and bilateral oophorectomy. Despite the advent of menopause treatment clinics, in many countries most women consult their own doctor.

The first major step for the clinician is to establish the diagnosis of the symptoms presented. With regard to psychologic and sexual complaints, the doctor needs full details of the presenting symptoms, their duration, and their association with the onset of the climacteric. Other menopausal complaints should be asked about. In the history-taking, symptoms suggesting other major disorders should be sought. These include major psychiatric disorders, especially depression and generalized anxiety disorder, marital problems and/or sexual dysfunction, and midlife crisis.[13] A personal developmental history will give some idea of the patient's coping style, personality, and vulnerability. Details of the woman's current environment and aspects of stress and support within this framework should be examined. Her attitudes and expectations of the menopause are also important. Information about factors that may affect her response to hormones, such as her responses to the oral contraceptive pill, postpartum depression, or premenstrual tension, should be sought. Organic aspects that may limit the use of hormones must be determined.

Many authors have drawn attention to the possible problems in the doctor-patient relationship that may produce barriers to free communication. Roberts[19] noted that doctors and patients may have qualitatively different ways of looking at the nature, context, and management of the menopause. Differences in gender and social background may produce a social distance that may make women less willing to share personal problems with their doctors. This is especially likely if the patient suspects that her doctor accepts the stereotype of the ''difficult''. or overanxious menopausal woman whose problems are basically physical or merely psychosomatic. Care must therefore be taken by the doctor to establish an empathic relationship with the patient.

Investigations

In the postmenopausal woman, plasma follicle-stimulating hormone and estradiol levels will help determine the degree of estrogen deficiency. This may be especially useful for the climacteric woman who has psychologic or sexual complaints but no vasomotor symptoms.

Therapy

An integrated approach to management is needed, aimed at reducing contributory hormonal, psychologic, and social stress, and promoting a positive adaptation to this life phase.

Explanation and Reassurance.—Whitehead[31] claims that this therapy was sufficient for 40% of women seeking help at menopause clinics. It is hoped that such discussions include the opportunity for the woman concerned to express her feelings. Since studies have shown that the woman with menopausal complaints may have fewer confiding relationships (see Chapter 9), the opportunity to discuss feelings, stress, and distress is particularly needed.

Hormone Therapy.—The aim of such therapy should be to provide an optimal hormonal background. Estrogen treatment in the estrogen-deficient woman is likely to improve psychologic and sexual functioning. A progestin must be added for those women with an intact uterus. The lowest dosage needed to reverse endometrial changes is recommended because of possible adverse psychologic and sexual effects. There may be fewer side effects if natural progesterone, or progestins chemically similar to this, are utilized. One month of therapy may be necessary before the patient detects change. Studies to date suggest that testosterone may be of benefit to the oopherectomized woman who has lost interest in sex.

Other Therapies.—Cognitive therapy strategies may be of use in helping the patient deal with stresses in her life.[21] These are aimed at helping the woman change her personal perception of events in her life. Such techniques may also help her to improve the quality of other social support relationships in her environment. Other counseling may be needed. For example, the woman with sexual problems frequently has a partner who is also dysfunctional.[23] Individual and couple counseling are often needed, since once dysfunction has been present for some time, negative expectations and sexual anxiety may prevent response to hormone therapy alone.

Finally, the benefit of patient support groups should be mentioned. Such groups can help women redefine their experience more positively, increase their social network, and learn from others' progress.

REFERENCES

1. Campbell S, Whitehead M: Oestrogen therapy and the menopause syndrome. *Clin Obstet Gynecol* 1977; 4:31–47.
2. Coope J: Double blind crossover study of estrogen replacement therapy, in Campbell S (ed): *The Management of the Menopause and Post-menopausal Years.* Lancaster, England, MTP Press Ltd, 1976, pp 159–168.
3. Coppen A, Bishop M, Beard RJ: Effects of piperazine oestrone sulphate on plasmatryptophan, oestrogens, gonadotrophins and psychological functioning in women following hysterectomy. *Curr Med Res Opin* 1977; 4:29–36.
4. Cullberg J: Mood changes and menstrual symptoms with different gestagen/estrogen combinations. *Acta Psychiatr Scand* 1972; [Suppl]236:1–86.
5. De Lignieres B, Vincens M: Differential effects of exogenous oestradiol and progesterone on mood in post-menopausal women: individual dose/effect relationship. *Maturitas* 1982; 4: 67–72.
6. Dennerstein L: Sexuality in the climacteric, in Notelovitz M, van Keep PA (eds): *Proceedings of the 4th International Congress on the Menopause.* Lancaster, England, MTP Press Ltd, in press.
7. Dennerstein L, Burrows GD: A review of studies of the psychological symptoms found at the menopause. *Maturitas* 1978; 1:55–64.

8. Dennerstein L, Wood C, Hudson B, et al: Clinical features and plasma hormone levels after surgical menopause. *Aust NZ J Obstet Gynecol* 1978; 18:202–205.

9. Dennerstein L, Burrows GD, Hyman G, et al: Menopausal hot flushes: A double blind comparison of placebo, ethinyl oestradiol and norgestrel. *Br J Obstet Gynaecol* 1978; 85: 852–856.

10. Dennerstein L, Burrows GD, Hyman GJ, et al: Hormone therapy and affect. *Maturitas* 1979; 1:247–259.

11. Dennerstein L, Burrows GD, Wood C, et al: Hormones and sexuality: Effect of estrogen and progesterone. *Obstet Gynecol* 1980; 56:316–322.

12. Dennerstein L, Laby B, Burrows GD, et al: Headache and sex hormone therapy. *Headache* 1978; 18:146–153.

13. Dennerstein L, Morse C, Gotts G, et al: The view from a PMS clinic, in Gise L, Strain L (eds): *Premenstrual Syndrome: New Findings and Controversies*. New York, Churchill Livingstone, Inc, 1985.

14. Dow MGT, Hart DM: Hormonal treatments of sexual unresponsiveness in postmenopausal women: A comparative study. *Br J Obstet Gynaecol* 1983; 90:361–366.

15. Fedor-Freybergh P: The influence of estrogens on the well-being and mental performance in climacteric and postmenopausal women. *Acta Obstet Gynecol Scand* [Suppl] 1977; 64:1–91.

16. George GCW, Beaumont PJV, Beardwood CJ: Effects of exogenous estrogens on minor psychiatric symptoms in postmenopausal women. *S Afr Med J* 1973; 47:2387–2394.

17. Hahn RG, Nachtingal RD, Davies TC: Compliance difficulties with progestin-supplemented oestrogen replacement therapy. *J Fam Pract* 1984; 18:411–414.

18. Hammarbäck S, Bäckström T, Holst J, et al: Cyclical mood changes as in the premenstrual syndrome during sequential estrogen—progestagen postmenopausal replacement therapy. *Acta Obstet Gynaecol Scand* 1985; 64:393–397.

19. Hepworth M: Sociological aspects of mid-life, in van Keep PA, Utian WH, Vermeulen A (eds): *The Controversial Climacteric*. Lancaster, England, MTP Press Ltd, 1981, pp 19–28.

20. Morrell MJ, Dixen JM, Carter CS, et al: The influence of age and cycling status on sexual arousability in women. *Am J Obstet Gynecol* 1984; 148:66–71.

21. Morse C, Dennerstein L: Thinking, feelings and symptoms. *Patient Management*. 1984; 8:111–116.

22. Paterson MEL: A randomised, double-blind, cross-over study into the effect of sequential mestranol and norethisterone on climacteric symptoms and biochemical parameters. *Maturitas* 1982; 4:83–94.

23. Sarrel PM: Sex problems after menopause: A study of fifty married couples treated in a sex counseling programme. *Maturitas* 1982; 4:231–237.

24. Semmens JP, Wagner G: Estrogen deprivation and vaginal function in postmenopausal women. *JAMA* 1982; 248:445–448.

25. Sherwin BB, Gelfard MN: Sex steroids and affect in the surgical menopause: A double-blind, cross-over study. *Psychoneuroendocrinology*. In press.

26. Sherwin BB, Gelford MM, Brender W: Androgen enhances sexual motivation in females: a prospective, crossover study of sex steroid administration in the surgical menopause. *Psychosom Med*. 1985; 47:339–351.

27. Studd JWW, Parsons A: Sexual dysfunction: The climacteric. *Br J Sex Med* 1977; December, pp 11–12.

28. Studd JWW, Chakravarti S, Oram D: The climacteric. *Clin Obstet Gynecol* 1977; 4:3–29.

29. Studd JWW, Collins WP, Chakravarti S, et al: Oestradiol and testosterone implants in the treatment of psychosexual problems in the postmenopausal woman. *Br J Obstet Gynecol* 1977; 84:314–315.

30. Tonge B: Unpublished M.D. Thesis. University of Melbourne, 1984.

31. Whitehead MI: The menopause. Part A: Hormone 'replacement' therapy—the controversies, in Dennerstein L, Burrows G (eds): *Handbook of Psychosomatic Obstetrics and Gynaecology*. Amsterdam, Elsevier Biomedical Press, 1983, pp 445–481.

32. Dennerstein L, Burows G: Psychological effects of progestins. *Maturitas* 1986; in press.

33. Collins A, Hanson U, Eneroth P: Post-menopausal symptoms and response to hormonal replacement therapy: Influence of psychological factors. *J Psychosom Obstet Gynecol* 1983; 2:227–233.

PART III

Adverse Effects of Hormone Replacement Therapy

CHAPTER **17**

Effects of Estrogen Replacement on Hepatic Function*

HOWARD L. JUDD, M.D.

IN HUMAN BEINGS it is now well established that estrogens, particularly those administered orally, have profound effects on hepatic function. In women, the implications of these responses in physiologic terms are unclear, but in other species these actions are essential for normal reproductive activity. For example, in birds' egg yolk, proteins provide nutrition to the developing embryo and fetus. As discussed by King et al.,[1] the synthesis of egg yolk proteins is regulated by estrogens. These proteins are synthesized in the liver of the mature female bird and transported through the circulation to the developing oocyte. These proteins consist of a complex group of molecules that includes various vitamin- and mineral-binding proteins, lipoproteins, phosphoproteins, and proteins normally regarded as typical constituents of the serum, such as serum albumin. Some are exclusively egg yolk proteins, such as vitellogenin and riboflavin-binding proteins, and are not found in the liver of mature males. Others are synthesized in the male bird at rates several-fold lower than in the female, such as low-density lipoproteins, while others are synthesized at rates similar to that of the female, such as serum albumin.

In amphibians, metamorphosis occurs during which morphologic, physiologic, behavioral, and biochemical changes are observed. Much of the research to define the biochemical changes during metamorphosis has been concerned with changes that take place with hepatic protein metabolism. Estrogens induce protein synthesis during prometamorphosis, prometamorphosis, and the metamorphic climax.[2] Some of these actions are presumably involved in the metamorphological process itself. Thus, in both birds and amphibians, some of the actions of estrogens on hepatic metabolism are definitely reproductive in nature.

In human beings, the same cannot be said. Estrogens clearly influence hepatic protein and lipid metabolism, but these actions do not appear to influence the reproductive activity of the mother or any function of the fetus. Estrogens enhance the production of carrier proteins, including sex hormone-binding globulin (SHBG), cortisol-binding globulin (CBG), thyroxine-binding globulin (TBG), transferrin, and ceruloplasmin.[3] These changes do not represent a medical hazard, but they do alter the results of the clinical laboratory tests that are used to determine serum levels of the substances bound to these carrier proteins.

Estrogens do influence the hepatic synthesis of other proteins that have been incrim-

*Work supported by USPHS Grants Ca 23093 and RR 865.

inated in causing or contributing to the occurrence of certain disease processes. For instance, hypertension may occur or be exacerbated in women receiving estrogen replacement therapy.[4] The elevation of blood pressure is usually reversible when the medication is discontinued. The problem is seen less frequently with estrogen replacement than with the use of oral contraceptives. Although increases of blood pressure have been reported, estrogen replacement has not been associated with an enhanced risk of cerebral vascular accidents.[5]

The mechanism responsible for this increase in blood pressure is believed to be related to the renin-angiotensin-aldosterone system.[6] Under physiologic conditions, renin substrate (angiotensinogen) is the rate-limiting step of the renin reaction.[7] Estrogen administration stimulates the hepatic synthesis of this protein. Associated with this are increases of angiotensin I formation and the secretion of aldosterone.[6]

Although all women who take a sufficient dosage of estrogen have increases in renin substrate levels, only a small percentage develop hypertension. There is also no difference in the absolute circulating levels of renin substrate in women with estrogen-induced hypertension and normotensive women receiving equal doses of the hormone.[8] Thus, the role of renin substrate in the genesis of estrogen-induced hypertension has been questioned. Recent work has shown that estrogen replacement therapy induces the synthesis and release of several forms of renin substrate that are electrophoretically and immunologically distinct from the predominant form of this plasma protein.[9] A large molecular weight form (more than 150,000 daltons) has a greater affinity for the enzyme renin than the predominant form. Circulating levels of this large form increase in women with estrogen-induced hypertension but not in normotensive subjects on the same dosage of medication. The induction of this large form is particularly profound following the administration of ethinyl estradiol.[10] These data suggest the induction of the synthesis of particular forms of renin substrate by estrogen may play an important role in the development of hypertension in some women receiving this form of therapy.

The administration of oral contraceptives increases the risk of overt venous thromboembolic disease and the occurrence of subclinical thrombosis that is extensive enough to be detected by laboratory procedures, such as ^{125}I fibrinogen uptake[11] and plasma fibrinogen chromatography.[12] In uncontrolled studies, thrombophlebitis has been reported with estrogen replacement therapy, whereas this association has not been present in controlled experiments.[13]

Both procoagulant and anticoagulant factors are present in blood to maintain its fluidity while permitting hemostasis with vascular injury. Estrogen exerts several effects on the clotting mechanism that may contribute to or be responsible for a generalized hypercoagulable state. Some of these effects are exerted through the action of estrogen on hepatic function. For example, the clotting factors VII, IX, X, and X complex are increased with estrogen administration.[14, 15] These factors are hepatic in origin. Estrogen replacement therapy can also lower anticoagulant factors, such as antithrombin III and anti Xa.[15] The former is of particular interest. It is hepatic in origin and inactivates thrombin, activated factor X, and other enzymes involved with the generation of thrombin. The potential importance of a reduction of antithrombin III during estrogen replacement therapy is suggested by the occurrence of thrombophilia (intravascular clotting) in subjects with a congenital deficiency of this factor.[16] A reduction of 20% or more has been found to be highly predictive of the occurrence of subclinical venous thromboembolic disease that is extensive enough to be detected by ^{125}I-fibrinogen uptake.[17] Administration of mestranol (up to 0.5 mg/day) has been shown to lower antithrombin III activity by 11% after two months, while ingestion of 1.25 mg/day of conjugated equine estrogens (the most frequently used preparation in the U.S.) was found to have no effect.[15] These findings presumably reflect differences in dosage, since 0.5 mg of mestranol should be equivalent to approximately 5 mg of conjugated estrogen.[18] These data indicate that the usual replacement doses of conjugated estrogen (less than 1.25 mg/day) do not affect antithrombin III activity and may explain the lack of evidence of an increased risk of thromboembolic disease with estrogen replacement therapy in contrast to that reported with oral contraceptives.

All studies have not confirmed the above-mentioned effects of estrogen replacement therapy on clotting parameters. These discrepancies likely result from investigators studying different estrogenic preparations. The relative potencies of these preparations are just now being defined. Until this definition is accomplished, it will be difficult to determine if discrepancies between studies are due to methodologic problems, the variable effects of the different types of estrogen preparations on clotting parameters, or the different potencies of the preparations.

Estrogen replacement therapy also influences hepatic lipid metabolism. An increased incidence of gallbladder disease has been reported with oral contraceptive usage and estrogen replacement therapy.[13, 19] Because bile saturation of cholesterol is between 75% and 90%, small increases can initiate precipitation, leading to stone formation. Increased amounts of cholesterol in bile is a common finding in gallbladder disease. Estrogen replacement increases the cholesterol fraction of bile.[20] Proposed mechanisms for this include increased turnover of body cholesterol and increased hepatic cholesterol synthesis. Cholesterol synthesis is regulated by the enzyme hydroxy-methyl-glutanyl-CoA-reductase, which is inhibited by chenodeoxycholate. A decrease of chenodeoxycholate and an increase of cholate are present in the bile of women receiving estrogen replacement. These changes in bile acids provide a possible explanation for the increased cholesterol in this fluid.

Circulating lipids are also influenced by estrogen replacement. Serum lipids are mostly bound to proteins, and the concentrations of the various types of lipoproteins correlate with the risk of heart disease. Low-density and very low-density lipoprotein levels correlate positively, while high-density lipoprotein concentrations correlate negatively. Estrogen replacement is associated with decreases of low-density lipoprotein cholesterol, reductions or no changes of very low-density lipoprotein (LDL), and increases of high-density lipoprotein (HDL) and triglycerides.[21] Recently, the heterogeneous nature of HDL has been recognized. The HDL fraction consists of several subfractions. The major ones, defined according to density, are the HDL_2 and HDL_3 subfractions.[22] It has been suggested that the HDL_2 subfraction may be a more effective epidemiologic discriminant of heart disease risk than total HDL. Estrogens have been shown to elevate the HDL_2 subfraction. This observation has been found in women who served as their own controls.[23]

Most earlier studies have assessed the effects of estrogen on total HDL or HDL_2 levels using study designs that compared the levels of lipoproteins in groups of women who were or were not using the hormone.[21, 24] The failure to control for other known determinants of HDL, such as degree of obesity, alcohol consumption, physical activity, and cigarette smoking, likely has influenced results, since it has been shown that estrogen and non-estrogen users may differ in characteristics other than just their lipid levels. For instance, women receiving exogenous estrogens have been found to be thinner than women not using the hormone.[25]

The effects of estrogens on lipoproteins are dose-dependent. Two mg of micronized estradiol given orally raises HDL_1 cholesterol and HDL_2 cholesterol levels by averages of 9% and 11%, respectively, in postmenopausal women treated for up to four months, while 4 mg results in increases of 19% and 21% for the same respective lipoprotein fractions.[23] When placebo and conjugated estrogen, 0.625 mg and 1.25 mg, were administered for 18 months the HDL fractions increased by 17%, 10%, and 18%, respectively.[26] The increases with estrogens were not statistically different from placebo.

In patients with familial defects of lipoprotein metabolism, estrogen replacement therapy has rarely been associated with massive elevations of plasma triglycerides, which have led to pancreatitis and other complications.[27] The effects of estrogen on circulating lipids are also believed to be related to changes in hepatic synthesis, although altered clearance of these substances may be involved.

The response of the liver to estrogens seems to be greater than other sites of action. This is particularly true of orally administered hormone. Dose-response studies using orally administered conjugated estrogen show subphysiologic or physiologic responses of the vaginal epithelium and urinary calcium excretion (an indirect marker of bone resorption) at estrogen doses that clearly exert supraphysiologic responses of hepatic markers of estrogen action.[28] The 0.15, 0.3, and 0.625 mg dosages of conjugated estrogen have no measurable effect on the percentage of superficial cells seen with vaginal cytology (Fig 17–1). Only the 1.25 mg dosage significantly increases this marker of estrogen action to a value intermediate between the percentages seen in women during the early and late follicular phases of their cycles. For the fasting urinary calcium/creatinine ratio, the 0.3, 0.625, and 1.25 mg dosages significantly suppress the ratios,

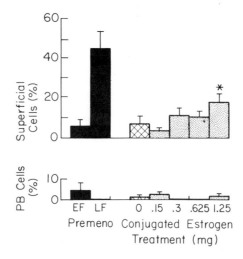

FIG 17–1.
Mean ± SE percentages of parabasal and superficial cells found by a vaginal cytologic technique in 21 postmenopausal women given various dosages of conjugated equine estrogens, each for six weeks. The results found in 15 premenopausal women during the early (*EF*) and late follicular (*LF*) phases of their menstrual cycles and in 15 additional postmenopausal women studied six weeks apart and given no therapy are shown for reference. The *T* represents values that are significantly different from premenopausal results, while the *asterisk* denotes values that are significantly different from baseline results in patients given conjugated estrogen. (From Geola FL, Frumar AM, Tartaryn IV, et al: Biological effects of various doses of conjugated equine estrogens in postmenopausal women. *J Clin Endocrinol Metab* 1980; 51:620. Used by permission.)

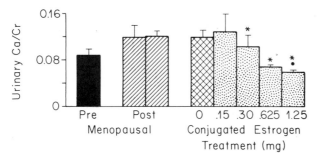

FIG 17–2.
Mean (± SE) urinary calcium/creatinine (*Ca/Cr*) in same groups of patients. (From Geola FL, Frumar AM, Tartaryn IV, et al: Biological effects of various doses of conjugated equine estrogens in postmenopausal women. *J Clin Endocrinal Metab* 1980; 51:620. Used by permission.)

but to values that are comparable to those observed in premenopausal women (Fig 17–2). These dosages increased the circulating concentrations of renin substrate, SHBG, CBG, and TBG to levels in excess of those observed in premenopausal women (Fig 17–3). Thus, orally administered doses of conjugated estrogen can exert physiologic effects on nonhepatic and pharmacologic responses of hepatic markers of estrogen actions.

Similar responses have been observed with orally administered ethinyl estradiol.[18] A dose response study of 5, 10, 20, and 50 µg of ethinyl estradiol showed significant elevations with all dosages of the percentage of superficial cells measured by a vaginal cytologic technique, but even the 50 µg dosage did not raise the percentage higher than that observed in premenopausal women (Fig 17–4). Significant suppressions of urinary calcium excretion with the 10, 20, and 50 µg dosages were observed; however, none

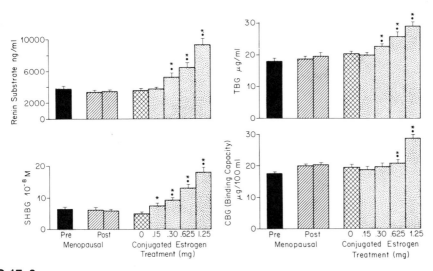

FIG 17–3.
Mean (±SE) serum renin substrate, SHBG, and TBG levels and binding capacity of CGB in the same groups. (From Geola FL, Frumar AM, Tartaryn IV, et al: Biological effects of various doses of conjugated equine estrogens in postmenopausal women. *J Clin Endocrinol Metab* 1980; 51:620. Used by permission.)

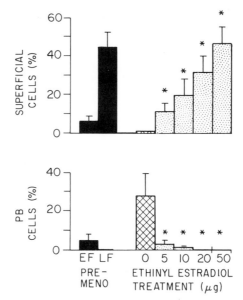

FIG 17–4.
Mean (±SE) for percentage of superficial and parabasal cells by vaginal maturation index in 20 postmenopausal women given various doses of ethinyl estradiol for four weeks each. Results in 20 premenopausal women during the early (*EF*) and late follicular (*LF*) phases of their menstrual cycles are shown for reference. See Fig 17–1 for symbols. (From Mandel FP, Geola FL, Lu JKH, et al: Biologic effects of various doses of ethinyl estradiol in postmenopausal women. *Obstet Gynecol* 1982; 59:673. Reprinted with permission from the American College of Obstetrics and Gynecology.)

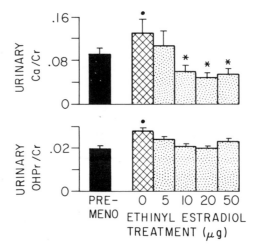

FIG 17–5.
Mean (±SE) urinary *Ca/cr* and hydroxproline/creatinine (*OHPr/Cr*) in same groups of patients. (From Mandel FP, Geola FL, Lu JKH, et al: Biological effects of various doses of ethinyl estradiol in postmenopausal women. *Obstet Gynecol* 1982; 59:673. Reprinted with permission of the American College of Obstetrics and Gynecology.)

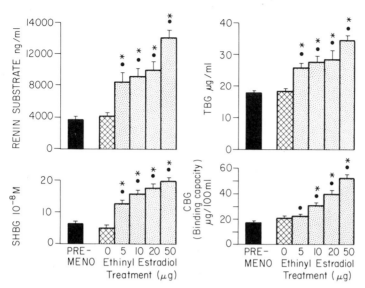

FIG 17–6.
Mean (±SE) serum levels of renin substrate, SHBG, and TBG, and serum binding capacity of CBG in the same groups. (From Mandel FP, Geola FL, Lu JKH, et al: Biological effects of various doses of ethinyl estradiol in postmenopausal women. *Obstet Gynecol* 1982; 59:673. Reprinted with permission of the American College of Obstetrics and Gynecology.)

of these dosages resulted in urinary calcium values that were significantly lower than those found in premenopausal women (Fig 17–5). In the same study, 5 μg of ethinyl estradiol doubled renin substrate levels and raised the levels of all the carrier proteins studied (Fig 17–6). All other doses of ethinyl estradiol had even greater actions on these hepatic proteins. Since the levels of these proteins are similar in pre- and postmenopausal women, these actions of ethinyl estradiol on hepatic protein metabolism must be considered pharmacologic and not physiologic responses.

Several factors could explain the enhanced responsiveness of the liver to orally administered conjugated estrogen and ethinyl estradiol. First, orally administered estrogens are absorbed by the intestines and delivered to the liver through the portal vein before entry into the general circulation. Since the volume of the general circulation is larger than the portal vasculature, and the liver partially metabolizes some estrogenic medications to less active forms, the concentration of active hormone present in the general circulation is said to be four to five times less than that in the portal circulation. Thus, more estrogen is presented to hepatocytes than the cells of other organs.

Second, during passage through the vascular system of an organ, the fraction of circulating estrogens that exits the vascular system, enters the interstitial space, and is presented to cells for action is much greater for the liver than for other organs.[29] Several factors influence the transport of steroid hormones from the circulation to the cells of an organ. These include capillary membrane permeability barriers, the anatomy of the microvascular of an organ, the plasma protein binding of steroids, and capillary transit time. Each of these will be discussed briefly.

In order for a steroid hormone to leave the vascular system, it must exit the capillary by passing between or through the capillary endothelial cells. The plasma membrane of these cells consists of a lipid-protein matrix. Studies indicate that steroids have different permeabilities to capillary endothelial cells. Two factors that influence the permeability characteristics of steroids are the lipid solubility and the polarity of the hormone. The latter is a function of the hydrogen bond-forming functional groups and the charged functional groups. In general, the polarity of a hormone appears to predict membrane permeability much better than lipid solubility does.

Using double-isotope, single-injection, tissue sampling methods, we have assessed the in vivo delivery of estrogens and estrogen conjugates into the uterus and liver during a single passage through these organs' capillary beds in pentobarbital-anesthetized female Sprague-Dawley rats.[29, 30] For studies of the uterus, the lower abdominal aorta and the right common iliac artery were surgically exposed. The latter was clamped, as was the left femoral artery. A mixture of (^{14}C) butanol (the reference substance) and ^{3}H-labeled test steroid was rapidly injected as a bolus into the lower abdominal aorta through a 27-gauge needle. Fifteen seconds after injection, the left uterine horn was resected. This time interval was sufficient for a single pass of the bolus through the uterine vasculature without recirculation. Influx into the liver was determined after injection into the portal vein immediately after ligation of the hepatic artery. Eighteen seconds after injection, the right major lobe was removed.

Uterine and liver tissues were processed, and the uterine influx index (UII) and liver influx index (LII) were calculated as described previously.[29–31] Both uterine and liver tissues were solubilized in 2.0 ml soluene-350 by equilibration at 50°C for about two hours. The tissue and injection solution samples were counted for double isotope (^{3}H and ^{14}C) liquid scintillation counting, and the UII or LII was computed as follows:

$$\text{UII or LII} = \frac{(^3\text{H}:^{14}\text{C}) \text{ dpm ratio in tissue}}{(^3\text{H}:^{14}\text{C}) \text{ dpm ratio in injectate}} \times 100$$

The UII or LII is equal to the ratio of the extraction *(E)* of the estrogen divided by the extraction of the butanol reference 15 and 18 seconds after injection. The *E* for butanol was measured previously, i.e., 77% and 84% in uterus and liver, respectively.[29, 31] Therefore, for the uterus, *E* = (UII) (0.77), and for the liver, *E* = (LII) (0.84).

Figure 17–7 shows the uterine extractions at 15 seconds following injection of radiolabeled estrogens in Ringer's lactate (protein free) into the lower abdominal aorta of the rat. In the absence of serum proteins, the injections allowed assessment of the influence of capillary membrane permeability barriers on hormone entry into this organ. The mean uterine extractions of estrone (E_1) and estradiol (E_2) were 101% and 97%, respectively, demonstrating that these steroids are freely diffusible through the uterine capillary endothelium. By contrast, the mean uterine extractions of estriol (E_3) and estetrol were significantly lower, at 39% and 35%, respectively. Low extractions were also found for the estrogen conjugates, estrone sulfate, estradiol glucuronide, and estriol glucuronide. These permeabilities did not completely parallel the lipid solubility of these steroids but did parallel the polarity of the compounds. These data reveal the prominent and, until recently, little-recognized impact of capillary endothelial cell permeability on the influx of circulating estrogens into this organ.

Conjugated estrogens are normally present in high concentrations in the circulation.[32] Although estrone sulfate can be converted by sulfatases found in endometrial cells to E_1, and this estrogen can be reduced by 17β hydroxylases present in the endometrium to E_2,[33] the uterus does not readily utilize this estrogen conjugate.[34] The low permeability of the uterine capillary endothelium to this steroid may explain this observation.

The second factor influencing the exit of circulating steroids into tissues is the anatomy of an organ's microvascular. Major differences exist in the microvascular of specific organs. For example, the microvascular permeability barrier in the uterus is the plasma membrane of the capillary endothelial cell. This barrier does not permit access of plasma proteins into the interstitial space of the uterus. In contrast, portal vein blood is delivered into the hepatic sinusoids. These are lined by cells whose plasma membranes are not intact, and large pores are present. These cells allow passage of substances such as steroids and proteins out of the sinusoids into the hepatic interstitial space. Thus, the microvascular permeability barrier of this organ is the plasma membrane of the hepatocytes.[35] Influx of steroids is related exponentially to the surface area of an organ's microvascular permeability barrier. The much larger hepatocyte surface area compared to the uterine capillary surface area should markedly enhance the transport of steroids into the liver as compared to the uterus. The impact of this difference in microvascular anatomy between the liver and the uterus should have profound impact on the influx of steroids into these organs.

Figure 17–8 shows the liver extractions of radiolabeled estrogens at 18 seconds following rapid portal vein injections in Ringer's lactate. In contrast to the uterus, all estrogens tested were highly diffusible through the liver sinusoids during a single pass, thus allowing enhanced estrogen action on hepatocytes to proceed. These data indicate that capillary membrane permeability is highly variable between the uterus and liver and is a very important factor in determining the action of circulating estrogens at the cellular level.

Plasma protein binding of steroids also influences the exit of steroids from the circulation. Steroids bind to albumin and to specific globulins. Albumin has a low binding affinity for steroids, but a high binding capacity, while specific globulins bind with a high affinity, approaching that of receptors, but they have a limited capacity. For more than 20 years, the existence of plasma protein binding of steroids has been recognized, and this has resulted in the concept that only the unbound fractions of circulating ste-

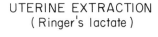

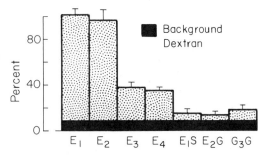

FIG 17–7.
The tissue extractions (percentage) in uterus of ^{3}H-labeled E_1, E_2, E_3, estrone sulfate *(E_1S)*, estradiol glucuronide *(E_2G)*, and estriol glucuronide *(E_3G)* in Ringer's solution relative to that of *(^{14}C)* butanol are shown. Data are mean ± SE (n = 4–8 animals/point). The tissue extraction of dextran refers to nonspecific isotope remaining in uterine capillaries at 15 seconds postinjection. (From Verheugen C, Pardridge WM, Judd HL, et al: Differential permeability of uterine and liver vascular beds to estrogens and estrogen conjugates. *J Clin Endocrinol Metab* 1984; 59:1128. Used by permission.)

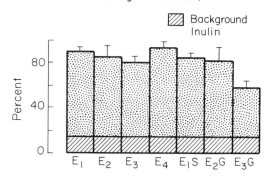

FIG 17–8.
Mean ($\pm$ SE) tissue extractions (percentage) in liver of ^{3}H-labeled estrogens in Ringer's solution relative to that of (^{14}C) butanol are shown. The tissue extraction of inulin refers to isotope remaining 18 seconds postinjection in liver capillaries. (From Verheugen C, Pardridge WM, Judd HL, et al: Differential permeability of uterine and liver vascular beds to estrogens and estrogen conjugates. *J Clin Endocrinol Metab* 1984; 59:1128. Used by permission.)

roids are available for entry into tissues. This fraction has been assessed by in vitro methods, usually using some type of dialysis membrane to determine the unbound, or so-called free, fraction.

Using our double-isotope, single-injection, tissue sampling methods, we have been able to examine in vivo the impact of plasma protein binding on the influx of steroids into specific organs of the rat. This is done by adding plasma proteins to the injection vehicle. Figure 17–9 shows the impact of plasma proteins on uterine uptake of radiolabeled estrogens. The addition of 4% albumin, the normal level found in humans, to Ringer's lactate resulted in a significant reduction of influx of E_2, a minimal effect on E_1, and none on estriol. These effects correspond to the dissociation constants of albumin for these estrogens.[36] The low influxes of the estrogen conjugates were not influenced by the addition of albumin to the injection vehicles. The addition of human pregnant sera to the injection vehicle allowed assessment of the impact of SHBG on hormonal influx. Significant reductions of influx of E_1 and E_2 were observed with the addition of human pregnant serum (high SHBG concentration and 4% albumin) when compared to that seen with 4% albumin alone. The degree of inhibition of extraction of E_2 and E_1 by the uterus were in accordance with the dissociation constants of SHBG for these respective estrogens.[37]

For the unconjugated estrogens, the percentages transported into the uterus, even in the presence of pregnant serum, were 22%–56%. These fractions greatly exceed the percentages of unbound estrogens.[31] Thus, some of the protein-bound fraction of circulating estrogens enter the uterus.

Since albumin and SHBG do not leave the circulation in a single pass through the uterus, it is likely that the estrogens leaving the circulation have dissociated from the protein during the time of transit through the capillary bed. The capillary transit time of an organ is the time required for a substance to pass from the organ's afferent to its efferent vessels and represents the interval that a substance is present in the capillary bed and thus available for transport. The capillary transit time of the uterus has not been

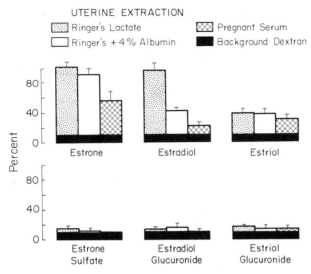

FIG 17–9.
Mean (±SE) tissue extractions of estrogens into uterus relative to radiolabeled butanol using Ringer's solution, Ringer's solution plus 4% bovine serum albumin, and pregnancy serum as the injection vehicles. Tissue extraction of dextran represents isotope remaining in uterine capillaries at time of tissue removal (method blank). (Verheugen C, Pardridge WM, Judd HL, et al: Differential permeability of uterine and liver vascular beds to estrogens and estrogen conjugates. *J Clin Endocrinol Metab* 1984; 59:1128. Used by permission.)

quantitated, but it is likely similar to that of skeletal muscle, approximately one to three seconds.[38] The half-times of estradiol dissociation from albumin is less than one second, probably milliseconds, while it is about seven seconds from SHBG.[39] Thus, dissociation of estrogens from plasma proteins likely occurs during the uterine capillary transit time and accounts for the influx of estrogens that appear to be bound to plasma proteins in in vitro assays into this organ.

For the liver, the capillary transit time is approximately five to ten seconds.[35] Estrogens bound to albumin or SHBG have a greater time to dissociate from these proteins and be unidirectionally transported into hepatocytes. Figure 17–10 shows the effects of 4% albumin and pregnant serum on the transport of radiolabeled estrogens into the liver. Only the transport of estrone sulfate was significantly lower with the addition of albumin, while the influxes of E_2, estrone sulfate, and estriol glucuronide were significantly reduced with pregnant serum when compared with the influxes observed with albumin alone. It should be noted that 36%–100% of these estrogens were transported out of the circulation into the liver in the presence of pregnant serum. These percentages far exceed those observed for the uterus, particularly the estrogen conjugates.

In summary, it appears that for the uterus, capillary membrane permeability is the most important factor influencing access of estrogens and their conjugates to this tissue, with plasma protein binding playing an additional role. This is strikingly different from the liver, in which estrogens and their conjugates are much more readily available for uptake, with capillary permeability and plasma protein binding playing only minor roles. For the estrogens we had studied, the percentages transported from pregnant serum into the liver were two- to sevenfold greater than those that were transported into the uterus.

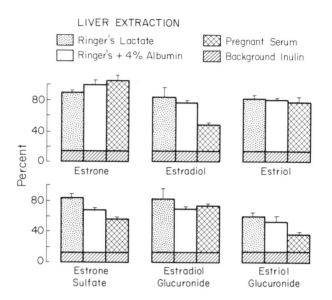

FIG 17–10.
Mean (±SE) tissue extractions of estrogens into liver relative to radiolabeled butanol using Ringer's solution, Ringer's solution plus 4% albumin, and pregnant serum as the injection vehicles. Tissue extraction of inulin represents isotope remaining in liver capillaries at time of tissue sampling (method blank). (From Verheugen C, Pardridge WM, Judd HL, et al: Differential permeability of uterine and liver vascular beds to estrogens and estrogen conjugates. *J Clin Endocinol Metab* 1984; 59:1128. Used by permission.)

This should also contribute to the enhanced responses of hepatic protein and lipid metabolism to circulating estrogens in comparison to other sites of action.

A third possible explanation for the enhanced actions of estrogens on hepatic as compared to nonhepatic markers is greater sensitivity of hepatocytes to estrogen action. To date, no in vitro studies have examined this issue and in vivo studies have been troubled by the variable responses of the liver to estrogens. The various hepatic markers of estrogen action have different sensitivities to these hormones. For the carrier proteins, SHBG is the most sensitive, with TBG next, and CBG the least (see Fig 17–3). Renin substrate is nearly as sensitive as SHBG, with increases of 65%–100% being recorded with administration of 0.625 mg of conjugated estrogen. Fortunately, the actions of estrogens on hepatic clotting factors are relatively insensitive. The 0.625 mg dosage of conjugated equine estrogen has never been shown to alter any of these factors in the circulation.

Hepatic lipid metabolism appears to be less sensitive than protein metabolism to estrogen action. Studies in which patients have been their own controls have shown increases in HDL cholesterol of 10% or less with the 0.625 mg dosage of conjugated estrogens.[26] These changes are not significantly different from the variation seen in untreated controls. Administration of conjugated estrogens vaginally up to 2.5 mg per day has also shown significant elevations of renin substrate and some of the carrier proteins, with no changes in total plasma cholesterol, triglycerides, or any of the lipoprotein fractions (Figs 17–11 and 17–12).[40]

In summary, the human liver continues to have certain vestigial responses to estrogen action which do not appear to have any identifiable role in reproductive function. With

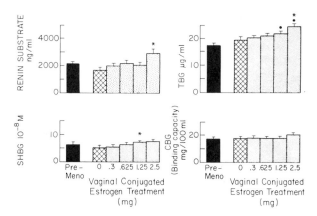

FIG 17–11.
Mean (±SE) levels of renin substrate, SHBG, and TBG, and serum binding capacity of CBG in 20 postmenopausal women given various doses of conjugated estrogen by vaginal creme with each dosage being given daily for four weeks. For reference, results in 20 premenopausal women are shown. See Figure 17–1 for symbols. (From Mandel FP, Geola FL, Meldrum DR, et al: Biological effects of various doses of vaginally administered conjugated equine estrogens in postmenopausal women. *J Clin Endocrinol Metab* 1983; 57:133. Used by permission.)

the possible exception of lipoprotein metabolism, the actions of estrogens on hepatic function in humans appear to be mainly deleterious and are thought to explain partially the occurrence of hypertension, intravascular coagulation, and cholelithiasis seen with this form of therapy.

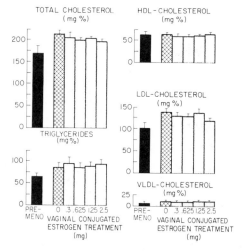

FIG 17–12.
Mean (±SE) levels of triglycerides and total and fractionated cholesterol in the same two groups. *HDL-cholesterol* = high-density lipoprotein cholesterol; *LDL-cholesterol* = low-density lipoprotein cholesterol; *VLDL cholesterol* = very low-density lipoprotein cholesterol. (From Mandel FP, Geola FL, Meldrum DR, et al: Biological effects of various doses of vaginally administered conjugated equine estrogens in postmenopausal women. *J Clin Endocrinol Metab* 1983; 57:133. Used by permission.)

REFERENCES

1. King CR, Udell DS, Deeley RG: Characterization of the estrogen-responsive domain of avian liver and cloning of double-stranded cDNA derived from estrogen-inducible RNA species. *J Biol Chem* 1979; 254:6781.
2. May FEB, Knowland J: Patterns of protein synthesis in livers of xenopus laevis during metamorphosis: Effects of estrogen in normal and thyrostatic animals. *Develop Biol* 1981; 82:158.
3. Mishell DR Jr: Current status of oral contraceptive steroids. *Clin Obstet Gynecol* 1976; 19:743.
4. Crane MG, Harris JJ, Windsor W III: Hypertension, oral contraceptive agents, and conjugated estrogens. *Ann Intern Med* 1971; 74:13.
5. Pfeffer RI, Van den Noort S: Estrogen use and stroke risk in postmenopausal women. *Am J Epidemiol* 1976; 103:445.
6. Laragh JH, Sealey JE, Ledingham JG, et al: Oral contraceptives: Renin, aldosterone and high blood pressure. *JAMA* 1967; 201:918.
7. Weir RJ, Briggs E, Mack A, et al: Blood pressure in women after one year of oral contraception. *Lancet* 1971; 1:467.
8. Eggena P, Barrett JD, Shionoiri H, et al: The influence of estrogens on plasma renin substrate, in Sambhi MP (ed): *Heterogeneity of Renin and Renin Substrate*. New York, Elsevier North-Holland, Inc, 1981, pp 256–60.
9. Eggena P, Hidaka H, Barrett JD, et al: Multiple forms of human plasma renin substrate. *J Clin Invest* 1968; 62:367.
10. Shionoiri H, Eggena P, Barrett JD, et al: An increase in high-molecular weight renin substrate associated with estrogenic hypertension. *Biochem Med* 1983; 29:14.
11. Sagar S, Stamatakis JD, Thomas DP, et al: Oral contraceptives, antithrombin III activity, and postoperative deep-vein thrombosis. *Lancet* 1976; 1:509.
12. Alkjaersig N, Fletcher A, Burstein R: Association between oral contraceptive use and thromboembolism: A new approach to its investigation based on plasma fibrinogen chromatography. *Am J Obstet Gynecol* 1975; 122:199.
13. Boston Collaborative Drug Surveillance Program: Surgically confirmed gallbladder disease, venous thromboembolism, and breast tumors in relation to postmenopausal estrogen therapy. *N Engl J Med* 1974; 290:15.
14. Von Kaulla E, Droegemueller W, Von Kaulla KN: Conjugated oestrogens and hypercoagulability. *Am J Obstet Gynecol* 1975; 122:688.
15. Bonnar J, Haddon M, Hunter DH, et al: Coagulation system changes in postmenopausal women receiving oestrogen preparations. *Postgrad Med J* 1976; 52(Suppl 6):30.
16. Egeberg O: Inherited antithrombim deficiency causing thrombophilia. *Thromb Diath Haemorrh* 1965; 15:516.
17. Stamatakis JD, Lawrence D, Kakkar VV: Surgery, venous thrombosis and anti-Xa. *Br J Surg* 1977; 64:709.
18. Mandel FP, Geola FL, Lu JKH, et al: Biologic effects of various doses of ethinyl estradiol in postmenopausal women. *Obstet Gynecol* 1982; 59:673.
19. Boston Collaborative Drug Surveillance Program: Oral contraceptives and venous thromboembolic disease, surgically confirmed gallbladder disease and breast tumors. *Lancet* 1973; 1:1399.
20. Heuman R, Larsson-Cohn U, Hammar M, et al: Effects of postmenopausal ethinylestradiol treatment on gallbladder bile. *Maturitas* 1979; 2:69.
21. Bradley DD, Wingerd J, Petitti DB, et al: Serum high-density-lipoprotein cholesterol in women using oral contraceptives, estrogens and progestins. *N Engl J Med* 1978; 229:17.
22. Cauley JA, LaPorte RE, Kuller LH, et al: Menopausal estrogen use, high density lipoprotein cholesterol subfractions and liver function. *Atherosclerosis* 1983; 49:31.
23. Wallentin L, Fahraeus L: High density lipoprotein subfractions during oral and cutaneous administration of 17β-estradiol to menopausal women. *J Clin Endocrinol Metab* 1983; 56:797.
24. Wallace RB, Hoover J, Barrett-Connor E, et al: Altered plasma lipid and lipoprotein levels associated with oral contraceptive and oestrogen use. *Lancet* 1979; 2:11.

25. Tikkanen M, Kuusi T, Vartianen E, et al: Treatment of postmenopausal hypercholesteremia with estradiol. *Acta Obst Gynecol Scand* [Suppl] 1972; 88:83.
26. Notelovitz M, Gudat JC, Ware MD, et al: Oestrogen-progestin therapy and the lipid balance of postmenopausal women. *Maturitas* 1982; 4:301.
27. Glueck CJ, Scheel D, Fishback J, et al: Estrogen-induced pancreatitis in patients with previously covert familial type V hyperlipoproteinemia. *Metabolism* 1972; 21:657.
28. Geola FL, Frumar AM, Tataryn IV, et al: Biological effects of various doses of conjugated equine estrogens in postmenopausal women. *J Clin Endocrinol Metab* 1980; 51:620.
29. Pardridge WM, Mietus LJ: Transport of protein-bound steroid hormones into liver *in vivo*. *Am J Physiol* 1979; 237:E367.
30. Laufer LR, Gambone JC, Chaudhuri G, et al: The effect of membrane permeability and binding by human proteins on sex steroid influx into the uterus. *J Clin Endocrinol Metab* 1983; 56:1282.
31. Verheugen C, Pardridge WM, Judd HL, et al: Differential permeability of uterine and liver vascular beds to estrogens and estrogen conjugates. *J Clin Endocrinol Metab* 1984; 59:1128.
32. Roberts KD, Rochefort JG, Bleau G, et al: Plasma oestrone sulphate concentration in postmenopausal women. *Steroids* 1980; 35:179.
33. Tseng L, Stolee A, Gurpide E: Quantitative studies on the uptake and metabolism of estrogens and progesterone by human endometrium. *Endocrinology* 1972; 90:390.
34. Holinka CF, Gurpide E: *In vivo* uptake of estrone sulfate by rabbit uterus. *Endocrinology* 1980; 106:1193.
35. Goresky CA, Rose CP: Blood-tissue exchange in liver and heart: The influence of heterogeneity of capillary transit times. *Fed Proc* 1977; 26:2629.
36. Westphal U: *Steroid-Protein Interaction*. New York, Springer-Verlag New York, 1971.
37. Dunn JF, Nisula BC, Rodbard D: Transport of steroid hormones: Binding of 21 endogenous steroids to both testosterone-binding globulin and corticosteroids-binding globulin in human plasma. *J Clin Endocrinol Metab* 1981; 53:58.
38. Sarelius IH, Damon DN, Duling BR: Microvasculature adaptions during maturation of striated muscles. *Am J Physiol* 1981; 241:4317.
39. Pardridge WM: Transport of protein-bound hormones into tissues *in vivo*. *Endocr Rev* 1981; 2:103.
40. Mandel FP, Geola FL, Meldrum DR, et al: Biologic effects of various doses of vaginally administered conjugated equine estrogens in postmenopausal women. *J Clin Endocrinol Metab* 1983; 57:133.

CHAPTER **18**

Menopause, Estrogen Treatment, and Carbohydrate Metabolism

WILLIAM N. SPELLACY, M.D.

THE USE OF ESTROGENS in the management of the menopausal woman has recently been through a three-phase cycle of "yes-no-yes" decision making by the medical profession. This has followed the acquisition of scientific knowledge giving a better understanding of the physiologic and pathologic processes involved. The woman with hot flushes and dyspareunia from an atrophic vagina clearly gets relief by using estrogen after the menopause, so physicians initially said "yes" to estrogen use. The realization that estrogen could induce breast and endometrial tissue to hyperplasia and neoplasia led to the "no" phase, when many physicians stopped advocating estrogen. A further understanding that estrogen retains bone calcium and prevents osteoporosis and serious bone fractures and their obvious morbidity and mortality, plus the realization that a cyclic progestin could put cells at rest by decreasing nuclear receptors for estrogen and therefore reduce the neoplasia risk, led to the present phase, in which physicians are once again saying "yes" to estrogen. With the resurgence of estrogen use for the menopausal woman, a search for other possible risks and benefits has begun.

There is a wide recognition that the use of oral contraceptives, which contain an estrogen and progestin steroid, is often accompanied by a deterioration of carbohydrate metabolism.[1] Extensive studies in this area have demonstrated that the effect is related to the high dose of steroids that are most often responsible.[1] Further studies of the mechanisms involved have demonstrated that a local tissue insulin receptor effect occurs and that estrogens tend to increase insulin receptor binding, whereas the progestins tend to decrease it.[2] Theoretically, one could therefore improve some cases of abnormal

TABLE 18–1.

Statistical Studies of Blood Glucose Levels in mg/dl Following an Oral Glucose Tolerance Test Performed Before and After Two Years of Menopausal Treatment with Estrogen (1.25 mg Premarin)

	CONTROL TEST					TWO-YEAR TREATMENT TEST				
		TIME AFTER GLUCOSE LOADING					TIME AFTER GLUCOSE LOADING			
TEST	Fasting	0.5 hr	1 hr	2 hr	3 hr	Fasting	0.5 hr	1 hr	2 hr	3 hr
Mean	85.1	119.8	101.9	89.8	78.1	86.0	130.7	110.1	97.4	73.5
SEM	2.5	5.8	5.8	4.1	4.7	1.3	6.8	6.7	6.6	6.6
t	0.39	1.42	1.27	1.08	0.71					
P	N.S.*	N.S.	N.S.	N.S.	N.S.					

*N.S. indicates not significant

TABLE 18–2.
Reports on the Effects of Estrogens on Carbohydrate Metabolism of "Normal" Menopausal Women

AUTHOR AND YEAR	NUMBER OF SUBJECTS	ESTROGEN USED	DURATION OF STUDY	TYPE OF TESTING	EFFECTS OF BLOOD GLUCOSE	OTHER
Jones & Mac-Gregor, 1936	10	Oestrin	3 mos	OGT*	Unchanged	
Buchler and Warren, 1966	4	Diethylstilbestrol, 5 mg qd	1 mo	OGT IVGT†	2/4 impaired, 1/4 same, 1/4 better	IVGT little changed
Sugawa et al., 1967	5	Estradiol 0.2 mg IM	—	Fasting	Unchanged	
Javier et al., 1968	9	Mestranol 75 MCG qd	1–10 mos	OGT	Impaired tolerance	
Goldman and Ovadia, 1969	30	Premarin 1.25 mg	3 mos	IVGT	Impaired tolerance	Decrease mean K value 1.74 to 1.45 $P <$ .005 return to normal post drug
Carter et al., 1970	4	Mestranol 1 mg Tid	5–36 mos	Fasting	Lower	Treated for breast cancer
Gow & Mac-Gillivray, 1971	20	Mestranol 20 MCG	4 mos	IVGT	Impaired tolerance	Returned to normal post drug
Ajabor et al., 1972	9	Premarin 1.25 mg	6 mos	OGT	Increased	No change in insulin, 3 received Enovid

Study	N	Treatment	Duration	Test*	Glucose	Insulin/Other
Spellacy et al., 1972	171	Premarin ethinyl estradiol mestranol	6 mos	OGT	Unchanged	Unchanged insulin levels
Notelovitz 1976	34	Premarin 1.25 mg	9 mos	OGT	Unchanged	Insulin unchanged
Syvalahti et al., 1976	10	Estriol succinate 2 mg or oestradiol valerianate 1–2 mg	—	Tolbutamide	Unchanged	
Rubio 1976	10	Estriol sucinate 6 mg	6 mos	OGT	Unchanged	
Larsson-Cohen and Wallentin, 1977	39	Ethinyl estradiol valerianate 2 mg	6 mos	OGT	EE-lower Fasting raised curve EV-None	EE-Elevated insulin and HGH EV-Insulin unchanged, elevated HGH
Thom et al., 1977	50	Premarin 1.25 mg oestradiol valerianate 20 mg	3 mos	OGT	P-Impaired 7 Improved 3 EV-None	
Spellacy et al., 1978	36	Premarin 1.25 mg	12 mos	OGT	Unchanged except elevated 1 hour value	Insulin levels unchanged
Natchtigall et al., 1979	84	Premarin 2.5 mg	10 yrs	—	Unchanged 2 hr pc	Also received provera 10 mg qd × 7

*OGT indicates oral glucose tolerance test
†IVGT indicates intravenous glucose tolerance test

carbohydrate metabolism with estrogen therapy alone, and likewise, such women would have a deterioration of their condition with the use of progestins. These data are therefore important to consider whenever exogenous female sex steroids are going to be used.

The metabolic studies during the use of sex steroids for the menopausal woman have been limited. There have been several studies of the effects of estrogens on carbohydrate metabolism in various laboratory animals.[3–9] In general, these have shown an improvement in blood glucose control in both the normal and experimentally induced hyperglycemic animal with estrogen treatments. This improved carbohydrate metabolism with estrogen use was contrasted by a deterioration seen with testosterone administration and no effect of progesterone.[5] Most of the early investigators attributed this effect to the suppression of the pituitary gland activity (FSH) by estrogen.[4]

In 1935 Mazer and associates noted that women treated with an estrogen (Theelin) had no change in blood glucose levels, whereas three diabetic women so treated had lowered blood glucose levels and less glucosuria.[10] Since then, a number of studies have been done on the effects of estrogens on carbohydrate metabolism in young women and menopausal women.

One such study involved the use of the conjugated estrogen, Premarin, in a dose of 1.25 mg. In this study, 12 menopausal women had an oral glucose tolerance test performed before and after two years of drug usage. The test involved the administration of 100 gm oral glucose after a ten-hour fast, and bloods were drawn fasting and at 30 minutes and one, two, and three hours after the glucose. Later the bloods were analyzed in duplicate for their glucose content. The drug was administered in a three-week-on-one-week-off cyclic manner without the addition of a progestogen. The results of this study are shown in Table 18–1. It can be seen that there were no significant alterations in any of the blood glucose values following two years of estrogen use.

The literature suggests that, for normal women of reproductive age, estrogens have tended to lower fasting glucose levels and have little effect on the glucose tolerance curve.[11, 12] This is in keeping with their ability to increase insulin receptor binding to insulin. The studies of menopausal women have been directed to two populations, namely, normal women and diabetics. Sixteen such studies of the normal menopausal woman are summarized in Table 18–2.[12–27] It can be seen that with ten drug groups there was no effect seen on the blood glucose levels if estrogens are used. In eight drug groups there was impairment of glucose tolerance resulting. In these studies, three groups were undergoing intravenous glucose tolerance testing, where some deterioration was noted with Premarin and mestranol.[14, 17, 19] One study by Ajabor et al. of six women, and one by Thom et al., showed higher glucose levels with Premarin therapy.[20, 26] In studies by Javier et al. and Gow and MacGillivray using mestranol, and in one by Larsson-Cohen and Wallentin using ethinyl estradiol, there were deteriorations noted.[16, 19, 25] These are both potent estrogens. In another report by Carter and co-workers, who had treated menopausal women who had breast cancer with very high doses of mestranol, they noted that the fasting blood glucose was lowered.[18] Buchler and Warren noted that diethylstilbestrol had a deteriorating effect on oral tolerance but little effect on intravenous glucose tolerance.[14] In four studies, plasma insulin levels were measured, and all of them report no change with estrogen therapy.[12, 20, 21, 23]

There have been several studies of the effects of estrogen treatment of the menopausal woman with diabetes mellitus, and these are listed in Table 18–3.[14, 26, 28–35] The results of these studies show that, generally, carbohydrate metabolism is unchanged or improved with the estrogen treatment in terms of either better blood glucose control or a

TABLE 18-3.
Reports on the Effects of Estrogens on Carbohydrate Metabolism in Menopausal Women with Diabetes Mellitus

AUTHOR AND YEAR	NUMER OF SUBJECTS	ESTROGEN USED	DURATION OF STUDY	TYPE OF TESTING	EFFECTS ON BLOOD GLUCOSE	OTHER
Collens et al., 1936	7	Amniotin, 100–400 rat Units qd	1 mo	Urine glucose	Unchanged	
Glen & Eaton, 1938	1	Dihydroxyoestrin, 10,000 mouse units	—	Blood	Lower	
Gessler et al., 1939	5	Estradiol Benzoate, 10,000 rat units Im qd	1–6 mos	Fasting blood	Lower 3/5 Unchanged 2/5	
Spiegelman, 1940	9	10,000 IU Estrogen Im 2×/week	5 mos	Insulin dose used	—	Less insulin needed
Lawrence & Madders 1941	5	Stilbestrol 1 mg qid	2 mos	Blood glucose & insulin dose used	Unchanged	
Cantilo, 1941	40	Estrin 5–15 mg 3×/week	—	Blood and urine glucose	Lowered	Also progesterone 1–100 mg 2×/week
Marcus & Glotzer, 1948	7	Estriol Benzoate 6000 rat units IM 2×/week	3 mos	Blood & urine glucose/insulin dose used	Lower	Less insulin needed
Nelson et al., 1963	9	Ethinyl estradiol 0.2 mg	—	Glucosuria	Unchanged	Estrogen plus cortisol increased glucosuria
Buchler and Warren, 1966	1	Diethylstilbestrol 5 mg qd	1 mo	Oral tolerance	Worse	
Thom et al., 1977	1	Premarin 1.25 mg	3 mos	Oral tolerance	Lowered	

decreased need for exogenous insulin. Indeed, in one long-term study, Hammond and co-workers found a statistically significant reduction in the frequency of diabetes in menopausal women treated with estrogen.[36]

Thus, the human studies published to date do not suggest any consistent adverse effects of physiologic-level replacement of estrogen on the carbohydrate metabolism of menopausal women. There appear to be no carbohydrate changes at low estrogen doses and adverse changes mainly at high doses with mestranol or ethinyl estradiol. Indeed, these data suggest that the menopausal woman with abnormal metabolism may benefit with such therapy and have an improvement in her glucose tolerance. These results are in agreement with those seen in the experimental animal, which demonstrate an increase in insulin receptor binding at the target tissues with estrogen treatment.[2] They also agree with data on the metabolism of human fat biopsies, which show that the cells from women respond better to insulin in terms of glucose transport compared to the fat cells from men.[37]

The recent trends suggest that the cyclic estrogen therapy should be accompanied with a shorter term of cyclic progestin treatment to reduce the potential for breast and endometrial neoplasia, due to the reduction of nuclear receptors for estrogen.[38] This further complicates the carbohydrate metabolic effects, since a number of the progestins have been shown to produce adverse carbohydrate metabolic effects.[1] In a three-month study using the sequential approach with mestranol and norethisterone or ethinyl estradiol and megestrol acetate, Thom and associates noted decreased glucose tolerance with both.[26] The progestins also affect lipid metabolism by reducing the levels of high-density lipoprotein (HDL) cholesterol.[39] Several studies have shown that medroxyprogesterone has a minimal effect on lipids, and therefore it seems to be an appropriate progestin to use in the menopausal woman.[40] While the long-acting form of medroxyprogesterone can alter carbohydrate metabolism,[41] it is less likely to occur with the low-dose short-term therapy used in the menopausal woman. Thus far, there have been few prospective studies of carbohydrate metabolism in normal and diabetic menopausal women receiving an estrogen-progestin replacement-type therapy. The one by Nachtigall and associates suggests no adverse effects.[22]

In summary, high-dose estrogen-progestin therapy to suppress ovulation in young women (oral contraceptives) has produced adverse effects on carbohydrate metabolism. The lower dose physiologic replacement of estrogens to menopausal women has tended to improve glucose tolerance, which is in keeping with the experimental evidence that estrogen increases insulin binding to its receptors. The use of estrogen-progestin mixtures in menopausal women has not been well studied, but the low dose and short cycle of use suggests that minimal adverse effects will be seen. This, coupled with other findings of increased bone density and less breast and endometrial neoplasia, points to a positive benefit-to-risk ratio. Animal studies suggest that estrogen given with other steroids such as etiocholanolone may provide improved carbohydrate benefits for diabetics at lower dosage and therefore lower risk.[42]

REFERENCES

1. Spellacy, WN: Carbohydrate metabolism in male infertility and female fertility-control patients. *Fertil Steril* 1976; 27:1132–1141.
2. Ballejo G, Saleem TH, Khan-Dawood FS, et al: The effect of sex steroids on insulin binding by target tissues in the rat. *Contraception* 1983; 28:413–422.
3. Barnes BO, Regan JF, Nelson WO: Improvement in experimental diabetes following the administration of Amniotin. *JAMA* 1933; 101:926–927.

4. Nelson WO, Overholser MD: The effect of oestrogenic hormone on experimental pancreatic diabetes in the monkey. *Endocrinology* 1936; 20:473–480.
5. Lewis JT, Foglia VG, Rodriguez RR: The effects of steroids on the incidence of diabetes in rats after subtotal pancreatectomy. *Endocrinology* 1950; 46:111–121.
6. Acevedo D, Migone A: Diabetes experimental y estrogenos. *Rev Cien Lima* 1952; 54: 1959–1962.
7. Houssay BA, Foglia VG, Rodriguez RR: Production or prevention of some types of experimental diabetes by estrogens or corticoids. *Arch Endocrinol* 1954; 17:146–164.
8. Basabe JC, Chieri RA, Foglia VG: Action of sex hormones on the insulinemia of castrated female rats. *Proc Soc Exp Biol Med* 1969; 130:1159–1161.
9. Paik SG, Michelis MA, Kim YT, et al: Induction of insulin-dependent diabetes by streptozotocin inhibition by estrogens and potentiation by Androgens. *Diabetes* 1982; 31:724–729.
10. Mazer C, Meranze DR, Israel SL: Evaluation of the constitutional effects of large doses of estrogenic principle. *JAMA* 1935; 105:257–263.
11. Talaat M, Habib YA, Higazy AM, et al: Effect of sex hormones on the carbohydrate metabolism and normal and diabetic women. *Arch Int Pharmacodyn Ther* 1965; 154:402–411.
12. Spellacy WN, Buhi WC, Birk SA, et al: The effect of estrogens on carbohydrate metabolism: Glucose, insulin, and growth hormone studies on one hundred and seventy-one women ingesting premarin, mestranol and ethyl estradiol for six months. *Am J Obstet Gynecol* 1972; 114:378–392.
13. Jones MS, MacGregor TN: Inhibitory effect of follicular hormone on the anterior pituitary in humans. *Lancet* 1936; 2:974–975.
14. Buchler D, Warren JC: Effects of estrogen on glucose tolerance. *Am J Obstet Gynecol* 1966; 95:479–483.
15. Sugawa T, Moriyama I, Hirooka C, et al: Observations on amino acid and protein metabolism with reference to the hormonal control in pregnancy. II. Effect of steroid hormone on glucogenesis of amino acid. *J Jap Obstet Gynecol Soc* 1967; 14:59–66.
16. Javier Z, Gershberg H, Hulse M: Ovulatory suppressants, estrogens, and carbohydrate metabolism. *Metabolism* 1968; 17:443–456.
17. Goldman JA, Ovadia JL: The effect of estrogen on intravenous glucose tolerance in women. *Am J Obstet Gynecol* 1969; 103:172–178.
18. Carter AC, Slivko B, Feldman EB: Metabolic effects of mestranol in high dose. *Steroids* 1970; 16:5–13.
19. Gow S, MacGillivray I: Metabolic, hormonal, and vascular changes after synthetic oestrogen therapy in oophorectomized women. *Br Med J* 1971; 2:73–77.
20. Ajabor LN, Tsai CC, Vela P, et al: Effect of exogenous estrogen on carbohydrate metabolism in postmenopausal women. *Am J Obstet Gynecol* 1972; 113:383–387.
21. Spellacy WN, Buhi WC, Birk SA: Effect of estrogen treatment for one year on carbohydrate and lipid metabolism in women with normal and abnormal glucose tolerance test results. *Am J Obstet Gynecol* 1978; 131:87–90.
22. Notelovitz M: The effect of long-term oestrogen replacement therapy on glucose and lipid metabolism in postmenopausal women. *S Afr Med J* 1976; 50:2001–2003.
23. Syvalahti E, Erkkola R, Punnonen R, et al: Serum growth hormone, serum immunoreactive insulin and blood glucose response to intravenous tolbutamide in postmenopausal women with and without natural oestrogen. *Ther Acta Pharm Toxicol* 1976; 38:177–185.
24. Rubio B: Efecto del succinato de estriol sobre la curva de tolerancia a la glucosa, en pacientes climatericas. *Mex Invest Med Int* 1976; 3:287–294.
25. Larsson-Cohn U, Wallentin L: Metabolic and hormonal effects of postmenopausal oestrogen replacement treatment. I. Glucose, insulin and human growth hormone levels during oral glucose tolerance tests. *Acta Endocrinol* 1977; 86:583–596.
26. Thom M, Chakravarti S, Oram DH, et al: Effect of hormonal replacement therapy on glucose tolerance in postmenopausal women. *Br J Obstet Gynaecol* 1977; 84:776–784.
27. Nachtigall LE, Nachtigall RH, Nachtigall RD, et al: Estrogen Replacement Therapy II: A prospective study in the relationship to carcinoma and cardiovascular and metabolic problems. *Obstet Gynecol* 1979; 54:74–79.
28. Collens WS, Slo-Bodkin SG, Rosenbliett S, et al: The effect of estrogenic substance on human diabetes. *JAMA* 1936; 106:678–682.

29. Glen A, Eaton JC: Insulin antagonism. *Q J Med* 1938; 31:271–291.
30. Gessler CJ, Halsted JA, Stetson RP: Effect of estrogenic substance on the blood sugar of female diabetics after the menopause. *J Clin Invest* 1939; 18:715–722.
31. Spiegelman AR: Influence of estrogen on the insulin requirement of the diabetic. *Am J Med Sci* 1940; 200:228–234.
32. Lawrence RD, Madders K: Human diabetes treated with oestrogens. *Lancet* 1941; 1: 601–602.
33. Cantilo E: Successful responses in diabetes mellitus of the menopause produced by the antagonistic action of sex hormones on pituitary activity. *Endocrinol* 1941; 28:20–24.
34. Marcus H, Glotzer S: Estrogens in diabetes. *NY State J Med* 1948; 48:1461–1464.
35. Nelson DH, Tanney H, Mestman G, et al: Potentiation of the biologic effect of administered cortisol by estrogen treatment. *J Clin Endocrinol Metab* 1963; 23:261–265.
36. Hammond CB, Jelovsek FR, Lee KL, et al: Effects of long-term estrogen replacement therapy I. Metabolic effects. *Am J Obstet Gynecol* 1979; 133:525–536.
37. Foley JE, Kashiwagi A, Chang H, et al: Sex differences in insulin-stimulated glucose tolerance transport in rat and human adipocytes. *Am J Physiol* 1984; 246:E211–E215.
38. Whitehead MI, Townsend PT, Pryse-Davies J, et al: Effects of estrogens and progestins on the biochemistry and morphology of the postmenopausal endometrium. *N Engl J Med* 1981; 305:1599–1605.
39. Knopp RH, Walden CE, Wahl PW, et al: Oral contraceptive and postmenopausal estrogen effects on lipoprotein triglyceride and cholesterol in adult female population: Relationships to estrogen and progestin potency. *J Clin Endocrinol* 1981; 53:1123–1132.
40. Hirvonen E, Mal konen M, Manninen V: Effect of different progestogens on lipoproteins during postmenopausal replacement therapy. *N Engl J Med* 1981; 304:560–563.
41. Spellacy WN, Mcleod AGW, Buhi WC, et al: The effects of medroxy progesterone acetate on carbohydrate metabolism: Measurements of glucose, insulin, and growth hormone after twelve months use. *Fertil Steril* 1972; 23:239–244.
42. Coleman DL, Leiter EH, Applezweig N: Therapeutic effects of Dehydroepiandrosterone metabolites in diabetes mutant mice (C57BL/KsJ-db/db). *Endocrinology* 1984; 115:239–243.

CHAPTER **19**

Breast Neoplasia

BRIAN E. HENDERSON, M.D.
RONALD K. ROSS, M.D.
MALCOLM C. PIKE, M.D.

THE HYPOTHESIS that exogenous hormones might be causally related to human breast cancer has developed, in large part, from epidemiologic and experimental studies that have linked endogenous levels of certain steroid and polypeptide hormones, especially estrogen and prolactin, to breast cancer risk.

Because of this evidence and the importance of breast cancer in terms of morbidity and mortality, there is reason for concern about the effects of cancer risk if the same or closely related hormones are administered for therapeutic purposes, for example, as oral contraceptives or estrogen replacement therapy in the menopause.

We begin this chapter by reviewing the epidemiologic and experimental data related to endogenous hormones and then review the rather large volume of epidemiologic information on exogenous hormones, especially hormone replacement therapy,[1] and human breast cancer. The epidemiologic risk factors related to endogenous endocrine hormones are shown in Table 19-1.

"ENDOCRINE" BREAST CANCER RISK FACTORS

Age at Menarche.—A significantly higher risk of developing breast cancer among women with an early age at menarche has been found in many case-control studies.[1, 2] Table 19-2 shows that menarche at age 12 or younger, compared to menarche at age 13 or older, translates into an approximately twofold increased risk of breast cancer in young women. The effect would be expected to decrease with increasing age[1] and it has been so reported.

In a subsequent study of these young women, we recorded not only age at onset of menstruation, but also age when "regular" menstruation was first established. For a fixed age at menarche, the establishment of regular menstrual cycles within one year of the first menstrual period more than doubled the risk of breast cancer when compared to those in whom it took more than five years for the menses to regularize.[3] A woman with early menarche (age 12 or younger) and rapid establishment of regular cycles had an almost fourfold increased risk of breast cancer when compared with a woman with late menarche (age 13 or older) and long duration of irregular cycles.

Age at Menopause.—The relationship between menopause and breast cancer risk has been known for some time.[4-6] The rate of increase in the age-specific incidence rate of breast cancer slows sharply at the time of menopause and the rate of increase in the

TABLE 19–1.

Epidemiologic Factors Associated With Increased Risk
of Breast Cancer

CATEGORY	RISK FACTOR
Anthropometric	Increased postmenopausal weight
Menstrual	Early age at menarche
	Late age at menopause
	Decreased frequency of artificial menopause
Reproductive	Nulliparity
	Late age at first full-term delivery

TABLE 19–2.

Relative Risk of Breast Cancer by
Age at Menarche in Women Aged
32 and Younger*

	AGE AT MENARCHE (YEARS)	
	− 12	13 +
Cases (n)	101	62
Controls (n)	128	142
Relative risk	1.8	1.0

*From Pike MC, Henderson BE, Casa-
grande JT, et al: Oral contraceptive use
and early abortion as risk factors for
breast cancer in young women. *Br J
Cancer* 1981; 43:72. Used by permission.

postmenopausal period is only about one sixth the rate of increase in the premenopausal period (Fig 19–1).

Trichopolous et al.[6] estimated that women whose natural menopause occurs before age 45 have only one half the breast cancer risk of those whose menopause occurs after age 55 (Table 19–3). Another way of expressing this result is that women with 40 or more years of active menstruation have twice the breast cancer risk of those with fewer than 30 years of menstrual activity. Artificial menopause, by either bilateral oophorectomy or pelvic irradiation, also markedly reduces breast cancer risk. The effect appears to be just slightly greater than that of natural menopause (defined as cessation of periods) (see Table 19–3). Feinleib[4] showed that a unilateral oophorectomy or a simple hysterectomy produced little change in risk.

Age at First Full-Term Pregnancy.—Two of the earliest known and most reproducible features of breast cancer epidemiology are the decreased risk associated with increased parity and the increased risk of single women.

MacMahon et al.[7] made a major advance in our understanding of the role of pregnancy in altering breast cancer risk through their analysis of an international collaborative case-control study. Single and nulliparous married women were found to have the same increased risk of breast cancer, which is approximately 1.4 times the risk of parous married women. Among married women in each country, parous women with breast cancer had fewer children than parous controls. MacMahon and his colleagues clearly demonstrated, however, that this protective effect of parity was totally due to a protec-

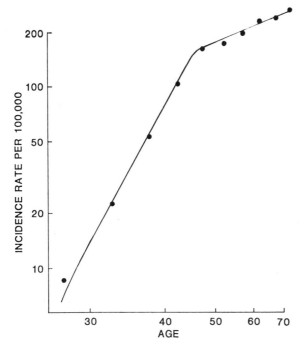

FIG 19–1.
Age-specific breast cancer incidence rates for U.S. white females 1969–1971.

tive effect of early age at first birth. Those women with a first birth occurring before age 20 had about one half the risk of nulliparous women (Table 19–4). Controlling for age at first birth, subsequent births had no influence on the risk of developing breast cancer (Table 19–5). Two recent studies in other populations have observed a small residual protective effect of an increasing number of births,[8–9] and this suggests that there may be certain circumstances in which multiparity does offer some further protection. The main protective effect is, however, undoubtedly associated with the first full-term pregnancy occurring at an early age.

In the study of MacMahon et al.,[7] incomplete pregnancies before the first full-term pregnancy did not have any protective effect. Recently, we found that a first-trimester abortion, whether spontaneous or induced, before the first full-term pregnancy was actually associated with an increase in the risk of breast cancer.[2] Abortions after the first full-term pregnancy did not carry any increased risk of breast cancer.

TABLE 19–3.

Relative Risk of Breast Cancer by Age of Menopause*

TYPE OF MENOPAUSE	AGE AT MENOPAUSE (YEARS)			
	≤44	45–49	50–54	≤55
Artifical menopause†	0.8	1.0	1.3	—
Natural menopause	1.0	1.3	1.5	2.0

*Derived from data in Trichopolous et al.[6]
†Bilateral oophorectomy.

Weight.—There is a strong relationship between weight and breast cancer risk. Table 19–6 shows the results of a study by deWaard et al.[10] in Holland. The relationship is critically dependent on age. For women younger than age 50 there is little or no increased risk associated with increased weight, but in the 60–69-year-old group, an increase in weight from less than 60 kg to 70 kg or greater increases the breast cancer risk by 80%. Similar results had been obtained in an earlier study of deWaard and Baanders-van Halewijn,[11] and have also been obtained by others.[12]

Whether this weight effect is one of excess weight (body fat?) or weight per se is not clear. Contradictory results have been reported on whether, for example, Quetelet's index (wt/ht^2) is correlated with breast cancer risk. Unadjusted weight appears to be as good an indicator of risk as any other function of weight and height.

TABLE 19–4.

Relative Risk of Breast Cancer by Age at First Birth*

AGE AT FIRST BIRTH (YEARS)	RELATIVE RISK
Nulliparous	1.0
≤19	0.5
20–24	0.6
25–29	0.8
30–34	0.9
≥35	1.2

*From MacMahon B, Cole P, Lin TM, et al: Age at first birth and cancer risk. *Bull WHO* 1970; 43:209. Used by permission.

TABLE 19–5.

Relative Risk of Breast Cancer by Number of Births After the First Birth, Adjusting for Age at First Birth*

NO. OF BIRTHS, AFTER THE FIRST	RELATIVE RISK
0	1.0
1	1.2
2	1.0
3	1.0
≥4	0.9

*From MacMahon B, Cole P, Lin TM, et al: Age at first birth and cancer risk. *Bull WHO* 1970; 43:209. Used by permission.

TABLE 19–6.

Relative Risk of Breast Cancer by Body Weight*

AGE AT DIAGNOSIS (YEARS)	WEIGHT (KG) ≤59	60–69	≤70
35–49	1.0	0.9	1.2
50–59	1.0	1.2	1.4
60–69	1.0	1.6	1.8

*Derived from deWaard F, et al.[10]

ESTROGEN LEVELS AND RISK OF BREAST CANCER

The breast cancer risk factors of early age at menarche and delayed age at menopause indicate that ovarian activity is an important determinant of risk.

Among all the hormones associated with ovarian activity, the estrogens, because of their important effects on the growth of breast epithelium and their important role in mammary tumor induction in rodents, have been the most extensively studied. Exogenous estrone (E_1), estradiol (E_2), and, under some conditions, estriol (E_3) increase the incidence of mammary tumors in mice and rats. They also increase the tumor yield and decrease the time to induction following administration of dimethylbenzanthracene. Removing the ovaries or administering an antiestrogenic drug has the opposite effect.[13]

Attempts to understand and quantify the role of estrogen in breast cancer development have been limited to some extent by our technical capability for measuring steroid hormones in human blood. For example, the techniques for measuring protein-bound and free estrogen fractions in undiluted human serum are relatively new. Prior to the development of this new technology, a few studies of estrogen levels in premenopausal patients and controls had been reported. England et al.[14] found a 15% average elevation of plasma total estrogens in patients with breast cancer and a similar increase was reported by Cole and his colleagues[15–16] for total urinary estrogens. Problems with other such studies have been discussed by Cole et al.; in particular, they pointed out that, in a number of studies, urine collection was neither done on a fixed day of the cycle nor in a similar manner for cases and controls.[15] They also noted that very close age matching is probably required in the premenopausal period.

The only substantial study of plasma estrogen levels in postmenopausal breast cancer cases and controls was reported by England et al.[14] They studied the estradiol levels in 25 cases and 25 controls, and found that, on average, the levels were 30% higher in cases. There have been at least five studies on urinary estrogens in postmenopausal cases and controls. Data on total estrogens from these studies[17–21] are given in Table 19–7. Taken together, these studies also support the finding of increased levels of estrogen found by England et al.[14]

Recent work on estrone production and metabolism shows that in postmenopausal women the major source of estrogens is extraglandular conversion of androstenedione to estrone and that the extent of this conversion is highly correlated with body weight.[22] Since body weight is an important risk factor for breast cancer in postmenopausal women, we must conclude that postmenopausal breast cancer cases should also have increased plasma levels of estrogens on this basis alone, and this may be the complete

TABLE 19–7.

Urinary Estrogens in Postmenopausal Women

STUDY (REF)	$E_1 + E_2$*		E_3*		$E_1 + E_2 + E_3$		$E_3/(E_1 + E_2)$	
	CASES	CONTROLS	CASES	CONTROLS	CASES	CONTROLS	CASES	CONTROLS
Arguelles et al. (17)	5.4†	3.8	7.0	7.1	12.4	10.9	1.5	1.8
Brown et al. (18)	2.1	1.7	5.8	4.1	7.9	5.8	2.8	2.4
Gronroos & Aho (19)	4.3	8.6	5.3	5.0	9.6	13.6	1.2	0.6
Marmorston et al. (20)	0.9	0.7	4.4	2.1	5.3	2.8	4.9	3.0
Persson (21)	2.9	2.8	6.1	3.3	9.0	6.1	2.1	1.2

*E_1, estrone; E_2, estradiol; E_3, estriol.
†Mg per 24 hours (different references give values in different units; values given here have been converted as accurately as possible to this common unit).

explanation of the increased estrogen levels of postmenopausal breast cancer cases discussed above. None of the six case-control studies of estrogen levels in postmenopausal women gave details of the weights of the women.

Recent findings by Siiteri et al.[23] and Moore et al.[24] emphasize the possible importance of bioavailable estrogen fractions in the etiology of breast cancer. Siiteri et al.[23] studied a small group of breast cancer cases and controls matched on age, weight, height, and menstrual status; they found the known relationship between obesity, reduced sex hormone-binding globulin (SHBG), and increased free E_2 in both cases and controls. They also found that some 'normal-weight' breast cancer patients with normal SHBG levels had an elevated percentage of free E_2. These results suggest that in breast cancer patients, free E_2 in serum may be elevated by factors unrelated to SHBG concentration.

Moore et al.[24] compared total and non-protein-bound estradiol levels in 38 postmenopausal women with breast cancer and in 38 controls of similar age and weight. Breast cancer cases had significantly higher levels of E_2 and non-protein-bound E_2 than controls, and significantly less SHBG. In fact, the level of non-protein-bound E_2 in cases was nearly four times that of controls. Unfortunately, cases and controls from this study were drawn from different populations, so interpretation of these results is difficult.

If elevated estrogens are important determinants of breast cancer risk, one would predict that teenage girls at increased risk of breast cancer would have higher estrogen levels. When comparing the plasma hormone levels of 36 daughters of young women with breast cancer and 36 daughters of control subjects, we found that the mean day 22 total serum estrogens (E_1 + E_2) were 27% higher in the patients' daughters.[25] Day 6 total serum estrogens were also elevated, but only by 13%. The patients' daughters did, however, have a clear excess of high values: 11 of 35 patients' daughters (31%) had values exceeding 10 ng/100 ml compared to only 3 of 31 control daughters (10%) (Fig 19–2). Findings of elevated urine estrogen levels in daughters of women with breast cancer compared to daughters of controls have been reported by others.[26] This elevation of estrogen levels is probably a consequence of the fact that the daughters of women with breast cancer had more regular menstrual cycles.

PROLACTIN LEVELS AND RISK OF BREAST CANCER

In recent years there has been intensive interest in the role of prolactin in breast carcinogenesis. Multiple pituitary isografts, which increase prolactin secretion, and hypothalamic lesions and drugs that stimulate prolactin secretion all increase the incidence of mammary tumors in rats and mice, while drug-induced suppression of prolactin release decreases the growth of established tumors. Both prolactin and ovarian hormones are needed to obtain optimal conditions for chemical transformation of breast epithelium and for growth of established or transplanted mammary tumors in rodents.[40]

We found a consistent elevation of plasma prolactin levels in daughters of young women with breast cancer compared to daughters of controls.[25] The most striking difference between the two groups of teenagers was obtained by considering the plasma levels of estrone plus estradiol (E_1 + E_2) and of prolactin together. Figure 19–2 shows the results for the specimens collected on day 6 of the menstrual cycle: values for 12 of the 34 patients' daughters fall above the line shown in the figure, compared to only 1 of the 30 daughters of controls. These prolactin results, referring to single, early morning blood samples, have been confirmed by Levin and Malarkey,[27] who found a 60%

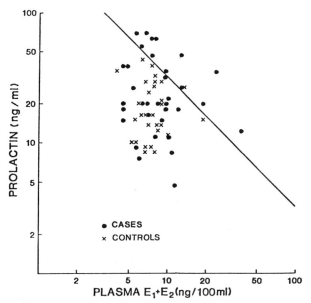

FIG 19–2.
Plasma prolactin and total estrogen (E_1 and E_2) on day 6 of the menstrual cycle in teenage daughters of breast cancer cases and controls. (From Henderson BE, et al: *N Engl J Med* 1975; 293:790. Used by permission.)

increase in the 24-hour mean prolactin level in young women with a family history of breast cancer compared to that of young women without this family history. One study found that prolactin levels were increased in other members of the family of breast cancer patients.[28]

A number of studies of prolactin levels in breast cancer patients and controls have been reported[29–33] (Table 19–8). In premenopausal women, all groups studied, except for Indians,[33] showed elevated prolactin levels in the cases. In postmenopausal women, although some studies report substantial elevations of prolactin in breast cancer cases,

TABLE 19–8.
Prolactin Levels in Breast Cancer Cases and Controls*

STUDY REFERENCE	POPULATION	PREMENOPAUSAL				POSTMENOPAUSAL			
		CASES		CONTROLS		CASES		CONTROLS	
29	U.K. whites	11.4*	(11)	9.7	(11)	—		—	
30	South African blacks	17	(12)	9.5	(84)	9.5	(14)	12.0	(28)
30	U.S. whites	29	(10)	12.5	(51)	19.0	(14)	13.0	(27)
30	Japanese	17.5	(11)	13.0	(12)	24.5	(11)	12.0	(16)
31	U.S. whites	17.9	(5)	13.1	(9)	7.5	(12)	10.4	(9)
32	U.S. whites	22.9†	(14)	9.1	(34)	13.5	(20)	4.9	(39)
		32.6‡	(21)			27.2	(17)		
33	Indians	22	(42)	31.0	(18)	17.0	(26)	20.0	(12)

*Published units for prolactin should be taken as applying only to the particular study and thus are not given. Figures in parentheses are number of cases/controls.
†Premastectomy and ‡ early postmastectomy values were separately reported in this study.

others report no differences. The finding of higher prolactin levels in post- compared to premastectomy breast cancer cases[32] suggests that any postdiagnosis case-control differences must be viewed with caution.

There is evidence that prolactin levels are lower in parous than in nulliparous women.[34, 35] In our study,[34] the mean early morning prolactin level of 88 nulliparous women was 35% higher than the mean value of their 62 parous sisters. This finding provides a hormonal basis for at least part of the protective effect of first full-term pregnancy and helps to explain the steady decrease in mean prolactin levels with age found by Vekemans and Robyn.[36]

PROGESTERONE AND RISK OF BREAST CANCER

We noted above that there is substantial evidence suggesting that elevated estrogen levels increase breast cancer risk. It has only recently been deduced that elevated levels of the other major ovarian hormone, progesterone, may also be an important factor in increasing breast cancer risk. In 1980, the "estrogen window hypothesis" was first proposed.[37] According to this hypothesis, "normal oestrogen stimulation and luteal inadequacy, characterized by diminished progesterone secretion, can explain the main epidemiological features of breast cancer" and "unopposed estrogen stimulation is the most favorable state for tumor induction." The basic assumption underlying this hypothesis was that progesterone would act as an antiestrogen on breast epithelium in much the same way as it does on the endometrium. In fact, it now appears that progesterone may be a mitogen to breast epithelium, and the totality of epidemiologic and experimental evidence suggests that more, not less, frequent ovulatory cycles are the major determinant of breast cancer risk.

The mitotic activity of breast epithelium varies markedly during the normal menstrual cycle, with peak activity occurring late in the luteal phase.[38] This suggests that progesterone, at least in the presence of estrogen, might induce mitotic activity in breast epithelium. This effect of progesterone would be in sharp distinction to its effect on endometrial tissue, where the peak mitotic activity is in the follicular phase of the cycle. It strongly agrees, however, with the experimental findings that progesterone induces ductal growth in rodent breast tissue,[39] and with Dao's conclusions[13] from his experimental studies that "the minimal hormonal combination necessary for initiation of carcinogenesis is . . . estrogen, and progesterone. It appears that . . . the target cell must be in an active proliferative state."

EXOGENOUS HORMONES AND BREAST CANCER

Oral Contraceptive Use in the Perimenopausal Period

Oral contraceptives have been widely used since the early 1960s. By 1978 the World Health Organization estimated that more than 80 million women throughout the world had been exposed to these drugs.[40] There is now a substantial body of literature on the relationship between oral contraceptive use and risk of breast cancer. Kelsey and Hildreth[41] recently summarized the results of 16 case-control and four cohort studies; as a group, these studies provide convincing evidence that oral contraceptives, when used during most of a woman's reproductive life, do not alter the risk of breast cancer. Likewise, most studies show little evidence of a trend of increasing risk with increasing duration of use. However, there have been a few studies that have demonstrated that certain subgroups of women using oral contraceptives may be at increased risk of breast cancer.

If breast tissue mitotic rate—and hence the amount of time spent in the luteal phase of the menstrual cycle—is a significant determinant of a woman's breast cancer risk, then combination-type oral contraceptives, which simulate the luteal phase of the cycle should, under certain circumstances, increase the risk of breast cancer. These circumstances will be those in which the woman's average breast-tissue mitotic activity, when taking the particular combination-type oral contraceptive, is greater than her average 'normal' breast-tissue mitotic activity. The late adolescent and perimenopausal periods, when anovular cycles are common, would be expected to provide just the right circumstances for increased risk from the combination-type pill. Five studies have reported specifically on the use of combination oral contraceptives around the time of the menopause.[42-46] All of these studies found some evidence of an elevated risk of breast cancer with such use, although the range of reported relative risks was wide (Table 19–9). In the first four studies, the excess risk was borne by women aged 46–50, while in the most recent study,[46] the excess risk was observed only in women older than 50. None of these studies reported on the possible risk-modifying effect of specific oral contraceptive formulations. In fact, the effects of different formulations of combination oral contraceptives on breast tissue mitotic activity are not known, but it may be presumed the combination oral contraceptives with higher doses of both estrogen and progestogen will have the greatest effect.

We recently found that long-term oral contraceptive use in the late adolescent period also carries with it a substantial increase in breast cancer risk.[47] However, two more recent studies have found different results. In one, increased risk of breast cancer was confined to use before first full-term pregnancy (FFTP)[48] and in the other, a larger population-based study, no difference in risk was reported for use at young ages or before FFTP.[49] Thus, for the moment, it is not clear whether combination oral contraceptives alter the risk of breast cancer when taken at a young age.

Estrogen Replacement Therapy and Breast Cancer

There are currently over 30 million postmenopausal women in the U.S. The advisability of long-term use of estrogen replacement therapy for such women remains con-

TABLE 19–9.

Breast Cancer Risk and Oral
Contraceptive Use During the
Perimenopausal Period

	RELATIVE RISK OF CURRENT USERS CF. NONUSERS	
	AGE AT DIAGNOSIS	
STUDY (REF)	41–45	46–50
Vessey (42)	0.7	2.4
Jick (43)	0.8	4.0
RCGP (44)	1.1	1.7
Brinton (45)	1.0	1.3
Hennekens (46)	0.6	0.8*

*The relative risk in women 50–55 was 3.8 (95% confidence interval = 1.6–9.0), compared to nonusers.

troversial. Concerns about the carcinogenic potential of estrogen replacement therapy have centered on the breast and endometrium.

Most early studies of the possible effects of estrogen replacement on the risk of breast cancer were uncontrolled follow-up studies. The most credible cohort study was done by Hoover et al.[50] Although they reported only a 25% excess of breast cancer in their cohort of menopausal estrogen users compared to the number expected based on general population rates (49 observed versus 39 expected), they did report a more substantial excess among women using high doses for a long time.

Early case-control studies that reported findings on menopausal estrogens and breast cancer were often limited by small numbers, by insufficient data on dose and duration of use, and by the definite possibility of bias. A new group of carefully conducted case-control studies have recently been published.[51-57] Five of these studies used healthy population control groups, three of which were drawn from pre-paid health program members,[52, 54, 55] one from breast cancer detection program subjects,[53] and one from retirement community residents[51] (Table 19–10). Four of these studies found moderate increases in risk of breast cancer (relative risks of 1.3 to 1.9) after long-term use. A fifth study included few long-term users but found a relative risk of 3.4 for *any* use of estrogen replacement therapy among women with spontaneous menopause.[52] Three of these five studies[51, 53, 54] also demonstrated an increasing breast cancer risk with increasing estrogen doses.

The two other recently reported studies[56, 57] used hospital controls as their comparison group and found no evidence to suggest that breast cancer risk was increased either overall or with long duration of use. One possible explanation for this is that hospital controls have more contact with the health care system and are therefore more likely to use elective drugs than the population as a whole.

Based on the best available data, it seems sensible to conclude that long-term use of estrogen replacement therapy in moderately high doses does carry with it a sizeable increase in breast cancer risk, that small doses for a short time convey no measurable increase in risk, and that the effects of smaller doses for long periods of time is not adequately studied but is unlikely to be substantial.

It has become increasingly popular in the U.S. to add a progestin in cyclic opposition to estrogen replacement in order to negate the carcinogenic effect of unopposed estrogen on the endometrium. However, the addition of a progestin may also have important effects on other components of the risk-benefit equation for estrogen replacement therapy. As noted above, progesterone may enhance mitotic activity in breast tissue, but no epidemiologic data are available on this point.

It is probable that certain subgroups of women may be relatively more susceptible to

TABLE 19–10.

Estrogen Replacement Therapy and Risk of Breast Cancer

STUDY (REF.)		EVER USE	LONG-TERM USE
Hoover	(50)	1.3	2.0
Ross	(51)	1.1	1.9
Jick	(52)	1.1	—
Brinton	(53)	1.2	1.3
Hoover	(54)	1.4	1.8
Hiatt	(55)	0.7	1.8

the carcinogenic effects of estrogens than others. The epidemiologic literature in this area is confusing. Some,[50–53] but not all,[54, 55] studies have found breast cancer risk following estrogen use to be enhanced in women with surgically-proven benign breast disease, especially if the estrogen use followed the diagnosis of the benign disease.[58] Some studies have found the greatest effect of estrogen in women with a natural menopause,[51, 52] while others have found the greatest effect among women having undergone oophorectomy.[50, 53, 55] Some studies have found higher relative risks of breast cancer in women who used estrogens and had a family history of breast cancer.[53, 54]

It is informative to compare the relative risks observed with various doses and durations of estrogen use, as reported by recent epidemiologic studies, to those expected using our recently published statistical model of breast cancer incidence.[59]

The model has the form

$$I(t) = a[d(t)]^{4.5}$$

where *I(t)* is the probability of being diagnosed with the cancer at age *t* (the incidence rate at age t) and *d(t)* is the "relevant age" of breast tissue. The *d(t)* incorporates the effects of age at menarche, age at first full-term pregnancy, and age at menopause. The model essentially assumes that "breast tissue aging" starts at menarche, moves regularly (at rate $f_0 = 1$) to first full-term pregnancy, and then slows to rate $f_1 (= 0.7)$ until menopause, when it slows further to rate $f_2 (= 0.1)$. The concept of "breast tissue aging" is associated closely with the cell kinetics of breast tissue "stem" cells; further details of and the procedure adopted for estimating the parameters of this model can be found in an article by Pike et al.[59]

Table 19–11 shows predicted relative risks for breast cancer at ages 55, 65, and 75 for various durations and doses of estrogen use beginning at age 50 for women with menarche at age 13, first full-term pregnancy at age 23, and menopause at age 50. The table presumes that, with use of 1.25 mg of conjugated estrogen, the aging rate f_1 continues at 0.7 for the duration of estrogen use, while with use of 0.625 mg of conjugated estrogen use, rate f_1 slows to 0.35. For example, for a 65-year-old woman with menarche at age 13, first full-term pregnancy at 23, and menopause at age 50, who did not use estrogen, the relevant breast tissue age d(65), can be calculated as follows:

$$d(65) = f_0(23 - 13) + 2.2 + f_1(40 - 23) + \\ (f_2 + f_1)(50 - 40)/2 + f_2(64 - 50) = 29.5$$

For the same woman who used 0.625 mg conjugated estrogen for 15 years beginning at menopause, the "relevant breast tissue age," d(65), can be calculated to be

$$d(65) = f_0(23 - 13) + 2.2 + f_1(40 - 23) + \\ (f_2 + f_1)(50 - 40)/2 + f_1(64 - 50)/2 = 33.0$$

and the relative risk can be calculated as

$$[a(33.0)^{4.5}]/[a(29.5)^{4.5}] = 1.66$$

Thus, by using estrogen replacement therapy for 15 years, the model would predict a 66% increase in risk of breast cancer by age 65. For the most part, these relative risk estimates are in line with those observed in epidemiologic studies.

The lifetime probability of developing breast cancer after long-term high-dose estrogen can be estimated using Third National Cancer Survey incidence rates as the baseline.[60] The approximate average relative risk for such use, based on a combination of

TABLE 19–11.

Predicted Relative Risks of Breast Cancer Compared to Nonusers by
Duration of Estrogen Use*

DURATION OF ESTROGEN USE	DOSE = 1.25 mg (f_1 = 0.7)	DOSE = 0.625 mg (f_1 = 0.35)
5	1.55	1.21
10	2.16	1.40
15	3.10	1.66

*Users and nonusers of estrogen were assumed to have had menarche at age 13, meno-
pause at age 50, and first full-term pregnancy at age 23.

all the epidemiologic case-control studies that used neighborhood controls for comparison, is 1.5. A woman undergoing menopause at age 50 who immediately begins estrogen therapy would increase her lifetime probability to age 80 of getting breast cancer
7.0%–9.6% if no latent period is required, to 9.2% allowing for a five-year latency,
and to 8.8% with a 10-year latency, assuming risk following exposure to be otherwise
unaffected. These are sizeable increases and carry with them sizeable increases in mortality. However, as noted elsewhere in this volume, this carcinogenic potential of long-
term estrogen use must be weighed in the context of other risks and benefits of estrogen
replacement therapy, especially the probable beneficial effects of replacement therapy
on the cardiovascular system.

REFERENCES

1. Pike MC, Henderson BE, Casagrande JT: Epidemiology of breast cancer, in Pike MC, Siiteri PK, Welsch CW (eds): *Banbury Report 8, Hormones and Breast Cancer*. Cold Spring Harbor, New York, Cold Spring Harbor Laboratory, 1981, p 3.
2. Pike MC, Henderson BE, Casagrande JT, et al: Oral contraceptive use and early abortion as risk factors for breast cancer in young women. *Br J Cancer* 1981; 43:72.
3. Henderson BE, Pike MC, Casagrande JT: Breast cancer and the oestrogen window hypothesis. *Lancet* 1981; ii:363.
4. Feinleib M: Breast cancer and artificial menopause: A cohort study. *J Natl Cancer Inst* 1968; 41:315.
5. Lilienfeld AM: Relationship of cancer of the female breast to artificial menopause and marital status. *Cancer* 1956; 9:927.
6. Trichopolous D, MacMahon B, Cole P: The menopause and breast cancer risk. *J Natl Cancer Inst* 1972; 48:605.
7. MacMahon B, Cole P, Lin TM, et al: Age at first birth and breast cancer risk. *Bull WHO* 1970; 43:209.
8. Thein-Hlaing Thein-Maung-Myint: Risk factors of breast cancer in Burma. *Int J Cancer* 1978; 21:432.
9. Tulinius H, Day NE, Johannesson G, et al: Reproductive factors and risk for breast cancer in Iceland. *Int J Cancer* 1978; 21:724.
10. deWaard F, Cornelis JP, Aoki K, et al: Breast cancer incidence according to weight and height in two cities of the Netherlands and in Aichi Prefecture, Japan. *Cancer* 1977; 40:1269.
11. deWaard F, Baanders-vanHalewijn E: A prospective study in general practice on breast cancer risk in postmenopausal women. *Int J Cancer* 1974; 14:153.
12. Lew EA, Garfinkel L: Variations in mortality by weight among 750,000 men and women. *J Chronic Dis* 1979; 32:563.
13. Dao TL: The role of ovarian steroid hormones in mammary carcinogenesis, in Pike MC, Siiteri PK, Welsch CW (eds): *Banbury Report 8, Hormones and Breast Cancer*. Cold Spring Harbor, New York, Cold Spring Harbor Laboratory, 1981, p 281.
14. England PC, Skinner LG, Cottrell KM, et al: Serum oestradiol-17β in women with benign and malignant breast disease. *Br J Cancer* 1974; 30:571.

15. Cole P, Cramer D, Yen S, et al: Estrogen profiles of premenopausal women with breast cancer. *Cancer Res* 1978; 38:745.
16. MacMahon B, Cole P, Brown JB, et al: Urine estrogens, frequency of ovulation and breast cancer risk: Case-control study in premenopausal women. *J Natl Cancer Inst* 1982; 70:247.
17. Arguelles AE, Hoffman C, Poggi UL, et al: Endocrine profiles and breast cancer. *Lancet* 1973; i:165.
18. Brown JB: Urinary oestrogen excretion in the study of mammary cancer, in Curie AR (ed): *Endocrine Aspects of Breast Cancer*. Edinburgh, E and S Livingstone, 1958.
19. Gronroos M, Aho AJ: Estrogen metabolism in postmenopausal women with primary and recurrent breast cancer. *Eur J Cancer* 1968; 4:523.
20. Marmorston J, Crowley LG, Myers SM, et al: Urinary excretion of estradiol and estriol by patients with breast cancer and benign breast disease. *Am J Obstet Gynecol* 1965; 92:460.
21. Persson BH, Risholm L: Oophorectomy and cortisone treatment as a method of eliminating estrogen production in patients with breast disease. *Acta Endocrinol* 1964; 44:15.
22. Siiteri PK, MacDonald PC: Role of extraglandular estrogen in human endocrinology, in Greep RO (ed): *Handbook of Physiology, Endocrinology,* vol II, Part I. Washington, DC, American Physiological Society, 1973, p 615.
23. Siiteri PK, Hammond GL, Nisker JA: Increased availability of serum estrogens in breast cancer: A new hypothesis, in Pike MC, Siiteri PK, Welsch CW (eds): *Banbury Report 8, Hormones and Breast Cancer*. Cold Spring Harbor, New York, Cold Spring Harbor Laboratory, 1981, p 87.
24. Moore JW, Clark GMG, Bulbrook RD, et al: Serum concentrations of total and non-protein-bound oestradiol in patients with breast cancer and in normal controls. *Int J Cancer* 1982; 29:17.
25. Henderson BE, Gerkins V, Rosario I, et al: Elevated serum levels of estrogen and prolactin in daughters of patients with breast cancer. *N Engl J Med* 1975; 293:790.
26. Trichopolous D, Brown JB, Garas J, et al: Elevated urine estrogen and pregnanediol levels in daughters of breast cancer patients. *J Natl Cancer Inst* 1981; 67:603.
27. Levin PA, Malarkey WB: Daughters of women with breast cancer have elevated mean 24-hour prolactin (PRL) levels and a partial resistance of PRL to dopamine suppression. *J Clin Endocrinol Metab* 1981; 53:179.
28. Kwa HG, Engelsman E, deJong-Bakker M, et al: Plasma prolactin in human breast cancer. *Lancet* 1974; i:433.
29. Cole EN, England PC, Sellwood RA, et al: Serum prolactin concentration throughout the menstrual cycle of normal women and patients with recent breast disease. *Eur J Cancer* 1977; 13:677.
30. Hill P, Wynder EL, Kumar H, et al: Prolactin levels in populations at risk for breast cancer. *Cancer Res* 1976; 36:4102.
31. Malarkey WB, Schroeder LL, Stevens VC, et al: Disordered nocturnal prolactin regulation in women with breast cancer. *Cancer Res* 1977; 37:4650.
32. Rose DP, Pruit BT: Plasma prolactin levels in patients with breast cancer. *Cancer* 1981; 48:2687.
33. Sheth NA, Ranadive KJ, Suraiya JN, et al: Circulating levels of prolactin in human breast cancer. *Br J Cancer* 1975; 32:160.
34. Yu MC, Gerkins VR, Henderson BE, et al: Elevated levels of prolactin in nulliparous women. *Br J Cancer* 1981; 43:816.
35. Kwa HG, Cleton F, Bulbrook RD, et al: Plasma prolactin levels and breast cancer: Relation to parity, weight and height, and age at first birth. *Int J Cancer* 1981; 28:31.
36. Vekemans M, Robyn C: Influence of age on serum prolactin levels in women and men. *Br Med J* 1975; i:738.
37. Korenman SG: Oestrogen window hypothesis of the aetiology of breast cancer. *Lancet* 1980; i:700.
38. Anderson JJ, Ferguson DJP, Raab GM: Cell turnover in the "resting" human breast: Influence of parity, contraceptive pill, age and laterality. *Br J Cancer* 1982; 46:376.
39. Dulbecco R, Henahan M, Armstrong B: Cell types and morphogenesis in the mammary gland. *Proc Natl Acad Sci USA* 1982; 79:7346.
40. World Health Organization: *Steroid Contraception and the Risk of Neoplasia, WHO Technical Report Series 619*. Geneva, World Health Organization, 1978.

41. Kelsey JL, Hildreth NG: *Breast and Gynecologic Cancer Epidemiology*. Boca Raton, Fla, CRC Press, Inc, 1983, p 30.
42. Vessey MP, Doll R, Jones K, et al: An epidemiological study of oral contraceptives and breast cancer. *Br Med J* 1979; 1:1752.
43. Jick H, Walker AM, Watkins RN, et al: Oral contraceptives and breast cancer. *Am J Epidemiol* 1980; 112:577.
44. Royal College of General Practitioners: Breast cancer and oral contraceptives: Findings in Royal College of General Practitioners study. *Br Med J* 1981; 1:2089.
45. Brinton LA, Hoover R, Szklo M, Fraumeni JF: Oral contraceptives and breast cancer. *Int J Epidemiol* 1982; 11:316.
46. Hennekens CH, Speizer FE, Lipnick RJ, et al: A case-control study of oral contraceptive use and breast cancer. *J Natl Cancer Inst* 1984; 72:39.
47. Pike MC, Henderson BE, Krailo MD, et al: Breast cancer in young women and use of oral contraceptives: Possible modifying effect of formulation and age at use. *Lancet* 1983; ii:926.
48. McPherson K, Neil A, Vessey MP, Doll R: Oral contraceptives and breast cancer (Letter). *Lancet* 1983; ii:1414.
49. Epidemiologic Studies Branch: Oral contraceptive use and the risk of breast cancer in young women. *MMWR* 1984; 33:25.
50. Hoover R, Gray L, Cole P, et al: Menopausal estrogens and breast cancer. *N Engl J Med* 1976; 295:401.
51. Ross RK, Paganini-Hill A, Gerkins VR, et al: A case-control study of menopausal estrogen therapy and breast cancer. *JAMA* 1980; 243:1635.
52. Jick H, Walker AM, Watkins RN, et al: Replacement estrogens and breast cancer. *Am J Epidemiol* 1980; 112:586.
53. Brinton LA, Hoover RN, Szklo M, et al: Menopausal estrogen use and risk of breast cancer. *Cancer* 1981; 47:2517.
54. Hoover R, Glass A, Finkle WD, et al: Conjugated estrogens and breast cancer risk. *J Natl Cancer Inst* 1981; 67:815.
55. Hiatt RA, Bawol R, Friedman GD, et al: Exogenous estrogen and breast cancer after oophorectomy. *Cancer* 1984; 54:139.
56. Kaufman DW, Miller DR, Rosenberg L, et al: Noncontraceptive estrogen use and the risk of breast cancer. *JAMA* 1984; 252:63.
57. Kelsey JL, Fischer DB, Holford JR, et al: Exogenous estrogens and other factors in the epidemiology of breast cancer. *J Natl Cancer Inst* 1981; 67:327.
58. Thomas DB, Persing JP, Hutchinson WB: Exogenous estrogens and other risk factors for breast cancer in women with benign breast disease. *J Natl Cancer Inst* 1982; 69:1017.
59. Pike MC, Krailo MD, Henderson BE, et al: 'Hormonal' risk factors, 'breast tissue age', and the age incidence of breast cancer. *Nature* 1983; 303:767.
60. Cutler JJ, Young JL (eds): *Third National Cancer Survey: Incidence Data. National Cancer Institute Monograph 41*. Washington DC, Government Printing Office, 1975.

CHAPTER **20**

Genital Neoplasia

HERBERT B. PETERSON, M.D.
NANCY C. LEE, M.D.
GEORGE L. RUBIN, M.B., B.S.

MUCH OF THE CONTROVERSY regarding the risks and benefits of estrogen replacement therapy centers around the relationship of estrogens to the development of cancer. Concerns regarding breast cancer have been addressed in Chapter 19. In this chapter, we present an overview of the relationship of estrogen therapy to the risk of developing genital neoplasms. As will be seen, substantially more information is available concerning endometrial cancer than is available for other genital tract cancers.

ENDOMETRIAL CANCER

Estrogens have been used in treating the menopause for approximately 50 years.[59] While estrogen replacement therapy in the U.S. declined somewhat in the mid to late 1970s, its use appears now to be increasing again. Approximately 749 million conjugated estrogen tablets were purchased in the U.S. during 1983 by an estimated 2.9 million women.[49] As early as 1923, Allen and Doisy[2] characterized estrogens as primary trophic sex hormones. Since that time, abundant information has become available that collectively demonstrates that unopposed estrogen therapy is associated with an increased risk of carcinoma of the endometrium when progestogens are not part of the treatment regimen. To consider this relationship in detail, we will first discuss the effects of steroid hormones on the endometrium. We will then detail currently available clinical, laboratory, and epidemiologic information concerning endogenous and exogenous estrogens and their impact on the risk of endometrial cancer. Finally, we will discuss strategies for reducing the risk of endometrial cancer when estrogen therapy is used.

Biologic Effects

Biochemical and morphological information is now available to help clarify the relationship between sex steroids and the endometrium. As will be seen, it is important to understand the effects of progestogens as well as the effects of estrogen in considering the impact of hormone replacement therapy on the risk of developing endometrial cancer. Both endogenous and exogenous estrogens must be considered in examining the biologic effects of hormone replacement therapy.

In premenopausal women, estradiol is the principle source of endogenous estrogen. In addition, androstenedione produced by the ovaries and the adrenals is converted peripherally to estrone. In postmenopausal women, the major source of endogenous estrogen is estrone. Estrone is obtained by peripheral conversion of adrenostenedione as produced by the adrenals and ovaries (85% and 15%, respectively). The major sources of exogenous estrogens for hormone replacement therapy in the United States are conjugated equine estrogens (Premarin*). These estrogens are a combination of the sulfates of estrone, equilin, and 17 α-dihydroequilin.

Several investigators[64, 72] have reported that estrogens diffuse across cell membranes and are bound in the cytoplasm to a specific receptor protein. The complex thus formed attaches to deoxyribonucleic acid (DNA) chromatin in the nucleus and then promotes ribonucleic acid (RNA) and protein synthesis. At the cellular level, estrogenic activity is dependent on the relative affinity for estrogen-receptor protein. Although estrogen receptors preferentially bind and retain estradiol relative to estrone,[80] the estrone in conjugated equine estrogens provides a potent stimulus to the postmenopausal endometrium.[92, 50] Thus, while estradiol is the most potent stimulator of cell biosynthesis, estrone has stimulatory effects as well. Whitehead[88] has shown that even reduced doses of conjugated estrogens (0.625 mg as opposed to 1.25 mg) are a potent stimulus to the endometrium. The most important direct consequence of estrogen stimulation of cell biosynthesis is that it may lead to endometrial hyperplasia.

The likelihood of developing hyperplasia appears to be related to the dose of estrogen prescribed.[9] Further, such hyperplasia can, in some women, progress to adenomatous and then atypical adenomatous hyperplasia, which has been reported to be premalignant.[8, 33, 28] Wentz[87] studied 115 women with hyperplasia of the endometrium; nearly 50% had developed adenocarcinoma during a two- to eight-year follow-up period. Of the 75 with adenomatous hyperplasia, 26.7% developed endometrial cancer, and 81.8% of the 22 women with atypical adenomatous hyperplasia developed cancer.

Progestogens are reported to modulate estrogen growth-promoting effects on the endometrium. They apparently do so by reducing the number of available estrogen receptors[79] and by producing 17-β estradiol dehydrogenase, which promotes conversion of estradiol to estrone.[66, 92] King and co-workers[50, 51] have demonstrated that addition of progestogens to the regimens of estrogen-treated postmenopausal women lowers the nuclear estradiol-to-estrone ratio relative to that for women treated with estrogen alone. Nordqvist[63] has shown that endometrial cells that are exposed to progesterone in vitro have reduced synthesis of DNA and RNA. Whitehead[92] has shown that in vivo stimulation of the postmenopausal endometrium by estrogens can be countered by progestogen treatment and that the progestogen effects are dependent on dose and duration.

Endogenous Estrogens

Some groups of women exposed to elevated, and often unopposed (by progestogens), levels of endogenous estrogens have been reported to be at increased risk of developing endometrial carcinoma. These women include those with (1) estrogen-producing ovarian tumors (granulosa-theca cell tumors), (2) polycystic ovary (Stein-Leventhal) syndrome, and (3) obesity, particularly after menopause. Women with diabetes, liver disease, or hypertension have also been reported to be at increased risk for endometrial cancer. Since 1922, when Schröder[69] first reported a case of endometrial cancer in a woman with an estrogen-producing ovarian tumor, numerous reports have suggested a relation-

*Use of trade names is for identification only and does not constitute endorsement by the Department of Health and Human Services or any of its agencies.

ship between granulosa-theca cell ovarian tumors and endometrial cancer. In a review by Braunstein,[7] 3%–23% of women with such ovarian tumors developed endometrial cancer and 22%–65% developed endometrial hyperplasia. Granulosa-theca cell tumors are similar to exogenous estrogen administration in that they result in high and sustained estrogen levels in tissues. Women with polycystic ovary syndrome, a condition characterized by anovulation, obesity, infertility, and hirsutism, appear to be at increased risk for developing endometrial cancer. Anovulation results in estrogen stimulation unopposed by progesterone. Jackson and Dockerty[45] and Chamlian and Taylor[13] reported on a total of 60 women with polycystic ovary syndrome; 19 (32%) developed endometrial cancer.

Obesity appears to increase the likelihood of endometrial cancer for both premenopausal[35] and postmenopausal women. In obese postmenopausal women, peripheral conversion of androstenedione to estrone in the absence of progestogens is thought to cause a reported two- to ninefold increased risk of endometrial cancer.[94, 24, 72] Siiteri and MacDonald[73] have determined that the rate of aromatization increases with body weight, since adipose tissue is rich in appropriate enzymes. Estrogen activity is dependent in part on the serum concentration of sex hormone-binding globulin (SHBG), which Nisker[62] has reported to be lower in obese women. Thus, obese women may have increased circulating estrogens which are, in turn, more available to tissues.

Numerous studies have identified diabetes, hypertension, and nulliparity or infertility as risk factors for endometrial cancer. We are not able here to review all of these, but the evidence suggests that obesity (which leads to increased circulating estrogens), anovulation (which results in unopposed estrogen stimulation), or both are frequent common denominators in these conditions.

Exogenous Estrogens

Clinical Studies

Ever since 1946, when Fremont-Smith et al.[25] reported the development of endometrial carcinoma in a 51-year-old woman who had been taking exogenous estrogens for six years, there has been concern that estrogen therapy increases the risk of endometrial cancer. Clinical studies of women with ovarian agenesis (Turner's syndrome)[22, 20] have described endometrial adenocarcinoma in women receiving estrogen therapy (DES) without cyclic progestogens. In one series, 3 of 24 women with ovarian agenesis who took estrogens for at least five years developed endometrial cancer.[20]

Epidemiologic Studies

Trends.—Reported rates for endometrial cancer in the U.S. remained essentially unchanged from the 1930s until about 1970.[17] Weiss et al.,[84] however, documented a sharp increase in the incidence of endometrial cancer during the early to mid 1970s at a time when use of exogenous estrogen therapy for the climacteric was increasing in the U.S. This increase was documented in a number of areas of the U.S. and found to rise up to 10% per year in certain areas. Subsequently, Austin and Roe[5] compared the incidence of endometrial cancer in the San Francisco Bay area between 1969 and 1975 with trends in estrogen sales and prescriptions. They found an increase in endometrial cancer incidence from 1969 to 1975. The peak of cancer cases, identified in 1975, corresponded with a peak in estrogen prescriptions that year (Fig 20–1). Concurrent with a decline in estrogen prescriptions between 1975 and 1979, there was a decline in endometrial cancer cases identified.

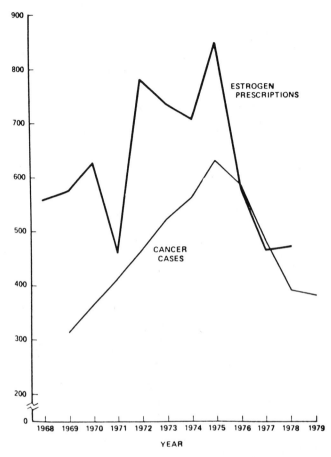

FIG 20–1.
Annual number of estrogen prescriptions to women ages 50–74, in western region sample, 1968–1978, and annual number of new cases of endometrial cancer among white women, ages 50–74, in the San Francisco-Oakland SMSA, 1969–1979. Source: RCE, California Department of Health Services; National Disease and Therapeutic Index, IMS America, Ltd. (From Austin DF, Roe KM: The decreasing incidence of endometrial cancer: Public health implications. *Am J Public Health* 1982; 72:65–68. Used by permission.)

Three other trend studies support a relationship between the use of exogenous estrogens and the incidence of endometrial cancer. Greenwald et al.,[31] using the New York State Tumor Registry, found a 68% increased incidence of endometrial cancer in the period 1960–1974, with 82% of this increase occurring during the last five years of the study. Jick et al.[47] reported data from the Commission on Professional and Hospital Activities that showed an increase from 70 cases of endometrial cancer per 100,000 woman-years at risk in 1970 to 135 per 100,000 woman-years at risk in 1975. Over the period 1975–1977, when U.S. national sales of noncontraceptive estrogens were declining, the incidence of endometrial cancer dropped 27%. Most recently, Marrett et al.,[56] using data from the Connecticut Tumor Registry, demonstrated little change in the risk of endometrial cancer between 1964 and 1969, a substantial increase in incidence during the next six years, and a decline in incidence between 1975 and 1979.

This temporal relationship does not constitute proof of a cause-and-effect relationship between exogenous estrogen use and endometrial cancer. Factors related to or unrelated to estrogen use per se may have contributed to the observed trends. For example, hysterectomy rates and screening techniques for endometrial cancer in the U.S. were not constant during the reported periods. It is unlikely, however, that such events entirely explain the remarkable parallel in the secular trends of estrogen use and endometrial cancer.

Case-Control Studies.—By the end of 1975, two case-control studies[74, 95] suggested that estrogen use resulted in an increased risk of endometrial cancer. Since then, at least 16 other case-control studies have supported similar conclusions. Most of these studies were conducted in the U.S., and most concerned use of the drug, Premarin, without concurrent use of progestogens. In general, these studies suggest that exogenous estrogen therapy is associated with a twofold to 15-fold increased risk of developing endometrial cancer as compared to no such therapy; more recent studies suggest risks at the lower end of the range. The increased risk is partly dependent on dose, duration, recency (time since last use), and latency (time since first use) of therapy.

Risk.—At least 18 case-control studies have been reported since the beginning of 1975 (Table 20–1). These suggest that estrogen therapy increases the risk of endometrial cancer from twofold to 12-fold for those who have ever used estrogen therapy (excluding those who used estrogens for contraception). For long-term users, this increased risk ranges from threefold to 15-fold. Compared with earlier studies, studies reported since 1980 generally suggest lower ranges for ever-users, with a two- to fourfold increase in risk.

The odds ratios, as approximations of the relative risks reported by these case-control studies, indicate that the risk of developing endometrial cancer in users is two to four times greater than that in nonusers. In absolute terms, however, the overall incidence

TABLE 20–1.

Risk Estimates from Case-Control Studies of Estrogen Replacement Therapy and Endometrial Cancer

STUDY		RELATIVE RISKS*	
AUTHOR	YEAR	EVER USERS	LONG-TERM USERS
Smith	1975	4.5	—
Ziel	1975	7.6	13.9
Mack	1976	5.6	8.8
Gray	1977	3.1	11.6
McDonald	1977	2.0	7.9
Wigle	1978	2.2	5.2
Horwitz	1978	12.0	—
Hoogerland	1978	2.2	6.7
Antunes	1979	6.0	15.0
Weiss	1979	7.5	8.2
Hulka	1980	—	4.2
Shapiro	1980	3.9	6.0
Jelovsek	1980	2.4	4.8
Spengler	1981	3.2	8.6
Stavraky	1981	4.2	14.4
Kelsey	1982	—	8.2
LaVecchia	1982	2.7	—
Henderson	1983	1.4	3.1

*Risk relative to never-users

of adenocarcinoma of the endometrium in women aged 50–74 years who have not taken estrogens is relatively low (estimated at 1 per 1,000 women per year).[86] Thus, a fourfold increased *relative* risk indicates an increase in *absolute* risk from 1 per 1,000 to 4 per 1,000 women per year.

Case-control studies have inherent methodologic problems that may distort the measure of association between the exposure and disease.[68] These include problems related to selection of cases and controls (selection bias) and differential recall of exposure information by cases and controls (recall bias). Another bias that may be present is called confounding. Confounding bias occurs when factors associated with both exposure (estrogen administration) and disease (endometrial cancer) are distributed unequally between cases and controls. Finally, chance must be considered as an explanation for findings.

Many of the case-control studies listed in Table 20–1 have attempted to minimize these biases. For example, Horwitz and Feinstein[41] suggested that the selection of cases in the case-control studies may have resulted in spuriously elevated risk estimates. They reasoned that estrogens may cause postmenopausal bleeding, which is more likely to lead to the detection of a previously undiagnosed uterine cancer. In a separate study, Horwitz and co-workers[42] reviewed necropsy data from Yale-New Haven Hospital (1918–1978) and Massachusetts General Hospital (1952–1978). They found that a large percentage of cases of endometrial cancer (67% and 52%, respectively) were undiagnosed before necropsy and that vaginal bleeding had not occurred in any of the 24 women whose disease was first diagnosed at necropsy. Their data suggest that some of the noted increased risks associated with estrogen use may, in fact, be related to a selection bias.

Hulka[43] and Shapiro[71] subsequently selected cases and controls in a fashion specifically to minimize the selection bias proposed by Horwitz and Feinstein. Their results suggest that selection bias does not entirely account for the observed association between estrogen use and endometrial cancer. The Shapiro and Hulka studies are among several that also controlled for confounding factors. Finally, in most of the studies reported in Table 20–1, sample sizes were large enough to make it unlikely that the increased relative risk estimates are due to chance.

Some of the case-control studies reported have strengthened the case for a causal relationship between estrogen therapy and endometrial cancer by establishing biologic plausibility through investigation of dose and duration responses and evaluating the effects of recency and latency of administration. Most of these studies suggest that the risk of endometrial cancer increases with increasing dose and duration of estrogen therapy. For example, Hulka[44] compared relative risks of developing endometrial cancer by dose of conjugated estrogens (0.625 mg or more versus less than 0.625 mg) over specified durations of use (more than 3½ years versus 3½ years or less). For long-duration users, she found that users of pills containing more than 0.625 mg conjugated estrogen had a greater risk of developing cancer than did users of preparations containing 0.625 mg or less. Neither high-dose nor low-dose users, however, had increased risks relative to either of two control groups when estrogen was used for only a short time (Table 20–2). At least eight additional investigators[57, 55, 29, 95, 93, 48, 71, 86] have shown that the risk of endometrial cancer increases with increasing duration of use. Approximately two years use appears to be required for an observed increased risk to develop. This short period is more consistent with estrogen playing a role as a promoter of endometrial cancer than with it acting as the initiator of carcinogenesis.[44]

TABLE 20–2.

Relative Risks of Endometrial Cancer for High- and Low-Dose Estrogen
Therapy by Duration of Use*

ESTROGEN THERAPY	NO. OF CASES	GYNECOLOGY CONTROLS		COMMUNITY CONTROLS	
		NO.	RR (95% CI)†	NO.	RR (95% CI)
Short-duration use‡					
No estrogen	125	118		172	
Low dose§	8	6	1.1 (0.4,3.4)	6	1.7 (0.6,5.1)
High dose‖	5	11	1.0 (0.3,4.1)	25	0.6 (0.2,1.6)
Long-duration use¶					
No estrogen	125	118		172	
Low dose	14	3	2.7 (0.7,10.9)	6	2.7 (1.0,7.4)
High dose	21	1	4.2 (0.8,22.8)	8	3.2 (1.2,8.4)

*From Hulka BS, Fowler WC Jr, et al: Estrogen and endometrial cancer: Cases and two
control groups from North Carolina, *Am J Obstet Gynecol* 1980; 137:92.
†Relative risks adjusted for age and four medical conditions with 95% confidence intervals
‡Use < 3.5 years
§Equivalent to ≤ 0.625 mg conjugated estrogen
‖ Equivalent to > 0.625 mg conjugated estrogen
¶Use ≥ 3.5 years

While there is consistency among studies regarding the impact of dose and duration
of therapy on the risk of developing endometrial cancer, there is some conflicting information regarding the effects of recency of estrogen therapy. Studies by Mack,[55] Wigle,[93] and Hulka[44] suggest that current users of estrogens have greater risks than past
users. In fact, Hulka[44] suggests that if more than two years have passed since a woman
last used estrogen, her risk is similar to that for a nonuser. In contrast, two other
studies[71, 86] suggest that the elevated risk of endometrial cancer persists for more than
two years after last use. There is no obvious explanation for the discrepancy in these
findings and further investigation is needed.

Relationship of Estrogen Therapy to Other Risk Factors for Endometrial Cancer

Ironically, some women who are at otherwise high intrinsic risk for endometrial cancer may be at little additional risk as a result of estrogen therapy. With regard to body
mass, three studies[43, 53, 74] suggest that obese women are at less additional risk of endometrial cancer from estrogen therapy than are nonobese women. Hulka et al.[44] have,
in fact, suggested that obese and hypertensive women have *no* additional increased risk
as a result of long-duration estrogen therapy. Their study used 256 cases, 224 gynecology controls, and 321 community controls; the findings on the study cases are particularly remarkable because they were consistent with the two separate control groups.

In contrast, LaVecchia et al.,[53] in a study of Italian women with endometrial cancer,
found that obese women using estrogen had a relative risk for endometrial cancer of
1.7, compared with obese women not using estrogen. The 70% increased risk associated
with estrogen use may have been due to chance, however (95% confidence interval:
0.9–3.2).*

If these findings are correct, they have a potentially important impact on estrogen-
prescribing practice. Holzman et al.[38] demonstrated in a survey of 50 physicians that

---

*When the 95% confidence interval includes 1.0, the result is not statistically significant at the
$P < .05$ level.

clinicians are least likely to prescribe exogenous estrogens for women with an otherwise high risk of endometrial cancer. Further investigation is needed to determine whether obese women or other women at high intrinsic risk for endometrial cancer are at any additional increased risk from estrogen therapy, and if so, to what extent this is true.

Cohort Studies.—Biases in case-control studies have caused some to question the validity of the findings of such studies in regard to estrogen and endometrial cancer.[41] At least five cohort studies[47, 34, 60, 28, 82] have evaluated the effect of noncontraceptive estrogen administration on the risk of developing endometrial cancer. Most of these studies involve a relatively small number of women with endometrial cancer but, in general, they support the findings of the case-control studies. Jick[47] examined the incidence of endometrial cancer in a large prepaid health plan in Seattle. Long-term users of estrogen who were 50–64 years of age and using estrogen at the time of diagnosis had an annual risk for endometrial cancer of 1%–3%, while never-users of estrogen had less than one tenth that risk. Jick also found that, as dose and duration of conjugated estrogen use increased, risk of endometrial cancer increased.

Hammond et al.[34] followed 301 women in North Carolina who received long-term estrogen therapy and 309 women who never received estrogen. All were followed for at least five years. Eleven women taking estrogen developed endometrial cancer, compared with three who did not take estrogen. Relative to the expected incidence of endometrial cancer from the Third National Cancer Survey, estrogen users had a ninefold increased risk of developing endometrial cancer.

Similarly, Gambrell[28] followed postmenopausal women at Wilford Hall USAF Medical Center for 2,872 patient-years of observation. The incidence of endometrial cancer for women using estrogen alone was 359 per 100,000 woman-years, compared with 248 per 100,000 in women not receiving estrogen. In contrast, Nachtigall[60] and Vakil[82] in two other cohort studies did not demonstrate any increased risk of endometrial cancer associated with estrogen therapy. Nachtigall followed 84 matched pairs of randomly chosen postmenopausal women in New York City for 10 years; one member of each pair received estrogen and the other received a placebo. Vakil studied 1,646 menopausal women undergoing estrogen treatment in Toronto. Interestingly, in the Vakil study, many estrogen users also concurrently used androgens or progestogens, and in Nachtigall's study, all estrogen users were treated with cyclic administration of progestogens. Both these studies are consistent with the contention that concurrent use of progestogens may moderate the increased risk of endometrial cancer associated with estrogen use alone. The potential effect of concurrent estrogen and progestogen therapy suggested by the Nachtigall and Vakil studies is supported by the Hammond[34] and Gambrell[28] studies. In the Hammond study, none of the 72 women treated with estrogen and progestogen developed cancer.

Gambrell found that estrogen-progestogen users had an incidence of endometrial cancer of 56 per 100,000 woman-years, much lower than the incidence of 359 per 100,000 among estrogen users alone and less than that observed in women not receiving any estrogen therapy (248 per 100,000 woman-years). Thus, the cohort studies, though limited by the small numbers of women developing endometrial cancer, generally support the case-control studies in suggesting a cause-and-effect relationship between exogenous noncontraceptive estrogens and development of endometrial cancer. In addition, however, they also suggest that the addition of progestogens to estrogen therapy regimens may modify this effect.

Behavior

Substantial evidence suggests that adenocarcinoma of the endometrium associated with estrogen use is generally of low stage and low grade and has fewer instances of myometrial invasion.[55, 57, 4, 44, 53, 14, 16, 81, 67, 23] Chu[14] studied 320 women with endometrial cancer; 284 of them had used estrogens for longer than one year. Chu found that 98% of estrogen users had stage 0 or I disease, compared with 88% of nonusers (Table 20–3). Similarly, 70% of estrogen users had no myometrial invasion, relative to 51% for nonusers. A greater proportion of users than nonusers had well-differentiated tumors, but unlike several other studies,[81, 67, 23, 16] the difference was not statistically significant.

Hulka,[44] however, cautioned that long-duration, continuous use of conjugated estrogens can result in more advanced tumors. In her study, she evaluated 256 women with invasive endometrial cancer. No excess cancer risk was noted for short-duration estrogen users, but women using estrogen for longer than 3½ years had an excess risk. The risk was highest for cancers that were stage IA grade 1 without myometrial invasion, but there was an increased relative risk of more advanced disease for long-term continuous (as opposed to cyclic) users. Progestogens were used by too few women in the study to evaluate their effect.

As might be expected, given these data, several reports suggest that users of estrogens who develop endometrial cancer have better survival than nonusers who develop cancer.[57, 16, 14, 23] Elwood and Boyes,[23] using actuarial methods, studied 494 women with endometrial cancer in British Columbia between 1969 and 1972 and found that estrogen users had survival rates at five years of 89.1%, compared with 73.5% for nonusers. Relative survival rates (rates after adjustment for expected deaths of women of the same age) were 94.2% for users and 81.3% for nonusers. Collins[16] found that estrogen users in Ontario with endometrial cancer had similar survival to estrogen users without cancer and had remarkably better survival than women with endometrial cancer who were not estrogen users (Fig 20–2).

TABLE 20–3.

Clinical Stage and Histologic Features of Endometrial Cancer in Women, by Estrogen Use*

CANCER FEATURES	ESTROGEN USERS (%)	ESTROGEN NONUSERS (%)
Stage:		
0, I	98	88
II	1	8
III	1	4
Differentiation:		
Good	90.7	84
Moderate	9.3	15
Poor	0	1
Degree of Myometrial Invasion:		
None	70.3	51
<50%	28.3	37
≥50%	1.4	12

*Adapted from Chu J, Schweid AI, Weiss NS: Survival among women with endometrial cancer: A comparison of estrogen users and nonusers. *Am J Obstet Gynecol* 1982; 143:569.

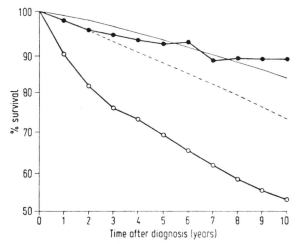

FIG 20–2.
Survival of women with endometrial cancer and a history of noncontraceptive estrogen use in Ontario, Canada. (From Collins J, Allen LH, Donner A, et al: Oestrogen use and survival in endometrial cancer, Lancet 1980; 2:961–963. Used by permission.)

Collins[15] has discussed several possible explanations for the association between estrogen use and improved survival following a diagnosis of endometrial cancer, including the following: (1) estrogen use may occur in healthier women; (2) estrogen use may lead to an earlier diagnosis, because women under therapy are more closely followed by physicians; (3) tumors associated with estrogen use may be hyperplasias, but are misdiagnosed as malignancies; and (4) tumors associated with estrogen use may be less aggressive. Collins concludes that the latter possibility is the most likely and offers the following unifying hypothesis:[15]

. . . endometrial cells undergo a random biochemical event and become initiated cancer cells; the administration of oestrogen leads to cell proliferation in the endometrium; when the administration of oestrogen coincides with the presence of initiated tumor cells, there is a higher probability of promoting those tumor cells to the stage of malignant neoplasia; oestrogens selectively promote those cells which have intact regulatory mechanisms including oestradiol receptors; and therefore oestrogen use is associated with tumors which are well differentiated. The association of endometrial cancer with oestrogen use does not become apparent before 3 to 5 years of exposure, implying that the initiating event is rare and/or the period of cell proliferation required is long. When oestradiol is withdrawn, the risk of endometrial cancer diminishes, implying that the initiating event may be dependent on subsequent exposure to oestrogen for its development to clinical cancer.

Reducing the Risks of Estrogen Therapy

Role of Progestogens

As early as 1965, Greenblatt[30] suggested that "administration of a progestational agent . . . the last five to ten days of a 20-day to 30-day course of an estrogen . . . will generally prevent the development of adenomatous hyperplasia. . . ." Information previously discussed concerning the physiologic effects of estrogens and progestogens on the endometrium give biologic plausibility to Greenblatt's statement. Since progestogens, as discussed, (1) suppress the amount of DNA synthesis in the endometrium,[92] (2) reduce the level of nuclear estrogen receptors in the endometrium,[79] and (3) increase the activity of estradiol and isocitric dehydrogenase,[66] it could be expected that progestogens might counteract the potent stimulus that estrogen may place on the endometrium.

Several studies have shown that this is indeed the case by demonstrating that progestogens can both prevent hyperplasia after estrogen treatment and reverse hyperplasia once it occurs. Paterson et al.[65] demonstrated in a prospective study of 745 women that unopposed estrogen causes hyperplasia in some women, but that women receiving, in addition, an appropriate dose and duration of progestogen therapy have a markedly reduced risk of hyperplasia. The 745 women studied had a total of 1,002 biopsy specimens. Of the 76 specimens from women receiving low-dose estrogen (including conjugated equine estrogens, 0.625 mg), 7% had cystic hyperplasia. The incidence of cystic hyperplasia was appreciably greater (14.8%) for women receiving high-dose estrogens (including conjugated equine estrogens, 1.25 mg) without progestogens added. By contrast, when progestogens were given with estrogens, only 1.2% of specimens had cystic hyperplasia. None of the 76 specimens from women on low-dose estrogen therapy developed adenomatous hyperplasia or atypical hyperplasia, but 4% on high-dose regimens did so. In contrast, only 0.6% of specimens from 366 women on combined estrogen-progestogen regimens developed adenomatous or atypical hyperplasia.

In a subsequent report from the same study population, Studd et al.[78] found that, of 855 women followed annually with endometrial biopsies for up to five years, women undergoing treatment with cyclical conjugated equine estrogens (Premarin, 0.625 mg) had a 7% incidence of cystic hyperplasia, while women taking higher doses (1.25 mg) had an incidence of 15%. When progestogen was added to high-dose therapy for seven days each cycle, however, the incidence of hyperplasia fell to 3%. Studd's report included women having subcutaneous implants of 50 mg estradiol. In 43 women so treated who did not take progestogen (norethisterone, 5 mg) as instructed, 56% developed hyperplasia. Increasing the duration of progestogen therapy afforded an increasing reduction in hyperplasia, and 40 women taking progestogen for 13 days per cycle did not develop hyperplasia at all.

Several reports demonstrate that progestogens can effectively treat endometrial hyperplasia once it develops. Wentz[87] found that 80 women with hyperplasia and 30 women with atypical hyperplasia had hyperplasia reversed after oral progestogen therapy (megesterol acetate 20 mg per day for six weeks or dimethisterone 100 mg per day for six weeks). Campbell[10] reported on 11 women with endometrial hyperplasia diagnosed before estrogen therapy and 22 women diagnosed during estrogen treatment. Following the diagnosis of hyperplasia, 23 of these women received estrogen and progestogen therapy. At repeat curettage approximately six months later, all but one had a normal endometrium. Progestogens used in the study were either norethisterone or medroxyprogesterone acetate. When a high-dose estrogen (including conjugated estrogens, 1.25 mg) regimen was used, 5 mg of progestogen was added, while only 2.5 mg was added for low-dose regimens (including conjugated estrogens, 0.625 mg). Gambrell[28] has reported on 258 patients with hyperplasia of the endometrium treated with progestogens. Progestogen treatment was successful in reversing hyperplastic endometrium to normal or atrophic endometrium in 93.8% of women. Gambrell noted that those with persistent hyperplasia had generally been treated with only seven days of progestogen each month, and he subsequently concluded that at least ten days of progestogen should be given to prevent or treat endometrial hyperplasia. This conclusion is consistent with recent reports by Studd[78] and Whitehead,[91] which suggest that 10–13 days of progestogen therapy per month may be necessary to prevent hyperplasia when estrogen is administered.

Because of concerns about possible side effects of progestogen therapy (discussed later), Whitehead et al.[92] investigated optimal doses and durations of progestogen therapy. They concluded that a minimum of seven days of progestogens is necessary for each month of estrogen therapy. However, they also concluded that duration of therapy is more important than dose of therapy and that, in fact, lower doses of progestogen than those often recommended could be used. This conclusion was reached by evaluating endometrial biopsy specimens for (1) suppression of DNA synthesis, (2) reduction of nuclear estradiol receptors, and (3) activities of estradiol and isocitric dehydrogenase and by finding similar effects after treatment with dl-norgestrel in doses of 150 and 500 μg daily and with norethindrone in doses of 1, 2.5 and 5 mg daily. Thus, they suggested that the lowest doses evaluated be used, i.e., 150 μg of dl-norgestrel or 1 mg norethindrone.

In a subsequent report, Whitehead et al.[90] provided further histologic and biochemical evidence that lower dose (i.e., lower than is often recommended) progestogens were effective in suppressing estrogen stimulation when the progestogens were given for ten days each month. Later, in a review of the literature, Whitehead[91] reiterated that the then currently recommended daily doses of norethindrone (10 mg) and norgestrel (500 μg) could be reduced without loss of protective effect. He also suggested that dosages of other progestogens, such as medroxyprogesterone acetate, could be reduced as well, but he cautioned that the minimum effective dose for all progestogens has yet to be determined.

Progestogens: Possible Side Effects

Presumably because of the reports noted, concomitant use of conjugated estrogens and progestogens has increased recently in the U.S. An estimated 12% of conjugated estrogen use was accompanied by use of medroxyprogesterone in 1983, relative to an estimated 5% in 1980.[49] Concern has been expressed recently, however, that progestogens may cause adverse effects in some women.

One undocumented but potentially important concern is the risk of cardiovascular disease. Certain progestogens have been shown to decrease plasma levels of high-density lipoproteins in a dose-dependent fashion,[6] lowering the ratio of high-density to low-density lipoproteins and thus increasing the risk of developing atherogenic cardiovascular disease. The potential effect of progestogens on the risk of cardiovascular disease is discussed in detail in Chapter 15. MacDonald has suggested that giving progestogens with estrogens may ". . . be tantamount to the addition of oral contraceptives to the treatment of postmenopausal women . . ." and that ". . . such treatment may create a more serious risk than the relatively low risk of endometrial carcinoma."[54] If this is true to an important degree, the risk of developing cardiovascular disease could offset the benefit of endometrial cancer prevention. In one recent Finnish study[37] of six women receiving medroxyprogesterone acetate, which is frequently used in the U.S., no adverse effects on lipoprotein metabolism were identified. A better characterization of the cardiovascular risks of different doses and durations of various progestogens in combination with estrogens is essential for a better determination of the risks and benefits of estrogen-progestogen therapy. This is especially true since the practice of combined therapy appears to be increasing.[49]

Other less-threatening side effects of progestogen therapy have been reported. These include breast tenderness, abdominal bloating, depression, and acne.[91] Whitehead et al.

have suggested that these symptoms are less frequent when the lower-dose progestogen regimen they recommend is employed. Almost all women experience some vaginal bleeding during progestogen therapy, with such bleeding occurring cyclically.

Whitehead[89] has studied the acceptability of combined estrogen and progestogen therapy. Of 76 women offered such therapy, four refused treatment because of anticipated monthly vaginal bleeding. Of the 72 women who began therapy, all had some vaginal bleeding. Ninety percent had withdrawal bleeding and 10% had breakthrough bleeding. However, the incidence of breakthrough bleeding associated with combined therapy was less than that recorded for women receiving high- or low-dose estrogen therapy without progestogen. Four women discontinued treatment because of their vaginal bleeding. The range for duration of therapy in the study was 2 to 49 months and the mean was 16 months.

Screening for Endometrial Cancer: When to Biopsy the Endometrium

Although progestogens appear to dramatically reduce the stimulatory effects of estrogen on the endometrium, they may not eliminate the risk of neoplasia.[11] Gambrell has observed that some focal areas of the endometrium may not respond to progestogens.[27] Thus, it is important to consider the need for endometrial sampling in women who are and who are not receiving cyclic progestogens while undergoing estrogen therapy.

Although there are no universally accepted recommendations for determining how often endometrial biopsies should be performed, useful guidelines have been developed.[1] For women undergoing estrogen-only treatment, endometrial biopsy is recommended before initiating therapy. In addition, such women should be considered candidates for annual endometrial biopsies. All women who have *unscheduled* vaginal bleeding during estrogen therapy, whether or not cyclic progestogens are used, should undergo endometrial biopsy.

As previously noted, most postmenopausal women receiving cyclic progestogens with estrogen therapy will undergo withdrawal bleeding. Such bleeding usually occurs about two days after progestogen therapy ceases and lasts for approximately three to four days. Consistent with the guidelines of the American College of Obstetricians and Gynecologists (ACOG), Gambrell[27] has suggested that women undergoing estrogen-progestogen therapy need not have endometrial biopsies at specified intervals when expected withdrawal bleeding occurs. However, when variations from the expected pattern occur, such as heavy flow or perimenstrual spotting, prompt endometrial sampling is warranted. In addition, he has advocated use of the ''Progestogen Challenge Test'' (PCT), discussed in the next section, to assist in identifying women at greatest risk of developing endometrial cancer.

When endometrial sampling is needed, how should it be accomplished? Diagnostic dilation and curettage (D & C) has traditionally offered the best opportunity for thorough sampling but entails operative and anesthetic risks.[32] Office curettage procedures using Randall or Novak aspiration cannulas have been reported to yield satisfactory tissue samples.[26] Grimes[32] has reviewed the risks and benefits of D & C compared to Vabra aspiration and concluded that both appear to provide adequate tissue specimens, although D & C may be more likely to detect polyps (which rarely contain malignancies). He notes further that cervical stenosis or large leiomyomas may preclude Vabra aspiration on an outpatient basis for some women, but office-based Vabra aspiration is an appropriate diagnostic test for most women. When specimens obtained through such procedures are inadequate, or if bleeding problems persist or recur after such a procedure, D & C under general anesthesia should be considered.[32] Clearly, the advantages and disadvantages of alternative approaches to endometrial sampling must be considered in relation to individual clinical circumstances.

Progestogen Challenge Test

In 1980, Gambrell[28] reported on use of the PCT to identify women at increased risk for adenocarcinoma of the endometrium. The PCT was administered using 5 mg norethindrone acetate (Norlutate) or 10 mg medroxyprogesterone acetate (Provera) for ten days per month to postmenopausal women undergoing estrogen therapy. Progestogens were continued for ten days each month for as long as withdrawal bleeding occurred. Subsequently, Gambrell suggested[27] that all women with intact uteri (whether or not on estrogen therapy) should have progestogens administered for 13 days each month for as long as there is withdrawal bleeding. When withdrawal bleeding ceases, he suggests that further progestogen be temporarily withheld but that thereafter the PCT be repeated each year. As noted, when using the PCT, Gambrell recommends endometrial sampling if unanticipated bleeding occurs.

Conclusion

In conclusion, there is substantial evidence from clinical, laboratory, and epidemiologic studies to suggest that exogenous estrogen administration is associated with an increased risk of endometrial cancer. This risk may have been overestimated in earlier studies. Most recent evidence suggests a twofold to fourfold increased relative risk, which results in an absolute increased risk of developing endometrial cancer from 1 per 1,000 in unexposed women to 4 per 1,000 women per year in exposed women. The risk of developing cancer is dose- and duration-dependent, with short-term use posing minimal if any increased risk. Women who develop endometrial cancer associated with estrogen use generally have tumors of low stage and grade. Progestogen therapy used for a minimum of seven to ten days per cycle and, when necessary, up to 14 days, appears to offset most of the excess risk associated with estrogen use.

Further studies are necessary to determine minimal effective progestogen doses and whether such doses carry any important cardiovascular risks for postmenopausal women. This information is critical for assessing whether adding progestogens increases or decreases overall health risks. Finally, endometrial sampling can be used to identify women at increased risk for endometrial cancer and can be incorporated into strategies for minimizing the risks of estrogen therapy.

OVARIAN CANCER

Little is understood about the causes of ovarian cancer. A better understanding is imperative, however, since ovarian cancer causes more deaths than any other female genital tract cancer.[21] There is some evidence that risk factors for certain ovarian cancers are similar to those for endometrial cancer. Both cancers are more common in western than in eastern countries and, in the west, are more common in white women than in women of black and other races. In addition, both tumors are more prevalent in nulliparous women. The shared risk factors give some plausibility to the possibility of shared etiologies.[85] There is thus some concern that estrogen therapy, which has been associated with an increased risk of endometrial cancer, may be associated with an increased risk of ovarian cancer as well. On the other hand, Stadel[76] proposed that menopausal estrogen therapy may actually decrease the risk of ovarian cancer by suppressing pituitary gonadotropin production, since a rise in such gonadotropins has been experimentally associated with ovarian carcinogenesis.

Weiss[83] noted a temporal association between two histologically related types of ovarian cancer—endometrioid and clear-cell tumors—and use of exogenous estrogen therapy (Table 20–4). He identified an increase in reported diagnoses of endometrioid and clear-cell tumors between 1969 and 1974 in San Francisco-Oakland and Detroit. Over the same period, the incidence of other epithelial ovarian cancers did not change. Weiss also noted that both endometrioid and clear-cell tumors bear a histologic resemblance to adenocarcinoma of the endometrium; he cautioned, however, that it was not until 1961 that the International Federation of Gynecology and Obstetrics established a classification for "endometrioid carcinoma of the ovary" and that the increased reported occurrence may simply reflect a greater awareness of the tumor. Before the cohort and case-control studies detailed below, this temporal relationship between exogenous estrogen therapy and endometrioid and clear-cell carcinoma of the ovary was the only evidence linking exogenous estrogens to a possible increased risk of ovarian cancer.

Cohort Studies

Hoover et al.[40] reported on the experience of 908 white women who were followed in a single gynecologic practice in Louisville, Kentucky, during 1939–1969. All had received conjugated equine estrogen (Premarin) therapy for at least six months. During the study period, eight women developed ovarian cancer, whereas 3.4 cases would have been expected. This yielded a borderline statistically significant elevated risk of 2.4 for the estrogen-treated group relative to the rate expected in the general population (derived from the Second and Third National Cancer Surveys). This excess risk of ovarian cancer in estrogen users was restricted to the 99 women in the study who took other estrogens in addition to Premarin (including other conjugated estrogens and diethylstilbestrol). Among women who used only Premarin, four developed ovarian cancer instead of the expected 2.8. The resultant 40% increased risk (relative risk: 1.4) for Premarin-only users was not statistically significant (95% confidence interval: 0.4–3.7).

The investigators found no increased cancer risk with increasing duration of estrogen use, but they did find an increased risk with increasing strength of estrogen dose usually used (Table 20–5). In the small group of women who had used diethylstilbestrol (DES)

TABLE 20–4.

Relative Frequency of Endometrioid and Clear-Cell Tumors of the Ovary in White Females*

| | PERCENTAGE OF TOTAL OVARIAN TUMORS | | |
AREA	1969–1970	1971–1972	1973–1974
San Francisco-Oakland	5.3	4.4	10.8
Detroit	3.9	6.8	7.4
Third National Cancer Survey	3.9†	—‡	—
Seattle-Tacoma	—	—	12.3§

*Adapted from Weiss NS: Exogenous estrogens and the incidence of neoplasms in tissues of mullerian origin, in Hiatt HH, Watson JD, Winsten JA (eds): *The Origins of Human Cancer. Cold Spring Harbor Conference on Cell Proliferation.* New York, Cold Spring Harbor Laboratory, 1977, vol 4, pp 413–422.
†Data for 1969–1971.
‡Data not available.
§Data for 1974 only.

TABLE 20–5.

Incidence and Relative Risks of Ovarian Cancer by Dose† and Duration of
Conjugated Estrogen Therapy in Menopausal Women, Louisville, Kentucky*

DOSE AND DURATION OF THERAPY	INCIDENCE		RELATIVE RISK (95% CI)§	
	OBSERVED	EXPECTED‡		
Usual dose (mg)				
0.3	3	1.8	1.7	(0.3–4.9)
0.625	3	1.2	2.5	(0.5–7.3)
1.25	2	0.3	6.7	(0.8–24.1)
Duration of use (years)				
≤5	6	2.1	2.9	(1.0–6.2)
>5	2	1.1	1.8	(0.2–6.6)
Total dose (mg)				
≤800	6	2.2	2.7	(1.0–5.9)
>800	2	1.0	2.0	(0.2–7.2)

*Adapted from Hoover R, Gray LA, Fraumeni JF Jr: Stilboestrol (Diethylstilbestrol) and
the risk of ovarian cancer, *Lancet* 1977; 2:533.
†In women who used various dosages, usual dose is listed.
‡Estimated from the Second and Third National Cancer Surveys.
§95% confidence interval.

for at least one year in addition to conjugated estrogens, ovarian cancer developed in
three women where only 0.1 cases of ovarian cancer would be expected, for a highly
statistically significant relative risk of 30. However, this finding was not confirmed in a
subsequent case-control study by Weiss,[85] which found no increased risk of ovarian
cancer after DES administration.

Case-Control Studies

Since 1975, at least six published case-control studies[3, 58, 36, 85, 19] and one additional
study (Centers for Disease Control, unpublished data), have examined the relationship
of noncontraceptive estrogen use to the risk of ovarian cancer (Table 20–6). All studies
were limited by having a relatively small number of ovarian cancer cases. None of the
studies found a statistically significant overall increased risk of ovarian cancer with use
of exogenous estrogen therapy. On the other hand, several of the studies identified
subgroups of women at possible increased risk.

Of the six published studies, only the one by Annegers et al.[3] demonstrated a protective effect, but that effect was possibly due to chance. The study examined risk factors
for epithelial ovarian cancers in 116 cases and 464 controls in Rochester, Minnesota.
For ever-users of an estrogen preparation (not limited to estrogens used for treatment of
the climacteric) the relative risk was a statistically significant 0.5 (a protective effect).
However, women using estrogens for at least six months had a relative risk of 1.0 (no
effect). When estrogen use was limited to conjugated equine estrogens (Premarin), those
who used Premarin for at least six months, compared with never-users, had a relative
risk of 0.7, which was not statistically significant.

Studies by McGowan et al.[58] and Hildreth et al.[36] showed no association between
noncontraceptive estrogen use and ovarian cancer. McGowan et al.[58] studied 197
women with epithelial ovarian cancers diagnosed in Washington, D.C., between 1974
and 1977, compared with 197 matched controls. Although risk estimates were not reported, the authors noted that noncontraceptive estrogen use was similar among cases

TABLE 20–6.
Case-Control Studies of Estrogen Replacement Therapy and Ovarian Cancer

STUDY	NO. OF CASES	NO. OF CONTROLS	RELATIVE RISK (95% CI)*		COMMENT
Annegers (1979)	116	464	0.7	(0.2–1.8)	Estrogen use may have included some premenopausal use. Risk = 1.0 for ≥6 mos. use.
McGowan (1979)	197	197	NS†		Use of noncontraceptive hormones "similar" between cases and controls
Hildreth (1981)	62	1,068	0.9	(0.5–1.6)	Risk unchanged after controlling for previous hysterectomy
Weiss (1982)	207	613	1.3	(0.9–1.8)	Dose, duration, and timing of estrogen use had no effect on risk. Risk increased to 3.1 (1.0–9.8) for endometrioid cancer
LaVecchia (1982)	135	437	1.0	(NS)	Risk increased to 2.3 (1.0–5.3) for endometrioid cancer
Cramer (1983)	173	173	1.6	(0.8–2.9)	Risk 2.0 (1.0–4.3) for natural menopause. Relative risk did not increase with increasing duration of use. Higher proportion of estrogen users among women with endometrioid cancer
Centers for Disease Control, unpublished	347	2,721	1.1	(0.7–1.5)	Risk increased to 1.5 (0.8–2.8) for women who had estrogen replacement therapy ≥5 years

*Relative to never-users. 95% CI, 95% confidence interval.
†Not stated.

and controls. Hildreth et al.[36] studied 62 epithelial ovarian cancer cases diagnosed in women ages 45–74 in seven Connecticut hospitals between 1977 and 1979, compared with 1,068 controls from the same hospital. They identified a relative risk of 0.9, which was not altered by controlling for previous hysterectomy status.

Weiss et al.[85] and Cramer et al.[19] both identified an overall modest increased risk of ovarian cancer in users of menopausal estrogens, although neither identified risks that were statistically significant. Weiss et al. reported on 207 cases of epithelial ovarian cancer among women aged 50–74 years. Cases were diagnosed in two counties of Washington state in 1976–1979 and four counties of Utah during 1975–1977. Women in the case group were compared with 613 controls from the same areas. Noncontraceptive estrogen use was defined as use for at least one year; compared with nonusers, users had a relative risk of 1.3 (or a 30% increased risk), with a 95% confidence interval of 0.9–1.8, suggesting that the increase may have been due to chance alone. The authors evaluated the relationship of dose, duration, and timing of estrogen therapy to ovarian cancer and found no effect, which decreases the likelihood of an important association.

Cramer et al. evaluated 215 white women in the Boston area who had a diagnosis of epithelial ovarian cancer during 1978–1981. The analysis for menopausal estrogen use was restricted to 173 cases and 173 controls, age 40 and older. Ever-users of menopausal estrogens had an increased relative risk of 1.6 (95% confidence interval: 0.8–2.9) compared with that for never-users; this increased risk was not statistically significant. However, when the analysis was further restricted to 92 cases and 92 controls who underwent natural (as opposed to surgical) menopause, the relative risk was a borderline statistically significant 2.0 (95% confidence interval: 1.0–4.3). As with the Weiss study, there was no statistically significant effect of duration of use on risk, although a relative risk of 2.8 associated with menopausal estrogen use for more than five years approached statistical significance. In addition, Cramer et al. identified a borderline statistically significant increased relative risk of 2.5 for cyclic (or nondaily) users as opposed to a risk of 1.2 for continuous users.

While no study has demonstrated a statistically significant overall increased risk for epithelial ovarian cancers associated with noncontraceptive use, studies by Weiss et al.,[85] LaVecchia et al.,[52] and Cramer et al.[19] suggest a possible increased risk for one particular type of epithelial cancer—endometrioid cancer of the ovary. Endometrioid tumors comprise an estimated 10%–20% of ovarian cancers.[18, 70] In the study of Weiss et al.,[85] 12 of 17 women with endometrioid carcinoma had taken estrogens for a relative risk of 3.1 (95% confidence interval: 1.0–9.8) but no relationship to dose or duration of use was noted. No relationship between estrogen use and clear-cell tumors (believed to be histogenetically related to endometrioid tumors) was found. Weiss et al. expressed concern that 44% of eligible women in their study could not be interviewed (primarily because of terminal illness or death), and that this may have biased the study results. The proportion of women with endometrioid cancer who were not interviewed was lower than that for other tumor types and hence thought not likely to account for the observed association. Endometrioid tumors accounted for only 17 of the 205 (8.3%) ovarian cancers in the study.

LaVecchia et al.[52] studied 135 women aged 40–69 years who had epithelial ovarian cancer, which was diagnosed in Milan, Italy, in 1978–1980, compared with 437 matched controls. All eligible cases and controls were interviewed. Although noncontraceptive estrogen use was not associated with an overall increased risk of ovarian cancer (relative risk: 1.0), estrogen users had a borderline statistically significant increased relative risk of 2.3 (95% confidence interval: 1.0–5.3) of developing endometrioid ovarian cancer. They also had a nonsignificant increased risk of 1.6 (95% confidence interval: 0.3–8.4) for developing clear-cell ovarian cancer.

Cramer et al.[19] found a higher (but not statistically significant) proportion of estrogen users among women with endometrioid and clear-cell cancers than among women having serous or mucinous tumors, but risk estimates were not reported.

Thus, there may be some association between exogenous estrogen use and development of endometrioid and possibly clear-cell cancers of the ovary. Each of the three epidemiologic studies that have specifically addressed endometrioid tumors reported an increased risk with estrogen use; however, all identified risks were of borderline statistical significance or were not statistically significant, suggesting that the findings may be due to chance alone.

Cancer and Steroid Hormone Study

Since data concerning menopausal estrogen use and the risk of ovarian cancer have not yet been published from the Cancer and Steroid Hormone Study, some preliminary results will be discussed in detail here. The Cancer and Steroid Hormone Study is a large, case-control study coordinated by the Division of Reproductive Health, Center for Health Promotion and Education, at the Centers for Disease Control, with support from the National Institute of Child Health and Human Development and the National Cancer Institute. Although designed primarily to examine the relationship between use of oral contraceptives and breast, endometrial, and ovarian cancer, information was collected on noncontraceptive estrogen use. Study participants were enrolled between December 1980 and April 1983 from the geographic areas of eight regional tumor registries of the Surveillance Epidemiology and End Results Centers of the National Cancer Institute. These are located in the urban areas of Atlanta, Detroit, Seattle, and San Francisco and the States of Utah, Iowa, Connecticut, and New Mexico.

The study methods have been described in detail elsewhere.[12] Briefly, a case was defined as a woman with histologically confirmed ovarian cancer newly diagnosed during the study period who resided in one of the eight areas at the time of the diagnosis. The control group consisted of women selected by randomly telephoning households in the same geographic areas.

We analyzed data on 347 women with ovarian cancer and 2,721 controls who were between the ages of 40 and 54 years. Logistic regression techniques were used to adjust the risk estimates for age, parity, oral contraceptive use, and menopausal status. We found that women who had ever used menopausal estrogens had no overall increased risk of developing ovarian cancer, compared with women who had never used them (relative risk, 1.1; 95% confidence interval, 0.7–1.5). However, like Cramer et al.[19] we found an increased risk of 1.5 for women who had used estrogens for five or more years, compared with women who had never used estrogens. The 50% increased risk, however, was not statistically significant and thus may be due to chance alone.

When we examined the risk of ovarian cancer by time since first use of estrogens—the latent period—we found that compared with never-users, women who had first used estrogens more than ten years before study enrollment had a nonsignificant increased risk of ovarian cancer of 1.3 (95% confidence interval: 0.6–2.8), while women who had first used estrogens more recently had a risk of 1.0. As with other studies on this issue, we are limited by the low numbers of women who have had long duration of use and long latent periods.

Our analysis, like those in the published studies, is limited by the small number of women with ovarian cancer. In addition, ours is limited by the enrollment cutoff at age 54. However, our results are consistent with the published findings in that we found no overall increased risk of ovarian cancer associated with estrogen use.

Conclusion

Few data are available to evaluate the relationship between hormone replacement therapy and ovarian cancer. Unlike the situation for endometrial cancer, there is no clinical or laboratory evidence to suggest an important relationship. Epidemiologic studies have been limited in study power because of the relatively small number of cases. Importantly, few women have been studied who have had long duration of use. Existing studies suggest no overall protective or strong harmful effect of hormone replacement therapy. Exogenous estrogens may possibly increase the likelihood of endometrioid cancer of the ovary, but further epidemiologic evidence will be necessary to determine if such a relationship exists.

CERVICAL CANCER

No data suggest that hormone replacement therapy has an important influence on the risk of developing cervical cancer. Trends in cervical cancer indicate that the incidence has decreased during the time period that hormonal replacement therapy has increased. It is unlikely, however, that there is any cause-and-effect relationship, since factors such as cancer screening are known to have played such an important role in this trend. To our knowledge, no epidemiologic studies have specifically evaluated the risk of cervical cancer associated with hormone replacement therapy.

CANCER OF THE FALLOPIAN TUBES

No reported studies suggest that hormone replacement therapy may increase the risk of cancer of the fallopian tubes. Weiss[83] has reported on the incidence of fallopian tube cancer in San Francisco-Oakland. During 1969–1975 there was no increase in cases of carcinoma of the fallopian tubes. The fact that the incidence of this rare tumor did not increase during a time of rising estrogen use suggests that there is probably no important relationship.

CARCINOMA OF THE VAGINA

While vaginal clear-cell adenocarcinoma in the United States has been reported in association with prenatal exposure to nonsteroidal estrogens, no theoretical reason or actual evidence supports any concern for a relationship between hormone replacement therapy and vaginal cancer.

CANCER OF THE VULVA

To our knowledge, the only reported study of hormone replacement therapy and the incidence of vulvar carcinoma was recently reported by Newcomb et al.[61] In that study, conducted among residents of Washington State, 37 women with in-situ tumors and 22 women with invasive vulvar tumors diagnosed during 1976–1979 were compared with controls from the same area. Women in the case group and the controls reported equal frequencies of menopausal estrogen use, thus suggesting that such use had no effect on the risk of developing vulvar malignancy.

SUMMARY

In summary, substantial clinical, laboratory, and epidemiologic evidence suggests that estrogen replacement therapy is associated with an increased risk of developing endometrial cancer that is generally of low stage and grade. There is good evidence to suggest that the excess two- to fourfold increased risk of endometrial cancer associated wtih exogenous estrogen use can, in many cases, be offset by concurrent progestogen therapy, but the overall health impact of estrogen-progestogen therapy needs further assessment. Whether or not progestogen therapy is used, endometrial sampling before and/or during therapy can minimize risk of disease. Little evidence is available to address the relationship of exogenous estrogens to development of ovarian cancer, but the information that is available suggests no large protective or harmful effect. The possibility that exogenous estrogens are related to one type of ovarian cancer—endometrioid cancer—exists and needs to be further evaluated. No evidence suggests that estrogen replacement therapy is related to any other reproductive tract malignancy.

REFERENCES

1. ACOG Technical Bulletin: Estrogen replacement therapy, American College of Obstetricians and Gynecologists, No. 70, June 1983.
2. Allen GR, Doisy EA: An ovarian hormone, a preliminary report on its localization, extraction, partial purification and action in test animals. *JAMA* 1923; 81:819.
3. Annegers JF, Strom H, Decker DG: Ovarian cancer: Incidence and case-control study. *Cancer* 1979; 43:723.
4. Antunes CMF, Stolley PD, Rosenshein MB, et al: Endometrial cancer and estrogen use. Report of a large case-control study. *N Engl J Med* 1979; 300:9.
5. Austin DF, Roe KM: The decreasing incidence of endometrial cancer: Public health implications. *Am J Public Health* 1982; 72:65.
6. Bradley DD, Wingard J, Petitti DB, et al: Serum high density lipoprotein cholesterol in women using oral contraceptives, estrogen and progestins. *N Engl J Med* 1978; 299:17.
7. Braunstein GD: The benefits of estrogen to the menopausal woman outweigh the risks of developing endometrial cancer, in Van Scoy-Mosher MB (ed): *Medical Oncology: Controversies in Cancer Treatment*. Boston, GK Hall Medical Publishers, 1981.
8. Campbell PE, Barter GA: The significance of atypical hyperplasia. *J Obstet Gynaecol Br Commonw* 1961; 68:688.
9. Campbell S, McQueen J, Minardi J, et al: The modifying effect of progestogen on the response of the postmenopausal endometrium to exogenous estrogens. *Postgrad Med J [Suppl]* 1978; 2:59.
10. Campbell S, Minardi J, McQueen J, et al: Endometrial factors: the modifying effect of progestogen on the response of the postmenopausal endometrium to exogenous estrogens. *Postgrad Med J* 1978; 54:59.
11. Campbell S, Whitehead M: Oestrogen therapy and the menopausal syndrome. *Clin Obstet Gynaecol* 1977; 4:31.
12. Centers for Disease Control Cancer and Steroid Hormone Study: Long-term oral contraceptive use and the risk of breast cancer. *JAMA* 1983; 249:1591.
13. Chamlian DL, Taylor HB: Endometrial hyperplasia in young women. *Obstet Gynecol* 1970; 36:659.
14. Chu J, Schweid AI, Weiss NS: Survival among women with endometrial cancer: A comparison of estrogen users and nonusers. *Am J Obstet Gynecol* 1982; 143:569.
15. Collins J: Oestrogen and endometrial cancer: A reappraisal. *J Royal Soc Med* 1981; 74:403.
16. Collins J, Allen LH, Donner A: Oestrogen use and survival in endometrial cancer. *Lancet* 1980; 2:961.
17. Cramer DW, Cutler SJ, Christine B: Trends in the incidence of endometrial cancer in the United States. *Gynecol Oncol* 1974; 2:130.
18. Cramer DW, Devesa SS, Welch WR: Trends in the incidence of endometrioid and clear cell cancers of the ovary in the United States. *Am J Epidemiol* 1981; 114:201.
19. Cramer DW, Hutchison GB, Welch WR: Determinants of ovarian cancer risk. I. Reproductive experiences and family history. *J Natl Cancer Inst* 1983; 71:711.
20. Cutler BS, Forbes AP, Ingersoll FM, et al: Endometrial carcinoma after stilbestrol therapy in gonadal dysgenesis. *N Engl J Med* 1972; 287:628.
21. DiSaia PJ, Creasman WT: *Clinical Gynecologic Oncology*. St Louis, The CV Mosby Co, 1984, p 286.
22. Dowsett JE: Corpus carcinoma developing in a patient with Turner's syndrome treated with estrogen. *Am J Obstet Gynecol* 1963; 86:622.
23. Elwood JM, Boyes DA: Clinical and pathological features and survival of endometrial cancer patients in relation to prior use of estrogens. *Gynecol Oncol* 1980; 10:173.
24. Elwood JM, Cole P, Rothman K, et al: Epidemiology of endometrial cancer. *J Natl Cancer Inst* 1977; 59:1055.
25. Fremont-Smith M, Meigs JV, Graham RM, et al: Cancer of endometrium and prolonged estrogen therapy. *JAMA* 1946; 131:805.

26. Gambrell RD Jr: Postmenopausal bleeding. *Clin Obstet Gynaecol* 1977; 4:129.
27. Gambrell RD Jr: Sex steroid hormones and cancer. *Curr Probl Obstet Gynecol* 1984; vol VII 14:26.
28. Gambrell RD Jr, Massey FW, Castaneda TA: Use of the progestogen challenge test to reduce the risk of endometrial cancer. *Obstet Gynecol* 1980; 55:732.
29. Gray LA Jr, Christopherson WM, Hoover R: Estrogens and endometrial cancer. *Obstet Gynecol* 1977; 49:385.
30. Greenblatt RB: Estrogen use and endometrial cancer. *N Engl J Med* 1965; 300:921.
31. Greenwald P, Caputo TA, Wolfgang PE: Endometrial cancer after menopausal use of estrogens. *Obstet Gynecol* 1977; 50:239.
32. Grimes DA: Diagnostic dilation and curettage: A reappraisal. *Am J Obstet Gynecol* 1982; 142:1.
33. Gusberg SB: The individual at high risk for endometrial cancer. *Am J Obstet Gynecol* 126:535, 1976.
34. Hammond CB, Jelovsek FR, Lee KL, et al: Effects of long-term estrogen replacement therapy: II. Neoplasia. *Am J Obstet Gynecol* 1979; 133:537.
35. Henderson BE, Casagrande JT, Pike MC, et al: The epidemiology of endometrial cancer in young women. *Br J Cancer* 1983; 47:749.
36. Hildreth NG, Kelsey JL, LiVolsi VA, et al: An epidemiologic study of epithelial carcinoma of the ovary. *Am J Epidemiol* 1981; 114:398.
37. Hirvonen E, Malkonen M, Manninen V: Effects of different progestogens on lipoproteins during postmenopausal replacement therapy. *N Engl J Med* 1981; 304:560.
38. Holzman GB, Ravitch MM, Metheny W, et al: Physicians' judgments about estrogen replacement therapy for menopausal women. *Obstet Gynecol* 1984; 63:303.
39. Hoogerland DL, Buchler DA, Crowley JJ, et al: Estrogen use—risk of endometrial carcinoma. *Gynecol Oncol* 1978; 6:451.
40. Hoover R, Gray LA, Fraumeni JF Jr: Stilboestrol (Diethylstilbestrol) and the risk of ovarian cancer. *Lancet* 1977; 2:533.
41. Horwitz RI, Feinstein AR: Alternative analytic methods for case-control studies of estrogens and endometrial cancer. *N Engl J Med* 1978; 299:1089.
42. Horwitz RI, Feinstein AR, Horwitz SM, et al: Necropsy diagnosis of endometrial cancer and detection bias in case-control studies. *Lancet* 1981; 2:66.
43. Hulka BS, Fowler WC, Kaufman DG, et al: Estrogen and endometrial cancer: Cases and two control groups from North Carolina. *Am J Obstet Gynecol* 1980; 137:92.
44. Hulka BS, Kaufman DG, Fowler WC Jr: Predominance of early endometrial cancers after long-term estrogen use. *JAMA* 1980; 244:2419.
45. Jackson RL, Dockerty MB: The Stein-Leventhal syndrome: Analysis of 43 cases with special reference to association with endometrial carcinoma. *Am J Obstet Gynecol* 1957; 73:161.
46. Jelovsek FR, Hammond CB, Woodard BH, et al: Risk of exogenous estrogen therapy and endometrial cancer. *Am J Obstet Gynecol* 1980; 137:85.
47. Jick H, Watkins RN, Hunter JR, et al: Replacement estrogens and endometrial cancer. *N Engl J Med* 1979; 300:218.
48. Kelsey JL, LiVolsi VA, Holford TR, et al: A case-control study of cancer of the endometrium. *Am J Epidemiol* 1982; 116:333.
49. Kennedy DL, Baum C, Forbes MB: Noncontraceptive estrogens and progestins: Use patterns over time. *Obstet Gynecol* 1985; 65:441.
50. King RJB, Campbell S, Whitehead MI, et al: Biochemical studies on endometrium from postmenopausal women receiving hormone replacement therapy. *Postgrad Med J* 1978; 54(2):65.
51. King RJB, Dyer G, Collins WP, et al: Intracellular estradiol, estrone, and estrogen receptor levels in endometria from postmenopausal women receiving estrogens and progestins. *J Steroid Biochem* 1980; 13:337.
52. LaVecchia C, Franceschi S: Noncontraceptive estrogen use and the occurrence of ovarian cancer. *J Natl Cancer Inst* 1982; 6:1207.
53. LaVecchia C, Franceschi S, Gallus G, et al: Oestrogens and obesity as risk factors for endometrial cancer in Italy. *Int J Epidemiol* 1982; 11:120.

54. MacDonald PC: Estrogen plus progestin in postmenopausal women. *N Engl J Med* 1981; 305:1644.
55. Mack TM, Pike MC, Henderson BE, et al: Estrogens and endometrial cancer in a retirement community. *N Engl J Med* 1976; 294:1262.
56. Marrett LD, Meigs JW, Flannery JT: Trends in the incidence of cancer of the corpus uteri in Connecticut, 1964–1979, in relation to consumption of exogenous estrogens. *Am J Epidemiol* 1982; 116:57.
57. McDonald TW, Annegers JF, O'Fallon WM, et al: Exogenous estrogens and endometrial carcinoma: case-control and incidence study. *Am J Obstet Gynecol* 1977; 127:572.
58. McGowan L, Parent L, Lednar W, et al: The woman at risk of developing ovarian cancer. *Gynecol Oncol* 1979; 7:325.
59. Mosher BA, Whelan EM: Postmenopausal estrogen therapy: A review. *Obstet Gynecol Surv* 1981; 36:467.
60. Nachtigall LE, Nachtigall RH, Nachtigall RD, et al: Estrogen replacement therapy II: A prospective study in the relationship to carcinoma and cardiovascular and metabolic problems. *Obstet Gynecol* 1979; 54:74.
61. Newcomb PA, Weiss NS, Daling JR: Incidence of vulvar carcinoma in relation to menstrual, reproductive, and medical factors. *J Natl Cancer Inst* 1984; 73:391.
62. Nisker JA, Hammond GL, Davidson BJ, et al: Serum sex-hormone-binding globulin capacity and the percentage of free estradiol in post menopausal women with and without endometrial carcinoma. *Am J Obstet Gynecol* 1980; 138:637.
63. Nordqvist S: The synthesis of DNA and RNA in normal human endometrium in short-term incubation in vitro and its response to oestradiol and progesterone. *J Endocrinol* 1970; 48:17.
64. O'Malley BW: Mechanism of action of steroid hormones. *N Engl J Med* 1971; 284:370.
65. Paterson MEL, Wade-Evans T, Sturdee DW, et al: Endometrial disease after treatment with oestrogens and progestogens in the climacteric. *Br Med J* 1980; 280:822.
66. Pollow K, Lubbert H, Boquoi E, et al: Studies on 17 β-hydroxy steroid dehydrogenase in human endometrium and endometrial carcinoma. *Acta Endocrinol* 1975; 79:134.
67. Robboy SJ, Bradley R: Changing trends and prognostic features in endometrial cancer associated with exogenous estrogen therapy. *Obstet Gynecol* 1979; 54:269.
68. Schlesselman JJ: *Case-Control Studies: Design, Conduct, Analysis.* New York, Oxford University Press, 1982.
69. Schröder R: Nordwestdeutsche gesellschaft fur gynakologie. *Zentralbl Gynakol* 1922; 46:193.
70. Scully RE: Recent progress in ovarian cancer. *Hum Pathol* 1970; 1:73.
71. Shapiro S, Kaufman DW, Slone D, et al: Recent and past use of conjugated estrogens in relation to adenocarcinoma of the endometrium. *N Engl J Med* 1980; 303:485.
72. Siiteri PK: Steroid hormones and endometrial cancer. *Cancer Res* 1978; 38:4360.
73. Siiteri PK, MacDonald PC: Role of extraglandular estrogen in human endocrinology, in *Handbook of Physiology.* Washington, DC, American Physiological Society, 1973, p 615.
74. Smith DC, Prentice R, Thompson DJ, et al: Association of exogenous estrogens and endometrial carcinoma. *N Engl J Med* 1975; 293:1164.
75. Spengler RF, Clarke EA, Woolever CA, et al: Exogenous estrogens and endometrial cancer: A case-control study and assessment of potential biases. *Am J Epidemiol* 1981; 114:497.
76. Stadel BV: The etiology and prevention of ovarian cancer. *Am J Obstet Gynecol* 1975; 123:772.
77. Stavraky KM, Collins JA, Donner A, et al: A comparison of estrogen use by women with endometrial cancer, gynecologic disorders, and other illnesses. *Am J Obstet Gynecol* 1981; 141:547.
78. Studd JW, Thom MH, Paterson MEL, et al: The prevention and treatment of endometrial pathology in postmenopausal women receiving exogenous estrogens, in Pasetto N, Paoletti R, Ambrus JL (eds): *Menopause and Postmenopause.* Lancaster, England, MTP Press Ltd, 1980, pp 127–139.
79. Tseng L, Gurpide E: Induction of endometrial estradiol dehydrogenase by progestins. *Endocrinology* 1975; 97:825.
80. Tseng L, Gurpide E: Nuclear concentration of estradiol in superfused slices of human endometrium. *Am J Obstet Gynecol* 1972; 114:995.

81. Underwood PB Jr, Miller CM, Kreuiner A Jr, et al: Endometrial carcinoma: The effect of estrogens. *Gynecol Oncol* 1979; 8:60.
82. Vakil DV, Morgan RW, Halliday M: Exogenous estrogens and development of breast and endometrial cancer. *Cancer Detect Prev* 1983; 6:415.
83. Weiss NS: Exogenous estrogens and the incidence of neoplasms in tissues of mullerian origin, in Hiatt HH, Watson JD, Winsten JA (eds): *The Origins of Human Cancer. Cold Spring Harbor Conference on Cell Proliferation,* Vol 4. New York, Cold Spring Harbor Laboratory, 1977, pp 413–422.
84. Weiss NS, Szekely DR, Austin DF: Increasing incidence of endometrial cancer in the United States. *N Engl J Med* 1976; 294:1259.
85. Weiss NS, Lyon JL, Krishnamurthy S, et al: Noncontraceptive estrogen use and the occurrence of ovarian cancer. *J Natl Cancer Inst* 1982; 68:95.
86. Weiss NS, Szekely DR, English DR, et al: Endometrial cancer in relation to patterns of menopausal estrogen use. *JAMA* 1979; 242:261.
87. Wentz WB: Progestin therapy in endometrial hyperplasia. *Gynecol Oncol* 1974; 2:362.
88. Whitehead MI, King RJB, McQueen J, et al: Endometrial histology and biochemistry in climacteric women during oestrogen and oestrogen/progestin therapy. *JR Soc Med* 1979; 72:322.
89. Whitehead MI, Minardi J, McQueen J, et al: Clinical considerations in the management of the menopause: The endometrium. *Postgrad Med J* 1978; 54[Suppl]:69.
90. Whitehead MI, Townsend PT, Pryse-Davies J, et al: Actions of progestins on the morphology and biochemistry of the endometrium of postmenopausal women receiving low-dose estrogen therapy. *Am J Obstet Gynecol* 1982; 142:791.
91. Whitehead MI, Townsend PT, Pryse-Davies J, et al: Effects of various types of dosages of progestogens on the postmenopausal endometrium. *J Reprod Med* 1982; 27[Suppl]:539.
92. Whitehead MI, Townsend BS, Pryse-Davies J, et al: Effects of estrogens and progestins on the biochemistry and morphology of the postmenopausal endometrium. *N Engl J Med* 1981; 305:1599.
93. Wigle DT, Grace M, Smith ESO: Estrogen use and cancer of the uterine corpus in Alberta. *Can Med Assoc J* 1978; 118:1276.
94. Wynder E, Escher G, Mantel N: An epidemiological investigation of cancer of the endometrium. *Cancer* 1966; 19:189.
95. Ziel HK, Finkle WD: Increased risk of endometrial carcinoma among users of conjugated estrogens. *N Engl J Med* 1975; 293:1167.

PART IV

Formulation and Pharmacology of Treatment

CHAPTER **21**

Pharmacology of Estrogens

RANDALL B. BARNES, M.D.
ROGERIO A. LOBO, M.D.

THE MAIN SOURCE of estrogen in premenopausal women is the dominant follicle and its subsequent development into the corpus luteum after ovulation.[1] During the reproductive years, cyclic estrogen production results in levels of estradiol (E_2) of about 40 pg/ml in the early follicular phase, about 250 pg/ml at mid cycle and 100 pg/ml during the midluteal phase.[2] Estrone (E_1) production during the menstrual cycle parallels that of E_2, with serum levels somewhat less than estradiol, varying from about 40 to 170 pg/ml. As the menopause approaches, follicular function declines, with decreases of both the length of the follicular phase and the concentrations of follicular and luteal-phase circulating estrogen. In response to these lowered estrogen levels, follicle-stimulating hormone (FSH) levels increase even in the presence of menstrual cyclicity.[3] Follicular development soon becomes inadequate as the climacteric approaches, and cycles lengthen and eventually become anovulatory. At the climacteric, the ovary fails to respond to gonadotropin stimulation, and estrogen deficiency results. Serum E_2 levels average only 13 pg/ml, while mean E_1 levels are typically about 30 pg/ml.[4, 5]

The physiologic consequences of estrogen deprivation in the menopause are diverse. Estrogen therapy has been shown to be effective in preventing or reversing some or all of those changes, including vasomotor instability, urogenital atrophy, and osteoporosis. In this chapter, estrogen metabolism in pre- and postmenopausal women will be reviewed and the pharmacology of the estrogen preparations commonly used for therapy of the menopause will be discussed.

ESTROGEN PRODUCTION

In premenopausal women, 95% or more of circulatory E_2 is secreted from the ovary containing the dominant follicle or corpus luteum.[1, 6] Peripheral conversion of E_1 to E_2 accounts for most of the remaining E_2 production.[1] The E_1 production in premenopausal women is more complex; E_1 circulates primarily as the 3-sulfo conjugate (E_1S). This reversible binding affords a large and stable pool of E_1. The principle source of E_1 is from the peripheral conversion of androstenedione and from the conversion of E_2. A very small quantity is secreted directly by the ovary and adrenal.

In the premenopausal woman about 1.2% of circulating androstenedione is converted in the fatty tissue peripherally to E_1. This conversion accounts for 10%–50% of E_1 production depending on the phase of the menstrual cycle.[5] In addition, about 15% of E_2 is converted peripherally to estrone, accounting for the remainder of estrone production.[1] Postmenopausally, the primary source of estrone is from the peripheral aromatization of androstenedione in the fatty tissue.[7] The primary source of androstenedione is the adrenal gland, about 95% of postmenopausal androstenedione production occurring in the adrenal gland and 5% in the ovaries. The conversion rate of androstenedione to estrone appears to be increased postmenopausally from 1.5% to 3%, although lower conversion rates have been reported.[8, 9] Increased conversion rates of androstenedione to E_1 correlate with increased body weight[8, 10] as well as with age. The site of aromatization may not be the adipocyte cell itself but the surrounding stromal tissue.[11] Thus weight loss may not result in decreased peripheral estrogen production in previously obese individuals. Peripheral conversion of testosterone and E_2 contribute minimally to E_1 production postmenopausally.[7]

Since E_2 is primarily the product of the developing follicle, in the menopause E_2 production is dramatically lowered, and the primary source of estradiol is from the peripheral conversion of E_1. Peripheral aromatization of testosterone makes a minor contribution of about 0.1%–0.2%, while there is little, if any, conversion of androstenedione to E_2.[7]

MECHANISMS OF ESTROGEN ACTION

Estrogens act at the cellular level by diffusion into the cytoplasm and subsequent binding to a specific nuclear-receptor protein. Previously, the binding of estrogen to its receptor was thought to occur in the cytoplasm followed by the translocation of the estrogen-receptor complex into the nucleus. More recent evidence suggests that, after estrogen enters the cell, it also binds directly with its receptor in the nucleus.[52] The estrogen-receptor complex then interacts with the nucleus chromatin, initiating m-RNA transcription. Subsequent protein synthesis on the ribosomes results in the expression of the estrogen effect on the target tissue.[12] The initial factors for the expression of estrogen action appear to be the amount of hormone available to diffuse into the cell and the affinity of the hormone-receptor complex for its nuclear binding site, expressed as its nuclear retention time. Of the naturally occurring estrogens, E_2 is the most potent and has the longest nuclear retention time, 6–24 hours. Weaker estrogens such as estriol (E_3) have a shorter nuclear retention time of one to four hours.[13] Both specifically protein-bound and unbound estrogens circulate in the blood, but it is generally accepted that only the unbound estrogen is available to diffuse across cell membranes and express biologic activity. The principle estrogen binding proteins are sex hormone binding globulin (SHBG) and albumin. However, a specific estrogen-binding protein has been described.

Of the estrogens, E_2 has the highest affinity for SHBG. About 38% of circulatory E_2 is specifically bound to SHBG, while 60% is loosely bound to albumin and 2%–3% is free to diffuse across cell membranes.[14] Estrone, E_3, and estrone-3-sulfate (E_1S) bind poorly to SHBG but have greater affinity for albumin than does E_2. Estrone-3-sulfate has the highest affinity for albumin, and more than 90% of it circulates bound to albumin.[15]

The concentration of unbound E_2 may be altered by changes in SHBG levels. It is known that estrogen therapy, pregnancy, and hyperthyroidism increase SHBG, while hypothyroidism, androgen excess, and obesity lower SHBG levels.[16, 17] Increased estrogen effects seen in obese postmenopausal women may be a result of increased unbound E_2 levels as well as from increased peripheral production of estrogens by aromatization.

ESTROGEN METABOLISM

Estrogen metabolism may be conceptualized in two stages. The first consists of the reversible interconversion of the principle circulating estrogens: E_1, E_2, and E_1S. The second consists of the irreversible oxidation of estrone and subsequent conjugation and excretion of those products (Fig 21–1).[18] Estradiol is converted to estrone by 17β-dehydrogenase in the liver[19] and other tissues. The conversion is reversible, but estrone formation is favored, as indicated by the percentage conversion of E_2 to E_1 (15%), which is greater than that of E_1 to E_2 (5%). Reversible metabolism of E_1 to E_1S occurs via sulfurylation in the liver and endometrium.[20] Estrone-3-sulfate is the principle circulating estrogen, with levels of about 1,000 pg/ml in the follicular phase and 1,800 pg/ml in the luteal phase.[21–23] Sixty-five percent of E_2 and 54% of E_1 are converted to E_1S, while 21% of E_1S is converted to E_1 and only about 1.5% is converted to E_2. It is thought that E_1S acts as a large, slowly metabolized estrogen pool, with 90% of its mass being bound to albumin. Although not biologically active, it is difficult to assess the importance of E_1S in producing the overall estrogen effect, since conversion to E_1

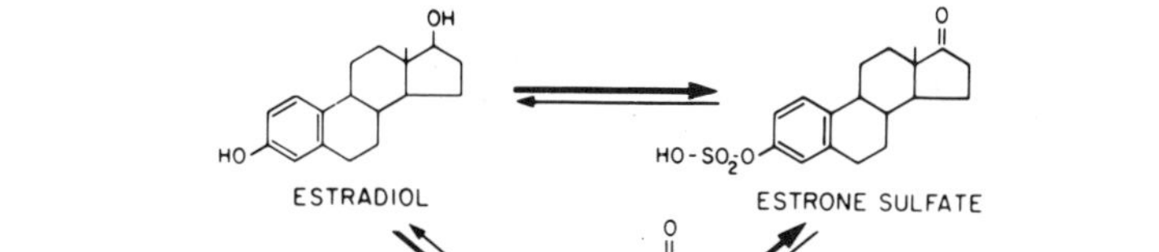

FIG 21–1.
Metabolism of the natural estrogens. Both estradiol and estrone exist in a reversible equilibrium with estrone sulfate, which may act as an inactive estrogen reservoir for both compounds. Once estrogen is metabolized to estrone by 17β-dehydrogenase, subsequent steps in degradation are principally oxidative. The A-ring hydroxylation produces catecholestrogens, which then may undergo methylation prior to excretion. D-ring hydroxylation produces mainly estriol with lesser amounts of the epiestriols. (From Quirk JG Jr, Wendel GD Jr: Biologic effects of natural and synthetic estrogens, in Buchsbaum HJ (ed): *The Menopause.* New York, Springer-Verlag, 1983. Used by permission.)

and E_2 has been documented to occur in target tissues such as the breast and may increase under certain conditions.[24]

Irreversible metabolism of estrogen proceeds primarily in the liver by oxidation of estrone.[25] Alterations of the "A" ring of the steroid nucleus results in the formation of catechol estrogens. This occurs by hydroxydation at the 2 or 4 positions, with 2-hydroxyestrone being the principle metabolite. Hydroxylation at the 16 position on the D ring results in the formation of estriol and its isomers, the epiestriols. There is no interconversion between products of A- and D-ring metabolism, each pathway being mutually exclusive. Estriol, the product of D-ring metabolism, is biologically a weak estrogen because of its short nuclear retention time. However, when given as a constant infusion in animals, its uterotropic effect is only slightly less than that of E_2.[26] The catechol estrogens are weakly estrogenic and have a very short half life.[27] They probably have only limited importance as circulating estrogens. Certain clinical situations such as obesity, hypothyroidism, and cirrhosis favor the metabolism of E_1 to E_3. Catechol estrogen formation by A ring metabolism is favored in states of weight loss, such as in anorexia nervosa and hyperthyroidism.

Although of limited importance as peripherally active estrogens, catechol estrogens are produced in the hypothalamus, where they may have important central nervous system effects. Catechol estrogens are competitive inhibitors of the enzymes tyrosine hydroxylase and catechol-o-methyl transferase. Thus they can modulate synthesis and degradation of the catecholamines, dopamine and norepinephrine. These neurotransmitters, in turn, may be important in the control of gonadotropin-releasing hormone (GRH) release.[28]

After "A" or "D" ring hydroxydation, estrogen metabolism proceeds in the liver and kidney by conjugation to glucuronides and sulfates, which are highly water soluble and are rapidly excreted by the kidney. The principle urinary estrogens are the conjugates of E_3 and 2-hydroxyestrone.[29] In addition to urinary excretion, there is a significant enterohepatic circulation of estrogen metabolites. When labeled E_2 or E_1 is injected, approximately one half is present in the urine excreted during the first 24 hours, while the remainder is found in bile.[30] The conjugated biliary estrogens undergo hydrolysis in the gut, and approximately 80% are reabsorbed. They are returned to the liver, where they may escape reconjugation and enter the systemic circulation, or they may be reconjugated and excreted in the urine or bile. Only about 10% of an injected estrogen will ultimately be lost in the feces. The enterohepatic circulation of estrogen metabolites may be an important factor in the prolonged effect of orally administered estrogens.[18]

PHARMACOLOGY OF ESTROGEN PREPARATIONS

Table 21–1 lists the estrogens commonly used in the treatment of the menopause. The metabolism and estrogenic effects of these compounds differ according to whether they are natural or synthetic estrogens and with their various routes of administration.

Synthetic Estrogens

Synthetic estrogens used for therapy of the menopause include ethinyl estradiol (EE_2); its C-3 methylated derivative, mestranol; its cylcophenyl ether, quinesterol; and the stilbene derivative, diethystilbestrol (DES). Ethinyl estradiol and DES are both rapidly and well absorbed by the intestinal tract. After ingestion of a 50 µg oral dose of EE_2,

TABLE 21–1.
Commonly Used Estrogen
Compounds

Natural and equine estrogens
    Estrones
        Conjugated equine estrogens
        Piperazine estrone sulfate
    Estradiols
        Micronized estradiol
        Estradiol valerate
Synthetic estrogens
    17α-ethinyl estrogens
    17α-ethinyl estradiol
    17α-ethinyl estradiol-3-methyl ether
        (mestranol)
    Stilbene derivatives
        Diethylstilbestrol

a blood level of about 400 pg/ml ensues. The inactive mestranol must be converted to EE_2 in the liver by demethylation of the C-3 hydroxy group. After ingestion of mestranol, maximum EE_2 levels are achieved in two to four hours.[31] As only about 50% of mestranol is demethylated, it has been estimated to have as little as half the potency of EE_2. After ingestion of EE_2, there is little initial metabolism through the liver. This is thought to be due to steric hindrance by the 17αethinyl group preventing 16αhydroxylation. With D-ring metabolism impeded, the main metabolite of EE_2 is the ethinyl equivalent of the catechol estrogen, 2-hydroxyesterone.[32, 33] A significant ethinyl estradiol sulfate pool, which is analogous to that of estrone sulfate, provides a large reservoir of hormone that can be activated by sulfate cleavage. This may explain in part ethinyl estradiol's long half life of 48 hours. Excretion of EE_2 is via gluco conjugates. Compared to natural estrogens, lesser amounts are excreted in the urine and greater amounts are excreted in the feces.[18] Quinesterol is an ester of EE_2 that has an extremely long half life, and therefore it has been prescribed on a once-a-week basis. Its metabolism rate is similar to the rate of EE_2.

Diethystilbestrol is conjugated to glucunorides prior to excretion in urine and feces. In addition, it undergoes extensive oxidation to products that can bind covalently to DNA and DNA-related proteins.[18]

Synthetic estrogens are distinguished from natural estrogens by their much greater potency. Although parallel dose response curves are not always obtained, EE_2 appears to be 75–1,000 times more potent on a per weight basis than conjugated equine estrogens (CEE) or piperazine estrone sulfate (ES) in terms of increasing the production of hepatic globulins: sex hormone-binding globulin (SHBG), renin substrate, corticosteroid-binding globulin, and thyroid-binding globulin. Diethylstilbestrol is 10–70 times more potent than ES in increasing hepatic globulins and four times more potent in the reduction of FSH levels.[34] The potential for adverse side effects afforded by ingestion of synthetic estrogens on hepatic globulins cannot be avoided by lowering the dose, since the minimum dose required for a therapeutic effect, such as normalization of the calcium/creatine ratio (10 μg), is greater than the minimum dosage that produced marked elevations in hepatic globulin production, 5 μg.[35] The route of administration also does not alter these hepatic effects. Vaginal administration of 50 μg of EE_2 results in circulating EE_2 levels equivalent to those achieved after oral ingestion of 10 μg of EE_2. The increase in SHBG is similar to that seen with the 10 μg oral dose.[36]

Natural Estrogens

The natural estrogens commonly used for treatment of the menopause are listed in Table 21–1. These compounds are most often administered orally. However, vaginal, subdermal, transdermal, and nasal administration have all been shown to be effective in achieving premenopausal serum levels of estrogen.

When given orally, both estrone sulfate, estradiol valerate, and micronized estradiol result in higher serum levels of E_1 and its conjugates than of E_2 (Figs 21–2 and 21–3).[37, 38] This rapid conversion of E_2 to E_1 occurs in the intestinal mucosa.[25] Further metabolism and conjugation occurs in the liver, with glucuronidation of up to 30% of the initial oral dose occurring in a single passage, followed by its rapid urinary and biliary excretion.[39] A measure of this "first passage" effect of oral estrogen is the increased concentrations of serum estrone-3-glucuronide which achieve levels of 10–100 nmol 14 hours after an oral dose.[39] Unusual but specific clinical problems related to this "first passage" effect have been well documented. In a subject with enhanced glucuronidation from chronic phenyltoin therapy, the ingestion of 1.25 mg of conjugated estrogen had little effect on serum E_1 or E_2 levels over 48 hours, while vaginal application of the same dose resulted in serum levels similar to those of other subjects.[40]

Maximum serum estrogen levels after ingestion of these estrogens are reached in about four to six hours.[41] Ingestion of 0.625 mg conjugated equine estrogen, 1.25 mg estrone sulfate, and 1 mg micronized estradiol result in similar maximum serum levels

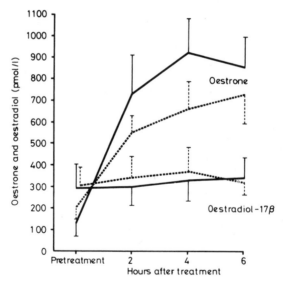

FIG 21–2.
Mean serum concentrations (± SE of mean) of estrone and estradiol-17β before and at two-hour intervals after oral piperazine estrone sulfate 1.5 mg *(dashes)* and estradiol valerate 2 mg *(solid line)* in postmenopausal women. (From Anderson ABM, Sklovsky E, Sayers L, et al: Comparison of serum oestrogen concentrations in postmenopausal women taking oestrone sulphate and oestradiol. *Br Med J* 1978; 1:140. Used by permission.)

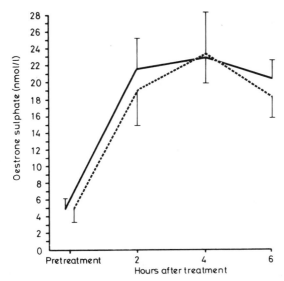

FIG 21–3.
Mean serum concentrations ($\pm$ SE of mean) of estrone sulfate before and at two-hour intervals after oral administration of 1.5 mg piperazine estrone sulfate *(dashes)* and 2 mg estradiol valerate *(solid line)* in postmenopausal women. (From Anderson ABM, Sklovsky E, Sayers L, et al: Comparison of serum oestrogen concentrations in postmenopausal women taking oestrone sulphate and oestradiol. *Br Med J* 1978; 1:140. Used by permission.)

of E_2 and E_1 of 30–40 pg/ml and 150–250 pg/ml, respectively (Table 21–2).[36] Significant levels of estrone are still present 24 hours after an oral dose, reflecting enterohepatic circulation and the slow metabolism of the E_1S pool. In addition to E_1S, CEE contain equilin sulfate (20%–25%) and other equine estrogens, which are also estrogenic in man. These equine estrogens differ from estradiol and estrone in that the B-ring of the steroid nucleus is unsaturated. After prolonged oral treatment with 1.25 mg CEE serum equilin levels reach a mean of 1.25 μg/ml. Levels can remain elevated for 13 weeks or more posttreatment due to storage and slow release from adipose tissue.[42] In addition, metabolism of equilin to equelenin and 17 hydroxy equelenin may contribute greatly to the estrogen stimulatory effect of CE therapy. For this reason, conjugated equine estrogens are, strictly speaking, not natural to human beings.

Although E_1 and its conjugates are the principle circulating estrogens, following ingestion of either estrone or estradiol preparations, the principle estrogen at the cellular and nuclear level appears to be E_2. Following estrogen ingestion, the E_2/E_1 ratio in the serum is less than 1, but the cytosolic E_2/E_1 ratio in the endometrium is greater than 1 for both the free and bound components. This reversal of the E_2/E_1 ratio is maintained in the nucleus also, suggesting that E_2 is the biologically active estrogen of significance despite its lower level in serum (Fig 21–4).[43] The increase in nuclear estradiol may be explained in part by its greater nuclear retention time, but the fact that in the free cytosolic fraction there is more E_2 than E_1 suggests active transport into the cell favoring E_2, or metabolism of E_1 to E_2 in the cytosol. Addition of a progestin alters this metabolism and the intracellular E_2/E_1 ratio approaches one.

With vaginal, transdermal or subdermal administration of estrogen compounds, the

TABLE 21–2.

Maximum Serum Estrogen Levels After Administration
of Various Estrogens*

DAILY ADMINISTRATION	DOSE	SERUM LEVELS ESTRADIOL (PG/ML)	ESTRONE (PG/ML)
ORAL			
Conjugated estrogens	0.6 mg	40	150
Piperazine estrone sulfate	0.6 or 1.2	34 or 42	125 or 250
Micronized estradiol	1.0	30	260
VAGINAL			
Conjugated estrogen	1.25 mg	25	120
SUBCUTANEOUS			
Estradiol pellet	25 mg (once)	50	40
TRANSDERMAL			
Transdermal therapeutic system	50 μg	60	50
Estrogen cream	5 gm	135	120

*From Lobo R, Mishell DR, Budoff PW, et al: *Estrogen Replacement Therapy,* Symposium Proceedings, San Francisco, May 9–10, 1984. Abbot Pharmaceuticals, Inc, p 9. Used by permission.

effects of gastrointestinal absorption are avoided, and serum estrogen levels more directly reflect the estrogen administered (Figs 21–5 and 21–6).[44] However, circulating levels of estrogen after vaginal administration are only about one fourth those seen with equivalent doses given orally.[45, 46, 36] With 0.3 mg CEE cream vaginally, no increase in systemic levels of estrogen are seen, but maturation of the vaginal epithelium occurs to a much greater extent and a vaginal effect has been documented that is equivalent to four times this dose given orally.[46] Micronized E_2 suspended in saline and administered vaginally results in a more rapid absorption than micronized E_2 in cream, with peak levels occurring at two and four hours respectively.[47, 48] Vaginal administration of 2 mg of micronized E_2 in cream is required to achieve the serum levels obtained by vaginal administration of 0.5 mg in saline.

Silastic vaginal rings impregnated with E_2 have also been shown to be an effective delivery system with relatively consistent E_2 levels of 100–150 pg/ml in serum over a period of three months.[49] Plasma E_1 and E_2 levels rise with increasing duration of vaginal estrogen therapy (Fig 21–7). This rise in circulatory estrogens correlates with increasing maturity of the vaginal mucosa (Fig 21–8) and may reflect enhanced transfer of estrogen across a healthy vaginal epithelium and/or increased vascularity in the estrogenized vaginal tissues.[39]

Subdermal, 25-mg estradiol pellets cause sustained serum E_2 levels in the 50–70 pg/ml range for three months that decline slowly to a mean of 37 pg/ml at six months.[50] This method has been documented to relieve vasomotor symptoms, allowing a relatively stable circulating level of E_2 with no changes occurring in hepatic globulins, and a reduction in urinary calcium/creatinine level to levels found in the premenopausal women.

Transdermal administration of E_2 with a patch applied to the skin provides controlled

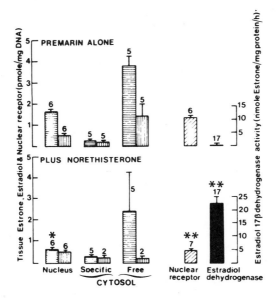

FIG 21–4.
Estrogen ratios in endometria and plasma from postmenopausal women receiving either Premarin alone *(top left)* or Premarin plus norethisterone *(bottom left)*. Results are expressed as mean ± SEM with the number observation at the top of each column. *Asterisk:* Students t-test $P < .005$. Double asterisk: students t-test $P < .001$. For other definitions, see Materials and Methods in the source: King RJB, Dyer G, Collins WP, et al: Intracellular estradiol, estrone and estrogen receptor levels in endometria from postmenopausal women receiving estrogens and progestins. *J Steroid Biochem* 1980; 13:377. Used by permission.)

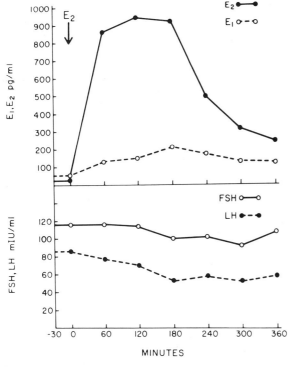

FIG 21–5.
Plasma E_1, E_2, LH, and FSH concentrations before and after the vaginal administration of 0.5 mg of micronized E_2. (From Schiff I, Tulchinsky D, Ryan KJ: Vaginal absorption of estrone and 17β-estradiol. *Fertil Steril* 1977; 28:1063. Used by permission.)

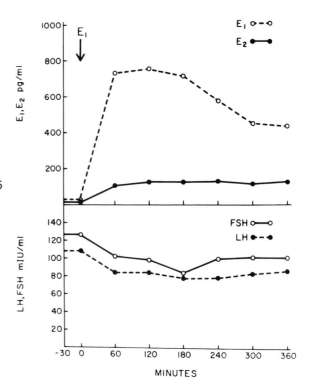

FIG 21–6.
Plasma E_1, E_2, LH, and FSH concentrations before and after the vaginal administration of 0.5 mg of E_1. (From Schiff I, Tulchinsky D, Ryan KJ: Vaginal absorption of estrone and 17β-estradiol. *Fertil Steril* 1977; 28:1063. Used by permission.)

diffusion of estradiol. Application of four such patches, each 4 cm in diameter and changed every three days, resulted in mean E_2 levels of 72 pg/ml and E_1 levels of 37 pg/ml after three weeks of therapy, with a significant reduction in vasomotor symptoms occurring in symptomatic women. As with the E_2 pellet, no effect on globulins occurs. However, the effects on calcium balance are less satisfactory, but this may be dose-related (Fig 21–9).[4]

Transdermal cream (Oestrogel) has been administered in Europe as a cream rubbed on the lower abdomen and thighs. About 5 gm of the cream creates E_2 levels of about 100 pg/ml within four to six hours (Fig 21–10).

Potency of Natural Estrogens

In comparing the potency of various oral preparations, the potency ratios for the undesirable hepatic effects are relatively constant for the natural estrogens, with CEE having more of a stimulatory effect than ES. However, as discussed earlier, the hepatic effects of synthetic estrogens are several orders of magnitude greater than those observed with the natural estrogens.[34, 35] Because of the excessive effects of synthetic estrogens on hepatic globulins, they are not recommended for estrogenic therapy in the menopause. While synthetic estrogen therapy is known to increase circulatory blood clotting factors, this is not observed with the natural estrogens. Thus, in contrast to the oral contraceptives that contain ethinyl estradiol, no increase in thrombosis has been reported with use of natural estrogens postmenopausally.

The mild increases in hepatic globulins seen with natural estrogens may be prevented entirely by avoiding oral administration (see Table 21–2). Estradiol delivered by a sub-

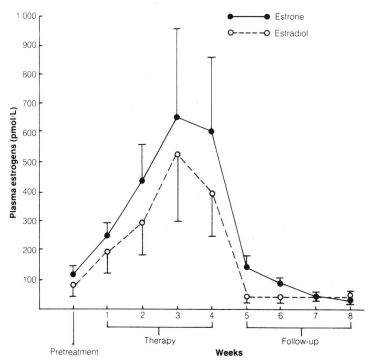

FIG 21–7.
Rise in mean plasma levels of estrone and estradiol demonstrates absorption in post-menopausal women using Premarin vaginal cream. (From Siddle N, Whitehead M: Flexible prescribing of estrogens. *Contemp Obstet Gynecol* 1983; 22:137. Used by permission.)

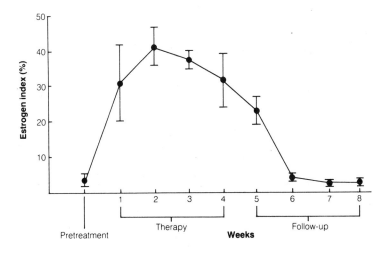

FIG 21–8.
Mean estrogen index peaks during week 2 in postmenopausal women using Premarin vaginal cream. (From Siddle N, Whitehead M: Flexible prescribing of estrogens. *Contemp Obstet Gynecol* 1983; 22:137. Used by permission.)

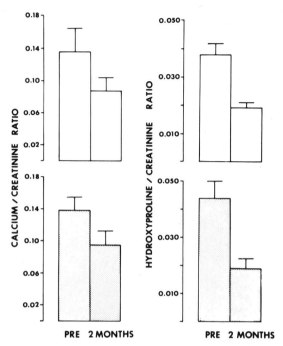

FIG 21–9.
Upper and lower panels show the mean ratios of urinary calcium/creatinine *(Ca/Cr)* and hydroxyproline/creatinine *(Cr)* in premenopausal control subjects and postmenopausal subjects. (From Laufer LR, DeFazio JL, Lu JKH, et al: Estrogen replacement therapy by transdermal estradiol administration. *Am J Obstet Gynecol* 1983; 146–533. Used by permission.)

dermal pellet or the transdermal therapeutic system can achieve therapeutic levels of estrogen, restore calcium/creatinine ratios to premenopausal levels and relieve hot flushes without adversely affecting hepatic globulins.[36, 51] However, the favorable increase in high-density lipoprotein cholesterol (HDL cholesterol) seen with oral therapy is also a hepatic effect, and this is not as consistently found with nonoral routes of administration. Nevertheless, if the dose and route of estrogen administration is carefully administered, it is presumed that this problem can be overcome. While an increase in HDL cholesterol may not occur with percutaneous therapy and administration of subdermal E_2 pellets has been shown to increase levels.[39, 50] If the correct dose of estrogen and its vehicle of administration is chosen, vaginal estrogen will give relief of vasomotor symptoms and normalize the calcium/creatinine ratio without any significant effect on hepatic globulins.[46]

Natural estrogens in the doses listed in Table 21–2 are effective in ameliorating postmenopausal symptoms. They produce serum estrogen levels similar to those in the early follicular phase and normalize the calcium/creatinine ratio to premenopausal levels with minimal effects on hepatic globulins. Although the minor alterations in hepatic globulins noted with oral therapy have not been shown to have clinical significance, they can be avoided entirely with oral ES in the lowest dose, vaginal CEE cream, and transdermal or subdermal E_2 preparations. Whether such preparations are, therefore, more desirable cannot be determined at present. Such decisions will require a more complete under-

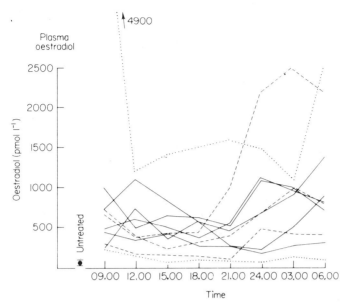

FIG 21–10.
Plasma estrone: pretreatment and during estrogel therapy. (———) 5 gm every night; (---) 5 gm alternate nights (applied on study night); (. . .) 5 gm alternate nights (none applied study night). (From Whitehead MI, Townsend PT, Kitchin Y, et al: Plasma steroid and protein hormone profiles in post-menopausal women following topical administration of oestradiol 17β, in Mauvais-Jarvis P, Vickers CFH, Wepierre J (eds): *Percutaneous Absorption of Steroids.* London, Academic Press Inc., 1980. Used by permission.)

standing of the effects of oral and nonoral estrogens on factors such as the lipoproteins and will require long-term clinical studies.

REFERENCES

1. Baird DT, Fraser IS: Blood production and ovarian secretion rates of estradiol-17β and estrone in women throughout the menstrual cycle. *J Clin Endocrinol Metab* 1974; 38:1009.
2. Kletzky OA, Nakamura RM, Thorneycroft IH, et al: Log normal distribution of gonadotropins and ovarian steroid values in the normal menstrual cycle. *Am J Obstet Gynecol* 1975; 121:688.
3. Sherman BM, Korenman SG: Hormonal characteristics of the human menstrual cycle throughout reproductive life. *J Clin Endocrinol Metab* 1975; 55:699.
4. Laufer LR, DeFazio JL, Lu JKH, et al: Estrogen replacement therapy by transdermal estradiol administration. *Am J Obstet Gynecol* 1983; 146:533.
5. Judd HL: Hormonal dynamics associated with the menopause. *Clin Obstet Gynecol* 1976; 19:775.
6. Lloyd CW, Lobotsky J, Baird DT, et al: Concentration of conjugated estrogens, androgens and gestagens in ovarian and peripheral venous plasma in women: The normal menstrual cycle. *J Clin Endocrinol Metab* 1971; 32:155.
7. Judd HL, Shamonki IM, Frumar AM, et al: Origin of serum estradiol in postmenopausal women. *Obstet Gynecol* 1981; 59:680.
8. Siiteri PK, MacDonald PC: Role of extraglandular estrogen in human endocrinology, in Greep RO, Astwood EB (eds): *Handbook of Physiology: Endocrinology.* Washington D.C., American Physiology Society, 1973, vol 2, part 1, p 45.
9. Longcope C: Metabolic clearance and blood production rates of estrogens in postmenopausal women. *Am J Obstet Gynecol* 1971; 111:778.

10. Meldrum DR, Davidson BJ, Tataryn IV, et al: Changes in circulating steroids with aging in postmenopausal women. *Obstet Gynecol* 1981; 57:624.
11. Ackerman GE, Smith ME, Mendelson CR, et al: Aromatization of androstenedione by human adipose tissue stromal cells in monolayer culture. *J Clin Endocrinol Metab* 1981; 53:412.
12. Eisenfeld AJ: Estrogen receptors. *Clin Obstet Gynecol* 1976; 19:767.
13. Clark JH, Hardin JW, McCormack SA: Estrogen receptor binding and growth of the reproductive tract. *Pediatrics* 1978; 62:1121.
14. Chung-Hsiu W, Motohashi T, Abdel-Rahman HA, et al: Free and protein bound plasma estradiol 17β during the menstrual cycle. *J Clin Endocrinol Metab* 1976; 43:436.
15. Rosenthal HE, Pietrzak E, Slaunwhite WR, et al: Binding of estrone sulfate in human plasma. *J Clin Endocrinol Metab* 1972; 34:805.
16. Anderson DC: Sex-hormone binding globulin. *Clin Endocrinol* 1974; 3:69.
17. Siiteri PI: Extraglandular oestrogen formation and serum binding of oestradiol: Relationship to cancer. *J Endocrinol* 1981; 89:119.
18. Quirk JG Jr, Wendel GD Jr: Biologic effects of natural and synthetic estrogens, in Buchsbaum HJ (ed): *The Menopause*. New York, Springer-Verlag, 1983.
19. Fishman J, Bradlow HL, Gallagher TF: Oxidative metabolism of estradiol. *J Biol Chem* 1960; 235:3104.
20. Pack BA, Tovar R, Booth E, et al: The cyclic relationship of estrogen sulfurylation to the nuclear receptor level in human endometrial curettings. *J Clin Endocrinol Metab* 1979; 48:420.
21. Loriaux DL, Ruder HJ, Lipsett MB: The measurement of estrone sulfate in plasma. *Steroids* 1971; 18:463.
22. Wright K, Collins DC, Musey PI, et al: A specific radioimmunoassay for estrone sulfate in plasma and urine without hydrolysis. *J Clin Endocrinol Metab* 1978; 47:1092.
23. Hawkins RA, Oakey RE: Estimation of oestrone sulfate, oestradiol-17β and oestrone in peripheral plasma: Concentrations during the menstrual cycle and in men. *J Endocrinol* 1974; 60:3.
24. Gurpide E, Stolee A, Tseng L: Quantitative studies of tissue uptake and disposition of hormones. *Acta Endocrinol* 1971:67 [Suppl 153]:247.
25. Buster JE: Estrogen metabolism, in Sciarra JJ (ed): *Gynecology and Obstetrics*. Philadelphia, Harper & Row, 1985.
26. Fishman J, Martucci CP: New concepts in estrogenic activity: The role of metabolites in the expression of hormone action, in Pasetto N, Paoletti R, Ambrus JL (eds): *The Menopause and Postmenopause*. Lancaster, England, MTP Press, 1980, p 43.
27. Merriam GR, Brandon DO, Kono S, et al: Rapid metabolic clearance of the catecholestrogen 2-hydroxyestrone. *J Clin Endocrinol Metab* 1980; 51:1211.
28. Fishman J, Norton B: Brain catecholestrogens: Formation and possible functions. *Adv Biosci* 1975; 15:123.
29. Fishman J: Role of 2-hydroxyestrone in estrogen metabolism. *J Clin Endocrinol Metab* 1963; 23:207.
30. Sandberg A, Slaunwhite WR: Studies on phenolic steroids in human subjects. II. The metabolic fate and hepato-biliary-enteric circulation of C^{14}-estrone and C^{14}-estradiol in women. *J Clin Invest* 1957; 36:1266.
31. de la Pena A, Chenault CB, Goldzieher JW: Radioimmunoassay of unconjugated plasma ethynylestradiol in women given a single oral dose of ethynylestradiol or mestranol. *Steroids* 1975; 25:773.
32. Bolt HW, Kappus H, Bolt HM: Ring A oxidation of 17α-ethynylestradiol in man. *Horm Metab Res* 1974; 6:432.
33. Bolt HM, Kappus H, Kasbohrer R: Metabolism of 17α-ethynylestradiol by human liver microsomes in vitro: Aromatic hydroxylation and irreversible protein binding of metabolites. *J Clin Endocrinol Metab* 1974; 39:1072.
34. Mashchak CA, Lobo RA, Dozono-Takano R, et al: Comparison of pharmacodynamic properties of various estrogen formulations. *Am J Obstet Gynecol* 1982; 144:511.
35. Mandel FP, Geola FL, Lu JKH, et al: Biologic effects of various doses of ethinyl estradiol in postmenopausal women. *Obstet Gynecol* 1982; 59:673.

36. Lobo R, Mishell DR, Budoff PW, et al: *Estrogen Replacement Therapy,* Symposium Proceedings, San Francisco, May 9–10, 1984. Abbot Pharmaceuticals, Inc, p 9.
37. Anderson ABM, Sklovsky E, Sayers L, et al: Comparison of serum oestrogen concentrations in post-menopausal women taking oestrone sulphate and oestradiol. *Br Med J* 1978; 1:140.
38. Yen SSC, Martin PL, Burnier AM, et al: Circulating estradiol, estrone and gonadotropin levels following the administration of orally active 17β-estradiol in postmenopausal women. *J Clin Endocrinol Metab* 1975; 40:518.
39. Siddle N, Whitehead M: Flexible prescribing of estrogens. *Contemp Obstet Gynecol* 1983; 22:137.
40. Englund DE, Johansson EDB: Plasma levels of oestrone, oestradiol and gonadotrophins in postmenopausal women after oral and vaginal administration of conjugated equine estrogens. *Br J Obstet Gynaecol* 1978; 85:957.
41. Whitehead MI, Townsend PT, Kitchin Y, et al: Plasma steroid and protein hormone profiles in postmenopausal women following topical administration of oestradiol 17β, in Mauvais-Jarvis P, et al (eds): *Percutaneous Absorption of Steroids.* New York, Academic Press, 1980, p 231.
42. Hammond CB, Maxson WS: Current status of estrogen therapy for the menopause. *Fertil Steril* 1982; 37:5.
43. King RJB, Dyer G, Collins WP, et al: Intracellular estradiol, estrone and estrogen receptor levels in endometria from postmenopausal women receiving estrogens and progestins. *J Steroid Biochem* 1980; 13:377.
44. Shiff I, Tulchinsky D, Ryan KJ: Vaginal absorption of estrone and 17β-estradiol. *Fertil Steril* 1977; 28:1063.
45. Deutsch S, Ossowski R, Benjamin I: Comparison between degree of systemic absorption of vaginally and orally administered estrogens at different dose levels in postmenopausal women. *Am J Obstet Gynecol* 1981; 139:967.
46. Mandel FP, Geola FL, Meldrum DR, et al: Biological effects of various doses of vaginally administered conjugated equine estrogens in postmenopausal women. *J Clin Endocrinol Metab* 1983; 57:133.
47. Rigg LA, Hermann H, Yenn SSC: Absorption of estrogens from vaginal creams. *N Engl J Med* 1978; 298:195.
48. Rigg LA, Milanes B, Villanueva B, et al: Efficacy of intravaginal and intranasal administration of micronized estradiol-17β. *J Clin Endocrinol Metab* 1977; 45:1261.
49. Stumpf PG, Maruca J, Santen RJ, et al: Development of a vaginal ring for achieving physiologic levels of 17β-estradiol in hypoestrogenic women. *J Clin Endocrinol Metab* 1982; 54:208.
50. Lobo RA, March CM, Goebelsmann U, et al: Subdermal estradiol pellets following hysterectomy and oophorectomy. *Am J Obstet Gynecol* 1980; 138:714.
51. Chetkowski R, Medrum D, Steingold K, et al: Biological effects of estradiol (E_2) administration by a transdermal therapeutic system (TTS), abstract. 32nd Annual Meeting of the Society for Gynecologic Investigation, Phoenix, Arizona, March 20–23, 1985, p 67.
52. Welshons WV, Krummel BM, Gorski J: Nuclear localization of unoccupied receptors for glucocorticoids, estrogens, and progesterone in GH_3 cells. *Endocrinology* 1985; 117:2140.

CHAPTER **22**

The Pharmacology of Progestogens

M. I. WHITEHEAD, M.B., B.S., M.R.C.O.G.
NICK SIDDLE, M.R.C.O.G.
GEOFFREY LANE, M.B., B.S., M.R.C.O.G.
MALCOLM PADWICK, M.B., B.S.
TIMOTHY A. RYDER, M.Sc., Ph.D.
JOHN PRYSE-DAVIES, M.D., F.R.C. Path.
R. J. B. KING, B.Sc., M.Sc., Ph.D., D.Sc.

IT IS NOW ALMOST ten years since the first retrospective, case-control studies[1-3] causally linked postmenopausal estrogen use with the development of endometrial carcinoma. The resultant publicity had many damaging effects, including loss of credibility for those within the medical profession who had advocated such treatment. Additionally, the lay public became suspicious of and disenchanted with exogenous estrogens, attitudes which remain to this day. However, not all the consequences of the publicity were adverse, because a major stimulus was applied to improve our understanding of the biologic effects of exogenous estrogens and thereby to develop safer but equally efficaceous regimens.

During the last eight years, various strategies have been suggested to reduce the risk of endometrial hyperstimulation with exogenous estrogen therapy. These have been discussed in detail elsewhere[4] and are now summarized.

POSSIBLE STRATEGIES FOR ENDOMETRIAL PROTECTION

Reducing The Estrogen Dose

Logically, reducing the estrogen dose will lower the degree of estrogen stimulation and minimize the risk of hyperplasia and carcinoma. However, dosage reductions are now known to reduce the beneficial effects of estrogens in relieving not only the physical and psychologic symptoms of the menopause but also in conserving postmenopausal bone mass. The bone-conserving effects of estrogens are increasingly being recognized as the major indication for long-term use, not only because the consequences of postmenopausal osteoporosis in terms of morbidity, mortality, and financial costs are appalling,[5] but also because adequate doses of exogenous estrogens are the most effective therapy for conserving bone mass.[6] Both types of beneficial effect are now known to be dose-dependent. Reductions in the daily dose of estradiol valerate (Trisequens, Novo Pharmaceuticals) from 4 to 2 mg daily are associated with a failure to relieve hot flushes completely,[7] and the 1 mg dosage exerts minimal bone-conserving activity.[8] Similar data are available for conjugated equine estrogens (Premarin, Ayerst Laboratories). A lowering in dose to 0.3 mg daily is associated, in our clinical experience, with a loss of suppression of vasomotor symptoms and does not appear to conserve bone mass as effectively as 0.625 mg daily.[9] Thus, the minimum effective bone-sparing doses of estradiol and conjugated estrogens are 2 mg and 0.625 mg daily, respectively, and at these dosages marked endometrial proliferation has been observed.[10–11]

Avoiding Estrone Preparations

It has been argued that because nearly all the retrospective, American epidemiologic studies associated mainly conjugated estrogens (65% of which is estrone sulphate) with an increase in risk of endometrial carcinoma, then this preparation must possess special carcinogenic properties[12] not present with the other estrogen formulations that contain estradiol or estriol. The assumption is that these latter preparations can be prescribed without a risk of endometrial hyperstimulation, but this assumption is incorrect. At equivalent dosages, estradiol causes the same degree of endometrial stimulation as conjugated estrogens,[11] with almost identical rates of hyperplasia.[10]

The degree of estrogenic stimulation being applied to the endometrium can be quantified by measurements of nuclear estradiol and cytoplasmic progesterone receptor.[13] Receptor levels during therapy with a variety of oral and parenterally administered estrogen preparations (oral conjugated estrogens, 0.625 and 1.25 mg; estradiol valerate, 2 mg; estrone sulphate, 1.5 mg; subcutaneous estradiol implant, 50 mg; and percutaneous estradiol cream, 3 mg) are illustrated in Figure 22–1.[11] Premenopausal proliferative and secretory-phase ranges are included for comparison. All preparations studied induced progesterone receptor and nuclear estradiol receptor levels to within the premenopausal proliferative phase range. Estrone sulphate (Ogen, Abbott Laboratories), 1.5 mg, and subcutaneous estradiol implants (Organon), 50 mg, produced hyperphysiologic levels of progesterone receptor. Conjugated estrogens, 1.25 mg, induced hyperphysiologic values for nuclear estradiol receptors. The levels of nuclear estradiol receptor with percutaneous estradiol cream (Oestrogel, Laboratories Besins-Iscovesco) were not significantly different from the proliferative phase range ($P > .01$). Thus all formulations apply a potent stimulus to the postmenopausal endometrium. The most likely explanation for this degree of stimulation is that even in the postmenopause, estradiol remains the predominant intranuclear estrogen within the endometrium.[14, 15] Estradiol is the most potent natural stimulator of cell biosynthesis;[16] thus, estrogen preparations that selectively increase plasma estradiol levels, such as those used in subcutaneous implantation, are likely to be associated with marked endometrial proliferation. Therefore, the high incidence of hyperplasia reported with estradiol implants, 56%,[17] might have been predicted.

At low dosages, less than 2 mg daily, estriol appears to have little proliferative effect upon the endometrium[18] and has therefore been recommended as the ideal estrogen for postmenopausal use.[19] However, it is doubtful whether such small estriol dosages actually impart an estrogenic stimulus, because, unlike all other estrogen preparations studied to date, low-dose estriol does not conserve bone mass and is no better than placebo at relieving acute vasomotor symptoms.[20] Unlike estradiol and estrone, estriol is not strongly bound to plasma proteins and globulins but circulates largely as the glucuronide. This facilitates rapid renal excretion.[21] Thus, an oral dose of estriol is absorbed and largely excreted within three hours. When administered at eight-hour intervals, estriol has been associated with the development of endometrial hyperplasia.[21]

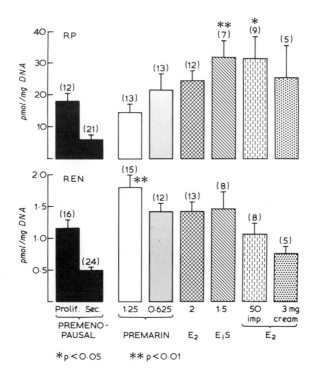

FIG 22–1.

Soluble progesterone receptor *(RP)* and nuclear estradiol receptor *(REN)* content of premenopausal *(solid bars)* and postmenopausal *(all other bars)* endometria. E_2 denotes estradiol valerate; E_1S, estropipate (piperazine estrone sulfate); E_2, subcutaneous estradiol implant (50 mg); E_2, percutaneous estradiol cream; *Prolif,* proliferative phase; and *Sec,* secretory phase. Results are expressed as means ± SEM. Figures in parenthesis denote numbers of observations. *P* values (Student's t-test) represent significant differences between premenopausal proliferative-phase levels and postmenopausal levels. (From Whitehead MI, Townsend PT, Pryse-Davies J, et al: Effects of estrogens and progestins on the biochemistry and morphology of the postmenopausal endometrium. *N Engl J Med* 1981; 305:1599–1604. Reprinted by permission of the *New England Journal of Medicine.*)

Continuous as Opposed to Cyclic Administration of Estrogens

In monkeys,[22] mice,[23] and rats,[24] prolonged estrogen exposure leads to a relatively refractory state within responsive tissues, the cells apparently down-regulating their response to the priming stimulus. Similar data are available for the postmenopausal woman. As the duration of estrogen stimulation is extended from 14 to 21 days, the nuclear estradiol receptor content of endometrial cells falls[13] and the estrogenicity of the vaginal epithelium (as measured by an estrogen index score) is reduced.[25] Furthermore, in one case-control study of endometrial carcinoma,[26] continuous administration of estrogens was associated with a slight, but not significant, reduction in risk for this malignancy as compared to cyclic therapy.

These observations led to the suggestion that continuous (every day) administration of estrogens might result in less endometrial stimulation than with cyclic therapy.[27] However, in a prospective study in which postmenopausal women received either continuous or cyclic conjugated estrogens, 0.625 mg daily in a double-blind fashion, the incidence of endometrial hyperplasia was similar in the two groups.[27] The incidence of hyperplasia with continuous therapy was 3.7 per 100 women-months, and with cyclic administration it was 4.5 per 100 women-months; this difference was not significant. Thus, continuous administration offered no advantage over cyclic therapy, and the authors concluded that the rate for the development of hyperplasia was unacceptably high in both groups.

Progestogen Addition to the Estrogen Therapy

The addition of a progestogen to the estrogen therapy has been shown to be protective to the endometrium. Prospective, histologic studies that monitored the endometrial response to exogenous estrogens and progestogens during a two-year period have reported an 18%–32% incidence of endometrial hyperplasia with estrogen therapy alone;[10] importantly, up to one third of the hyperplasias were of the more sinister atypical variety that carries a higher risk of subsequent malignant change. The incidence of hyperplasia was significantly reduced to 3%–4% when progestogens were added for seven days each calendar month.[10] Extending the duration of progestogen administration to ten days reduced the incidence of hyperplasia still further, to 2%,[17] and maximum protective effects were obtained with 12–13 days progestin exposure, the incidence of hyperplasia being zero.[17] The incidence of endometrial carcinoma with combined estrogen-progestogen regimens is also reduced, and not only to below that recorded with unopposed estrogens, but also to below that observed in untreated women. The incidence rates for endometrial carcinoma in the untreated population seen at Wilford Hall USAF Medical Center in 1975–1979 were 242.2 per 100,000 women; in the estrogen users, it was 434.4 per 100,000 women, and with combined estrogen-progestogen therapy it was 70.8 per 100,000 women.[28] The difference between the estrogen-progestogen users and the estrogen-users was highly significant ($P < .0001$).

BENEFITS AND RISKS OF PROGESTOGEN THERAPY

To support the argument for the widespread use of progestogens, it is necessary to show that the benefits outweigh the disadvantages. Concern has been expressed that progestogen addition might negate the beneficial effects of estrogens upon the symptomatic and psychologic status and might reduce the bone-conserving effects. Additionally, certain types of progestogens, particularly the testosterone and 19-nortestosterone derivatives, have been linked during oral contraceptive therapy with an increased incidence of arterial disease and hypertension,[29, 30] adverse affects that are possibly mediated through suppression of high-density lipoprotein (HDL) cholesterol.[31] Obviously, it is pointless to add a progestogen to protect against the development of endometrial carcinoma if such an addition antagonizes the beneficial effects of estrogens upon the cardiovascular system[32] and increases the death rate from myocardial infarction.

Thus, the ''ideal'' progestogen for addition to postmenopausal estrogens should antagonize only the undesirable estrogenic actions upon the endometrium, and perhaps also upon breast tissue. The beneficial effects of estrogens should not be negated. Different types of progestogens appear to cause dissimilar psychologic and metabolic effects, and the route of administration is likely to influence the risk of adverse effects. Importantly, the majority of progestogen-induced side effects appear to be dose-related and the minimum effective dosage should be prescribed. In the search for the ''ideal'' progestogen, the type, route of administration, and dose of progestogen must be considered. These will now be discussed in detail.

PHARMACOLOGY OF PROGESTOGENS
Classification

Progestogens can be classified in a variety of ways: the classification presented here (Table 22–1) is based upon structure and is modified from Brotherton.[33] The earliest progestogens to be used clinically were derivatives of testosterone and 19-nortestosterone. In addition to their progestogenic actions, these compounds, not surprisingly, also possess varying degrees of androgenic and, to a lesser extent, estrogenic activity. More recently, derivatives of progesterone have become available: their potency has been enhanced by the addition of a halogen molecule.

Potency

The most comprehensive assessment of potency has been undertaken using the McPhail Scale in the Clauberg Test.[34] The results are shown in Table 22–2. In this test, immature female rabbits weighing 800–1,000 gm are estrogen-primed and then receive a progestogen, either orally or subcutaneously, for five days. They are killed on the sixth day. Progestogens increase endometrial proliferation in rabbits, which can be graded using the McPhail Scale. In this assessment, the most potent progestogens are the halogenated derivatives of progesterone, cyproterone acetate and chlormadinone acetate, followed by the progesterone derivative, medroxyprogesterone acetate (MPA), and then by a 19-nortestosterone derivative, norgestrel. The validity of extrapolating the data obtained from this type of assessment to the human postmenopausal situation has been questioned.[35] In rabbits, progestogens increase endometrial cell proliferation, but in human beings, they are added to postmenopausal estrogens to oppose the stimulatory effects of estrogens and to decrease mitotic activity. Identical comments apply to the Greenblatt Test,[36] which, although performed in humans, assesses the ability of progestogens to maintain the endometrium: the antiestrogenic effects of progestogens are not determined in the Greenblatt Test. The most appropriate bioassay available for assessing the antiestrogenic effects in humans is most probably the Kaufmann Test.[37] However, this assay requires castrates with an intact uterus, of whom there are few, and the results, being purely descriptive, are difficult to quantitate scientifically.

TABLE 22–1.
Structural Classification of Progestogens*

PARENT COMPOUND	DERIVATIVE
Progesterone	Medroxyprogesterone acetate
	Megestrol acetate
	17-α Hydroxyprogesterone caproate
Halogenated progesterone	Chlormadinone acetate
	Cyproterone acetate
Retroprogesterone	Dydrogesterone
19-norprogesterone	Gestonorone caproate
Testosterone	Dimethisterone
19-nortestosterone	Ethynodiol diacetate
	Lynestrenol
	Norethindrone
	Norethynodrel
	Norgestrel

*From Brotherton J: *Sex Hormone Pharmacology*. London, Academic Press, 1976, pp 1–78. Used by permission.

TABLE 22–2.

Potency of Various Progestogens*

STEROID	SUBCUTANEOUS	ORAL
Progesterone	1	1
Cyproterone acetate	250	1,000
Chlormadinone acetate	75	333
Medroxyprogesterone acetate	75	333
L-norgestrel	66	
Megestrol acetate	2	400
Norethisterone acetate	25	330
Norethisterone	12	100
Ethynodiol diacetate	7.5	100
Dimethisterone	2.5	100
Lynestrenol	2.5	33
Norethynodrel	2.5	33
Gestonorone acetate	25	33
Dydrogesterone	25	7.5
17-hydroxyprogesterone acetate	1	1

*From Neumann F: Chemische Konstitution und pharmakolishe Wirkung, in Langecker H (ed): *Hanbuche der Experimentellen Pharmakologie, Band XXII Die Gestagne.* New York, Springer-Verlag New York, 1968, pp 680–1025. Adapted from Brotherton et al.[33] Used by permission.

Notwithstanding these reservations, the McPhail Scale in the Clauberg Test clearly illustrates two important points. First, different classes of progestogens possess vastly dissimilar potencies, with the halogenated-progesterone derivatives being the most potent and the 19-nortestosterone derivatives being the least potent. Second, different routes of administration give quite dissimilar results. For example, dydrogesterone, a retroprogesterone, is much more potent when administered subcutaneously than when given orally; conversely, megestrol acetate, a progesterone derivative, gives exactly opposite results.

Routes of Administration

Numerous studies have reported on the metabolic pathways of the synthetic progestogens after oral and/or parenteral administration.[38–41] While of interest to the pharmacologist, these data are of only limited value to the clinician because the biologic effects of the parent steroid and the metabolic products were not determined; and the plasma levels were not correlated with the end-organ response, Thus, it is not known whether different routes of administration achieve dissimilar therapeutic responses, and these studies will not be considered further.

The situation with progesterone is different, because elevations of plasma levels to within the secretory-phase range after progesterone administration would strongly suggest a therapeutic effect in terms of secretory transformation within an estrogen-primed endometrium. It has been established that progesterone is well absorbed after rectal and vaginal[42] and also oral administration.[43] Again, comparisons of the metabolic and biologic effects with different routes of administration are conspicuously lacking from the literature. Indeed, we can find only one report addressing this issue, and this study was performed in premenopausal women. Ottoson et al.[44] administered single 100-mg doses of progesterone either orally or as intramuscular injections to four women during the follicular phase of the ovulatory cycle. The serum levels of progesterone were two to three times higher with the intramuscular as compared to the oral route. The latter was associated with a more pronounced rise in deoxycorticosterone and comparisons of the ratio of deoxycorticosterone to progesterone with the two routes of administration are shown in Figure 22–2. Little change was observed with the intramuscular route; conversely, with the oral route, the deoxycorticosterone/progesterone ratio increased very significantly and quickly following progesterone ingestion.

These alterations with the oral route almost certainly represent rapid gut and liver metabolism. The intramuscular mode of administration avoids a "first-pass" hepatic effect and, in consequence, progesterone metabolism is decreased: thus, the circulating concentrations of the parent compound are higher and those of the metabolites, such as deoxycorticosterone, are lower. The very profound effects of hepatic metabolism after oral administration of progesterone are further illustrated in Figure 22–3. These data show the plasma levels of progesterone and its metabolites, 20-αdihydroprogesterone, 17-hydroxyprogesterone, and pregnanediol-3α-glucuronide, in postmenopausal women following oral administration of progesterone (Utrogestan, Laboratoires Besins-Iscovesco), 100 mg at 9:00 A.M. and 200 mg at 9:00 P.M. for five days. Pretreatment values (Days 1–2) for the parent compound and its three metabolites were significantly increased by therapy and surged further, during the 24-hour profile performed on Day 7, following additional progesterone administration, 200 mg, at 9:00 P.M. The peak mean factorial increase for progesterone was 34; for 20-αdihydroprogesterone, it was 15; for 17-hydroxyprogesterone, it was 7; and for pregnanediol-3α-glucuronide, it was 75. Thus, with the oral route, rapid and significant metabolism occurs, and oral administration of progesterone has now been associated with significant conversion to deoxycorticosterone in postmenopausal women.[45]

The biologic and clinical consequences of this rapid hepatic metabolism remain to be elucidated. However, we believe that if certain classes of progestogens, such as the testosterone and 19-nortestosterone derivatives, modulate lipid and lipoprotein metabolism in an adverse manner and reduce HDL cholesterol, then we predict that these effects are likely to be more pronounced with oral, as compared to parenteral, therapy.

The studies of oral progesterone reported here[43–45] all agree that wide interpatient variation in absorption occurs and peak values for progesterone can vary as much as threefold between individuals. Identical data are available for certain synthetic progestogens such as medroxyprogesterone acetate (MPA).[36, 41, 46] This variation in absorption and attainment of maximal plasma concentrations is of crucial importance clinically and the consequences will be discussed further below.

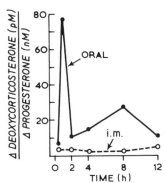

FIG 22–2.
The mean ratio between the increase in deoxycorticosterone and progesterone $\left(\dfrac{\Delta\ \text{deoxycorticosterone}}{\text{progesterone}}\right)$ in plasma after oral and intramuscular administration of 100 mg of progesterone in four women in the follicular phase of the cycle. (From Ottoson UB, et al: *Br J Obstet Gynaecol* 1984; 91:1111–1119. Used by permission.)

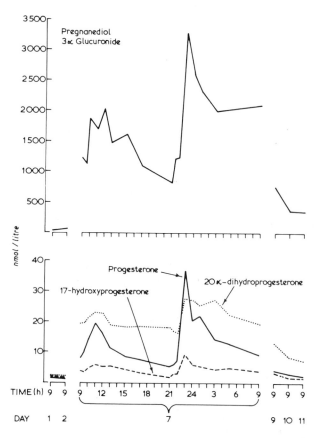

FIG 22–3.

Mean concentrations of progesterone, pregnanediol 3α-glucuronide, 17-hydroxyprogesterone, and 20α-dihydroprogesterone in the peripheral plasma of postmenopausal women before, during, and after administration of oral progesterone. Pretreatment, *Days 1 and 2;* after five days of treatment with 100 mg progesterone at 9 hours and 200 mg at 21 hours, *Day 7;* and posttreatment, *Days 9–11.* (From Padwick M, Endacott J, Matson C, et al: Absorption and metabolism of oral progesterone when administered twice daily. *Fertil Steril,* in press. Used by permission.)

PROGESTOGEN EFFECTS UPON THE ENDOMETRIUM

Cellular responses within the endometrium can be determined histologically and biochemically.

Histology

Histologic evaluation includes assessments using the conventional light microscope and also the transmission electron microscope. As stated previously, progestogen addition to postmenopausal estrogens protects against the development of endometrial hyperplasia.[10, 17] These early studies were performed with dosages of norethindrone of 2.5–5 mg daily and of dl norgestrel, 500 μg daily. Subsequently, we have reported that smaller doses of norethindrone and dl norgestrel, 1 mg and 150 μg, are equally protective.[11, 47] We now present our most recent data, which include evaluation of even lower daily dosages of norethindrone and dl norgestrel, which are both 19-nortestosterone derivatives. We also present data for oral progesterone, for MPA, which is a progesterone derivative, and for dydrogesterone, which is a retroprogesterone.

Endometrial biopsies were obtained from postmenopausal women receiving conjugated estrogens, 0.625 mg or 1.25 mg daily, continuously (for 365 days each year) with varying doses of norethindrone, dl norgestrel, oral progesterone, MPA or dydrogesterone added for the first 12 days of each calendar month. All patients had received therapy for a minimum of three months. The biopsies were obtained using either a Vabra suction curette or at conventional dilatation and curettage under general anesthesia. All tissue was immediately placed into aceto-alcohol for subsequent examination by the same pathologist. The methodology has been described in detail elsewhere.[11, 48–49] Fragmented, isthmic, or endocervical tissue that was considered unreliable for assessment was discarded.

Proliferative endometrium was defined as that which was identical to endometrium obtained during the proliferative phase of the ovulatory cycle. Nonsecretory endometrium was identical to proliferative endometrium, except that no mitotic figures were observed. We regard this as indicating that the added progestogen is exerting an antimitotic effect and reducing cell proliferation. Early and late secretory endometrium showed appearances identical to those seen between days 17 and 21 or 22 and 26 of the ovulatory cycle, respectively. Atypical hyperplasia was defined as tissue showing nuclear atypia, with gland "crowding," and "back-to-back" gland formation. Preliminary data from these studies have been published elsewhere.[11, 47–49]

The histologic results are shown in Table 22–3. The numbers of samples showing the various histologic patterns are stated, together with details of the numbers of samples in which tissue was obtained in quantities insufficient for reliable assessment. Thus, for example, with norethindrone 0.35 mg daily, no endometrial sample showed atypical hyperplasia; two specimens were of a proliferative pattern; 14 samples showed nonsecretory features; 26 biopsy specimens exhibited early secretory changes; and one sample showed late secretory changes. Two biopsies were deemed unreliable for assessment.

Our interpretation of these data is as follows. We regard the presence of atypical hyperplasia as indicating that the estrogen stimulation is not effectively opposed by the added progestogen. Thus, 75 μg dl norgestrel, 100 mg oral progesterone, 5 mg MPA are inadequate for routine use. One biopsy obtained from a woman who received dydrogesterone, 20 mg daily, showed atypical hyperplasia, but subsequent investigation revealed that this patient had experienced irregular bleeding prior to commencing treatment, and we believe that the hyperplasia is likely to have predated therapy. All other samples obtained from women receiving 20 mg dydrogesterone daily showed early secretory features. In our opinion, proliferative endometrium also indicates an inadequate progestational response, and therefore, we have reservations about the widespread use of norethindrone, 0.35 mg, and dydrogesterone, 5 mg.

The norethindrone data illustrate, par excellence, the wide interpatient variation in response to progestogens and the problem that this poses for the clinician. With norethindrone, 0.35 mg daily, only 2 of the 43 samples suitable for assessment exhibited proliferative features, the other 41 showing evidence of progestational activity. Norethindrone, 0.7 mg daily, was not associated with either proliferative or hyperplastic endometrium, and therefore is a dosage that, in our opinion, can be recommended for widespread use. However, in those 41 patients whose biopsies revealed evidence of progestational activity with 0.35 mg daily, an increase in dose to 0.7 mg is likely to be unnecessary and may increase the risk of adverse effects. What is needed is a simple

TABLE 22–3.

Endometrial Histology in Postmenopausal Women Receiving Conjugated Estrogens (Premarin), 0.625 mg or 1.25 mg Daily, With Progestogens Added for 10–12 Days Each Calender Month

TYPE OF PROGESTOGEN ADDED TO ESTROGEN	ATYPICAL HYPERPLASIA	PROLIFERATIVE ENDOMETRIUM	NONSECRETORY ENDOMETRIUM	EARLY SECRETORY ENDOMETRIUM	LATE SECRETORY ENDOMETRIUM	INSUFFICIENT SAMPLE	TOTAL SAMPLES EXAMINED
Norethindrone							
0.35 mg	—	2	14	26	1	2	45
0.7 mg	—	—	6	18	1	1	26
2.5 mg	—	—	2	24	6	2	34
5.0 mg	—	—	2	11	—	—	13
dl norgestrel							
75 µg	3	1	5	9	1	—	19
150 µg	—	1	3	11	—	—	15
500 µg	—	1	6	13	3	—	23
Oral progesterone							
100 mg	3	1	—	1	3	1	9
200 mg	—	—	4	11	1	—	16
300 mg	—	—	2	9	3	—	14
Medroxyprogesterone acetate							
2.5 mg	—	3	6	12	—	9	30
5.0 mg	1	1	2	9	2	2	17
10 mg	—	—	3	20	1	5	29
Dydrogesterone							
5 mg	—	1	4	5	1	—	11
10 mg	—	—	1	19	1	—	21
20 mg	1	—	—	9	—	—	10

test to enable the clinician to determine which patients will respond adequately to very low progestogen dosages and those patients in whom the dosage needs to be increased. Until such a test is developed, our interpretation of these data is that the minimum effective daily dose of norethindrone is 0.7 mg; of oral progesterone, 300 mg; of MPA, 10 mg; and of dydrogesterone, 10–20 mg. The dl norgestrel data are more difficult to interpret, but 75 μg is clearly inadequate.

Transmission Electron Microscopy.—Progestogens induce the formation of certain fine structural features, which include nucleolar channel systems, giant mitochondria, and basal glycogen. Data for norethindrone at doses of 1, 2.5, 5, and 10 mg and dl norgestrel, at doses of 150 and 500 μg, daily, have been published previously;[11] the low dosages were as effective as the higher at inducing these features. Further (unpublished) data for norethindrone are now available, and 75% of samples with 0.35 mg daily and 90% of samples with 0.7 mg daily exhibit these features (unpublished).

The ultrastructural data for oral progesterone[48] and dydrogesterone[49] have also been published previously. In summary, the minimum effective dosage of oral progesterone was 300 mg daily; dydrogesterone at 10 and 20 mg daily produced similar good responses. The MPA results show that 2.5 mg induces suboptimal induction of these features and that 5 and 10 mg daily produce similar results with approximately 85% of samples showing these features.[60]

Biochemistry

Within the endometrium, estrogen stimulation promotes cell proliferation (mitotic effect) and increases DNA synthesis in both glandular and also stromal tissue. This can be quantitated by measuring the incorporation of radioactive thymidine into newly formed DNA. The cells that are actively dividing are thereby labeled and can be counted. Estrogens also promote the formation of their own receptor proteins. These proteins combine with the steroid, and the receptor-estrogen complex then translocates through the cell cytoplasm into the nucleus. Occupation of the appropriate genome by the steroid-receptor complex modifies protein transcription and translation, and cellular biosynthesis is thereby modulated.

Progestogen addition results in a reduction in DNA synthesis and nuclear estradiol-receptor content. Thus, progestogens antagonize the stimulatory effects of estrogens. This antimitotic or antiproliferative effect can be determined by measuring the suppression of DNA synthesis and nuclear estradiol receptor content. In addition, progestogens are responsible for changes in the patterns of intracellular protein production, changes which are classified as secretory effects. These effects are mediated, at least in part, by the induction of various enzymes, such as estradiol 17-β and isocitric dehydrogenases.

We have measured DNA synthesis, nuclear estradiol receptor levels, and the activities of estradiol and isocitric dehydrogenases in endometrial tissue removed from postmenopausal women during estrogen therapy alone with either conjugated estrogens, 0.625 mg or 1.25 mg daily, and during combined estrogen-progestogen therapy with the various types and dosages of progestogens stated in Table 22–3. The methodology and the majority of the data have been published previously, and the interested reader is referred to these articles for the results for norethindrone and dl norgestrel,[11] oral progesterone,[48] and dydrogesterone.[49] In summary, these biochemical results showed good agreement with the histologic data referred to previously, and low dosages of norethindrone and dl norgestrel were as effective as the higher doses at reducing DNA synthesis and nuclear

estradiol receptor content and at inducing the activities of estradiol and isocitric dehydrogenases. The minimum effective dosages of oral progesterone and dydrogesterone
that are required to elicit biochemical responses to within the secretory-phase range were
300 mg and 10–20 mg daily, respectively.

The biochemical data for MPA are now published,[60] and the results for DNA synthesis and induction of the activities of estradiol dehydrogenase are presented in Figures
22–4 and 22–5. Data from the premenopausal proliferative and secretory phases are
included for comparisons. Synthesis of DNA in endometrial glandular epithelium (labeling index) was significantly reduced by all three dosages of MPA as compared to
conjugated estrogen therapy alone. However, more samples showed optimal DNA
suppression as the dose of MPA was increased from 2.5 mg to 5 mg to 10 mg daily.
These results again illustrate the wide interpatient variation in response. In our opinion,

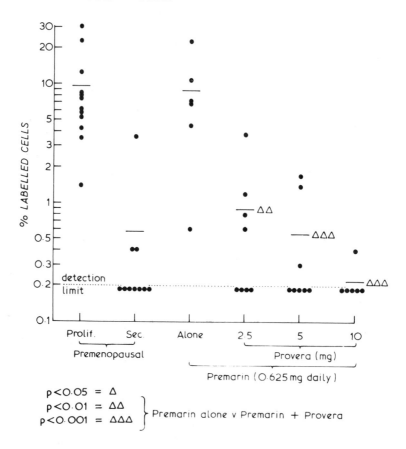

FIG 22–4.
Epithelial DNA synthesis (labeling index) in the
endometrium of postmenopausal women treated
with conjugated equine estrogens (Premarin)
0.625 mg daily continuously, either alone or with
medroxyprogesterone acetate (Provera), 2.5 mg,
5 mg, or 10 mg daily, added for 12 days each
calendar month. Proliferative *(Prolif)* and secretory *(Sec)* phase ranges are included for comparison. Means are shown. (From Lane G, Siddle
NC, Ryder TA, et al: Is Provera the ideal progesterone for addition to postmenopausal estrogen
therapy? *Fertil Steril* 1986; 45:345–352. Used by
permission.)

ESTRADIOL DEHYDROGENASE

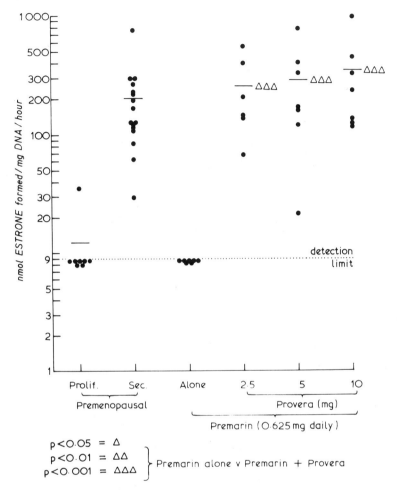

FIG 22–5.
Estradiol dehydrogenase activity in the endometrium of postmenopausal women treated with conjugated equine estrogens (Premarin) 0.625 mg daily continuously either alone or with medroxyprogesterone acetate (Provera) 2.5 mg, 5 mg, or 10 mg daily added for 12 days each month. For abbreviations and explanations of results, see Legend to Fig 22–4. (From Lane G, Siddle NC, Ryder TA, et al: Is Provera the ideal progesterone for addition to postmenopausal estrogen therapy? *Fertil Steril* 1986; 45:345–352. Used by permission.)

the most likely explanation for this is the variation in plasma levels referred to previously,[39, 41, 46] which in turn indicates variation in absorption and metabolism of MPA. From a clinical viewpoint, where maximal endometrial protection is required in all patients, the 10 mg dose has to be recommended. Similar responses were observed for suppression of nuclear estradiol receptor content (data not shown).

Induction of estradiol dehydrogenase activity is shown in Figure 22–5. Again, premenopausal proliferative and secretory-phase values are included for comparisons. All three doses of MPA resulted in induction of dehydrogenase activity to within the secretory-phase range.

CLINICAL IMPLICATIONS OF THE ENDOMETRIAL DATA

As stated previously, the benefits of progestogens have to be shown to outweigh the disadvantages before they can be recommended for widespread addition to postmenopausal estrogen therapy.

It is clear from the histologic and biochemical data that progestogens have to be administered for at least 12 days each month to afford adequate endometrial protection against the development of hyperplasia and carcinoma.[17, 47] Extending the duration of administration is potentially disadvantageous, given that the majority of progestogen-mediated effects are dose-related. However, it is also clear from the data presented here that the dosages of certain progestogens can be greatly reduced without a loss of protective effect. At present, we recommend the addition of 0.7 mg norethindrone, or 150 μg dl norgestrel, or 300 mg oral progesterone, or 10–20 mg dydrogesterone, or 10 mg MPA daily for 12 days each month.

Are there differences between these doses of these progestogens in terms of adverse effects upon the physical, psychologic, and metabolic (including cardiovascular and bone) status of postmenopausal women? Regrettably, there are few answers to these questions at present. Combined estrogen-progestogen therapy incorporating 250 μg levo-norgestrel daily exerts a less beneficial effect on mood, mastalgia, and breast size than estrogen alone.[50, 51] Our clinical experience would support these data, because with dl norgestrel 500 μg daily, (equivalent to 250 μg levo-norgestrel), approximately 10% of our patients experience a "premenstrual tension-like" syndrome during the progestogen phase of treatment (unpublished observations). However, in our experience, reducing the dose to 150 μg dl norgestrel daily results in a reduction in the frequency and intensity of these adverse changes. Sadly, no data from properly conducted, prospective studies are available on the physical and psychologic changes caused by the dosages of the progestogens that we are currently recommending for addition to postmenopausal estrogen therapy.

The current information on the effects of combined estrogen-progestogen therapies on plasma lipid and lipoprotein moieties is likewise deficient. The metabolic effects of progestogens are clearly dose-related,[31, 52] but, in general, the published studies have tended to use progestogen dosages greatly in excess of those required. For example, Hirvonen et al.[53] compared the effects of MPA, 10 mg daily, with those of dl norgestrel, 500 μg daily, and norethindrone, 10 mg daily, when added to postmenopausal estrogens. MPA 10 mg daily caused significantly less depression of HDL cholesterol than either of the 19-nortestosterone derivatives, and therefore Hirvonen et al.[53] argued that MPA was the progestogen of choice for addition to postmenopausal estrogens. We believe that these conclusions are invalid, because it is now known that lower dosages of norethindrone, 1 mg daily, cause virtually no changes in HDL cholesterol values;[54] and this dose appears endometrial protective. Data comparing the effects of oral progesterone, 300 mg daily, and levo-norgestrel, 120 μg daily, are available.[55] Oral progesterone, 300 mg, caused less suppression of HDL cholesterol, and particularly the HDL_2 subfraction, than 120 μg levo-norgestrel: whether reducing the dose of norgestrel still further to 75 μg levo-norgestrel (equivalent to 150 μg dl norgestrel) would minimize these effects is unknown. Likewise, no data are available on the effects of dydrogesterone, 10–20 mg daily, on lipid metabolism.

We believe it unlikely that progestogen addition will negate the beneficial effects of estrogens on bone metabolism. Two prospective studies, incorporating either 10 mg MPA daily[56] or 1 mg norethindrone daily,[57] have reported that combined estrogen-progestogen regimens, started soon after the menopause, actually slightly increase bone mass when prescribed for ten years[56] and two years.[57]

SUMMARY

There can be no doubt that exogenous estrogens are highly effective in relieving not only the acute symptoms of ovarian failure, such as vasomotor instability and vaginal dryness, but also in conserving postmenopausal bone mass. The beneficial effects have been dealt with in full elsewhere in this book. The major concern of exogenous estrogen use remains the genesis of premalignant and malignant change in vulnerable end-organs, especially the endometrium.

Various strategies have been proposed to try to overcome this potential hazard and these strategies have been reviewed. We believe that progestogen addition is the only sensible approach, and the intracellular mechanisms, whereby progestogens antagonize estrogen stimulation, are understood much better today than five years ago. Progestogens should be administered for at least 12 days each month to confer maximum endometrial protection, but concern has been expressed that progestogens, per se, will cause undesirable physical, psychologic, and metabolic effects.

Different types of progestogens possess dissimilar potencies. The halogenated progesterone derivatives, on a weight-for-weight basis, are the most potent: the 19-nortestosterone derivatives appear to be the least potent. It is probable that the biologic consequences of progestogens will depend not only upon the type, but also upon the route of administration. We predict that the metabolic effects of progestogen addition will be most marked with the oral route and least marked with parenteral administration. It is not known whether it will be possible to develop parenterally administered progestogen preparations for use in postmenopausal women. Certainly, estrogens can be administered subcutaneously as implants, transvaginally or percutaneously as creams, and also percutaneously from skin patches with minimal disturbances to hepatic function.[58, 59] Could the same be achieved for progestogens?

Minimum effective daily dosages of certain types of progestogens have now been established in terms of endometrial protection. Regrettably, few data are available on the physical, psychologic, and metabolic effects of these progestogen dosages. Norethindrone, 1 mg, and MPA, 10 mg, appear to cause minimal lipid disturbances and do not oppose the beneficial effects of estrogens on bone mass. Oral progesterone, 300 mg, causes few lipid disturbances. More research is urgently needed to determine which of these progestogens is most suitable for addition to postmenopausal estrogens.

ACKNOWLEDGMENTS

We are indebted to L. Peachey for help with the transmission electron microscopy; to J. Minardi, V. Williams, and O. Young for their nursing help; to R. Johnston, D. Leach, and S. Murdoch for the preparation of the autoradiograms. The financial assistance of Ayerst Laboratories, Laboratoires Besins Iscovesco, Upjohn (U.K. Ltd), Duphar Laboratories, and the Imperial Cancer Research Fund Laboratories is gratefully acknowledged. The help of J. Horn and H. Kenna in preparing this manuscript is much appreciated.

RFERENCES

1. Smith DC, Prentice R, Thompson D, et al: Association of exogenous estrogens and endometrial cancer. *N Engl J Med* 1975; 293: 1164–1167.
2. Ziel H, Finkle W: Increased risk of endometrial carcinoma among users of conjugated estrogens. *N Engl J Med* 1975; 293:1167–1170.
3. Mack T, Pike M, Henderson B, et al: Estrogens and endometrial cancer in a retirement community. *N Engl J Med* 1976; 294:1262–1267.
4. Whitehead MI, Lane G, Siddle NC, et al: Avoidance of endometrial hyperstimulation in estrogen-treated postmenopausal women. *Semin Reprod Endocrinol* 1983; 1:41–53.
5. Stevenson JC, Whitehead MI: Postmenopausal osteoporosis. *Br Med J* 1982; 285:585–588.
6. Christiansen C, Christiansen MS, McNair P et al: Prevention of early postmenopausal bone loss: Controlled 2-year study in 315 normal females. *Eur J Clin Invest* 1980; 10:273–279.
7. Christensen MS, Hagen C, Christiansen C, et al: Dose-response evaluation of cyclic oestrogen/gestagen in postmenopausal women. *Am J Obstet Gynecol* 1982; 144:873–879.
8. Christiansen C: Oestrogens and osteoporosis. Presentation to the Oslo Society of Gynaecologists. Oslo, Norway, 1981.
9. Genant HK, Cann CE, Ettinger B, et al: Quantitative computer tomography of vertebral spongiosa. A sensitive method for detecting early bone loss after oophorectomy. *Ann Intern Med* 1982; 97:699–705.
10. Whitehead MI, King RJB, McQueen J, et al: Endometrial histology and biochemistry in climacteric women during oestrogen and oestrogen/progestin therapy. *J R Soc Med* 1979; 72:322–327.
11. Whitehead MI, Townsend PT, Pryse-Davies J, et al: Effects of estrogens and progestins on the biochemistry and morphology of the postmenopausal endometrium. *N Engl J Med* 1981; 305:1599–1604.
12. Ziel HK, Finkle WD: Association of estrone and the development of endometrial cancer. *Am J Obstet Gynecol* 1976; 124:735–740.
13. King RJB, Whitehead MI, Campbell S, et al: Effect of estrogen and progestin treatments on endometria from postmenopausal women. *Cancer Res* 1979; 39:1094–1101.
14. King RJB, Dyer G, Collins WP, et al: Intracellular estradiol, estrone and estrogen receptor levels in endometria from postmenopausal women receiving estrogens and progestins. *J Steroid Biochem* 1980; 13:377–382.
15. Whitehead MI, Lane G, Dyer G, et al: Oestradiol: The predominant intranuclear oestrogen in the endometrium of oestrogen-treated postmenopausal women. *Br J Obstet Gynaecol* 1981; 88:914–918.
16. King RJB, Mainwaring WIP: *Steroid Cell Interactions*. London, Butterworths, pp 288–373, 1974.
17. Studd JWW, Thom MH, Paterson MEL, et al: The prevention and treatment of endometrial pathology in postmenopausal women receiving exogenous oestrogens, in Pasetto N, Paoletti R, Ambrus JL (eds): *The Menopause and Postmenopause*. Lancaster, England, MTP Press Ltd, pp 127–139, 1980.
18. Myrhe E: Endometrial response to different estrogens, in Lauritzen C, van Keep PA (eds): *Frontiers of Hormone Research, vol 5. Estrogen Therapy, the Benefits and Risks*. Basel, S Karger AG, pp 126–143, 1978.
19. Follingstad AJ: Estriol: The forgotten estrogen. *JAMA* 1978; 239:29.
20. Lindsay R, Hart DM, Maclean A, et al: Bone loss during oestriol therapy in postmenopausal women. *Maturitas* 1979; 1:279–285.
21. Englund DE: Oestrogen treatment and the menopause. *Acta Univ Upsaliensis* 1979; 335.
22. Hisaw FL, Hisaw FL Jr: Action of estrogen and progesterone on the reproductive tract of lower primates, in Young WC, Corner GW (eds): *Sex and Internal Secretions*. Baltimore, Williams & Wilkins Co, vol 1, pp 556–589, 1961.
23. Lee AE: Cell division and DNA synthesis in the mouse uterus during continuous oestrogen treatment. *J Endocrinol* 1972; 55:507.
24. Katzenellenbogen BS, Ferguson ER: Anti-estrogen action in the uterus: Biological ineffectiveness of nuclear-bound estradiol after antiestrogen. *Endocrinology* 1975; 97:1.
25. Dyer G, Young O, Townsend PT, et al: Dose-related changes in vaginal cytology after topical conjugated estrogens. *Br Med J* 1982; 284:789.

26. Feinstein AR, Horowitz RI: A critique of the statistical evidence associating estrogens with endometrial cancer. *Cancer Res* 1978; 38:4001–4007.
27. Schiff I, Sela HK, Cramer D, et al: Endometrial hyperplasia in women on cyclic or continuous estrogen regimens. *Fertil Steril* 1982; 37:79–85.
28. Gambrell RD: Clinical use of progestins in the menopausal patient. *J Reprod Med* 1982; 27:531–538.
29. Kay CR: The happiness pill? *J R Coll Gen Pract* 1980; 30:8–19.
30. Meade TW, Greenberg G, Thompson SG: Progestogens and cardiovascular reactions associated with oral contraceptives and a comparison of the safety of 50 and 30μg oestrogen preparations. *Br Med J* 1980; 280:1157–1161.
31. Larsson-Cohn U, Wallentin L, Zador G: Plasma lipids and high density lipoproteins during oral contraception with different combinations of ethinyl oestradiol and norgestrel. *Horm Metab Res* 1979; 11:437–440.
32. Ross RK, Paganini-Hill A, Mack TM, et al: Menopausal oestrogen therapy and protection from ischaemic heart disease. *Lancet* 1981; 1:858–860.
33. Brotherton J: *Sex Hormone Pharmacology*. London, Academic Press, pp 1–78, 1976.
34. Neumann F: Chemische Konstitution und pharmokalishe Wirkung, in Langecker H (ed): *Hanbuch der Experimentellen Pharmakologie, Band XXII Die Gestagne*. New York, Springer-Verlag New York, 1968, pp 680–1025.
35. Whitehead MI, Siddle NC, Townsend PT, et al: The use of progestins and progesterone in the treatment of climacteric and postmenopausal symptoms, in Bardin CW, Milgrom E, Mauvais-Jarvis P (eds): *Progesterone and Progestins*. New York, Raven Press, pp 281–298, 1982.
36. Greenblatt RB, Jungck EC, Barfield WE: A new test for efficiency of progestational compounds. *Ann N Y Acad Sci* 1958; 71:717–724.
37. Kaufman C: Unwandlung der Uterusschleimhaut einer kastrierten Frau aus dem atrophishen Stadium in das sekretorischen Funktion durch Overialhormone. *Zentralbl Gynekol* 1932; 56:2058.
38. Nilsson S, Victor A, Nygren K-G: Plasma levels of d-norgestrel and sex hormone binding globulin during oral d-norgestrel medication immediately after delivery and legal abortion. *Contraception* 1977; 15:87–93.
39. Laatikainen T, Nieminen U, Adlercreutz H: Plasma medroxyprogesterone acetate levels following intramuscular or oral administration in patients with endometrial adenocarcinoma. *Acta Obstet Gynecol* Scand 1979; 58:95–99.
40. Sall S, DiSaia P, Morrow CP, et al: A comparison of medroxyprogesterone serum concentrations by the oral or intramuscular route in patients with persistent or recurrent endometrial carcinoma. *Am J Obstet Gynecol* 1979; 135:647–650.
41. Mazzei T, Scarselli G, Ciuffi M, et al: Oral medroxyprogesterone acetate pharmacokinetics. *Chemiotherapia* 1983; 2:222–225.
42. Nillius SJ, Johansson EDB: Plasma levels of progesterone after vaginal, rectal or intramuscular administration of progesterone. *Am J Obstet Gynecol* 1971; 110:470–477.
43. Whitehead MI, Townsend PT, Gill DK, et al: Absorption and metabolism of oral progesterone. *Br Med J* 1980; 280:825–827.
44. Ottoson U-B, Carlstrom K, Damber J-E, et al: Serum levels of progesterone and some of its metabolites including deoxycorticosterone after oral and parenteral administration. *Br J Obstet Gynecol* 1984; 91:1111–1119.
45. Ottoson U-B, Carlstrom K, Damber J-E, et al: Conversion of oral progesterone into deoxycorticosterone during postmenopausal replacement therapy. *Acta Obstet Gynecol Scand* 1984; 63:577–579.
46. Cornette JC, Kirton KT, Duncan GW: Measurement of medroxyprogesterone acetate by radioimmunoassay. *J Clin Endocrinol Metab* 1971; 33:459–466.
47. Whitehead MI, Townsend PT, Pryse-Davies J, et al: Effects of various types and dosages of progestogens on the postmenopausal endometrium. *J Reprod Med* 1982; 27(8):539–548.
48. Lane G, Siddle NC, Ryder TA, et al: Dose-dependent effects of oral progesterone on the oestrogenised postmenopausal endometrium. *Br Med J* 1983; 287:1241–1245.
49. Lane G, Siddle NC, Ryder TA, et al: Effects of dydrogesterone on the oestrogenised postmenopausal endometrium. *Br J Obstet Gynecol* 1986; 93:55–62.

50. Dennerstein L, Burrows GD, Hyman GJ, et al: Some clinical effects of oestrogen/progestogen therapy in surgically castrated women. *Maturitas* 1979; 2:19–28.
51. Dennerstein L, Burrows GD, Hyman GJ, et al: Hormone therapy and affect. *Maturitas* 1979; 2:247–259.
52. Notelowitz M: Carbohydrate metabolism in relation to hormonal replacement therapy. *Acta Obstet Gynecol Scand [Suppl]* 1982; 106:51–56.
53. Hirvonen E, Malkonen M, Manninen V: Effects of different progestogens on lipoproteins during postmenopausal replacement therapy. *N Engl J Med* 1981; 304:560–562.
54. Christiansen C, Christensen MS, Grande P, et al: Low-risk lipoprotein pattern in post-menopausal women on sequential oestrogen/progestogen treatment. *Maturitas* 1984; 5:193–199.
55. Fahraeus L, Larsson-Cohn U, Wallentin L: L-norgestrel and progesterone have different influences on plasma lipoproteins. *Eur J Clin Invest* 1983; 30:447–453.
56. Nachtigall LE, Nachtigall RH, Nachtigall RD, et al: Estrogen replacement therapy. 1: A 10-year prospective study in relationship to osteoporosis. *Obstet Gynecol* 1979; 53:277–281.
57. Christiansen C, Christensen MS, Transbol I: Bone mass in postmenopausal women after withdrawal of oestrogen/progestogen therapy. *Lancet* 1981; 1:459–461.
58. Campbell S, Whitehead MI: Potency and hepato-cellular effects of oestrogens after oral, percutaneous and subcutaneous administration, in van Keep PA, Utian W, Vermeulen A (eds): *The Controversial Climacteric*. Lancaster, England, MTP Press Ltd, pp 103–125, 1982.
59. Padwick ML, Endacott J, Whitehead MI: Efficacy, acceptability and metabolic effects of transdermal estradiol in postmenopausal women. *Am J Obstet Gynecol* 1985; 152:1085–1091.
60. Lane G, Siddle NC, Ryder TA, et al: Is Provera the ideal progestogen for addition to postmenopausal estrogen therapy? *Fertil Steril* 1986; 45:345–352.

CHAPTER **23**

Therapeutic Regimens

DONNA SHOUPE, M.D.
DANIEL R. MISHELL, JR., M.D.

WITH THE STEADY improvement in medical care and resultant increase in life expectancy, about one third of a woman's life is now spent postmenopausally. During this estrogen-deficient period, as shown in the previous chapters, estrogen replacement therapy should improve the quality of her life by preventing symptoms of dysuria, urinary frequency and incontinence, pruritus, hot flushes,[1, 2] sleeping disturbances,[1, 2, 3] dyspareunia, and vaginal atrophy. Estrogen replacement therapy has also been shown to contribute to the menopausal woman's sense of well-being.[1] In addition, estrogen has been shown to increase the length of a woman's life by decreasing her chance of dying from osteoporotic hip fracture[4–10] or myocardial infarction.[4, 71]

Despite numerous studies documenting the benefits of estrogen replacement, there is a relative paucity of studies that can be used to determine the optimal type, dosage, duration, and route of administration of estrogen. Even less information is available regarding the effects of various dosages and types of progestogens, when used in conjunction with estrogen, upon the symptoms and metabolic changes ameliorated by estrogen alone.

The use of unopposed estrogen treatment in the postmenopausal woman is associated in a dose-dependent manner with the development of endometrial hyperplasia.[12–16] Furthermore, the use of oral estrogen for more than five years has been well-documented to be associated with an increased risk of developing adenocarcinoma of the endometrium.[12] Since progestins inhibit the replenishment of estrogen receptors in the endometrium and have an antimitotic activity, their use in combination with estrogen should reduce this risk. It has been etablished that the addition of progestational therapy to both cyclic[13, 17–19] and continuous[20] estrogen replacement regimens prevents the development of estrogen-induced endometrial hyperplasia. It has been shown that the addition of a progestin to estrogen replacement therapy significantly reduces the chance of developing endometrial cancer and may actually reduce the incidence below that of untreated women.[21, 22] For this reason, in postmenopausal women with the uterus intact, progestins are usually added to the estrogen treatment regimen. Although the reduction of endometrial hyperplasia is dependent on the number of days that progestin is administered each month, it has not been established which type, dose, or duration of progestin treatment is optimal to prevent the estrogen-increased number of endometrial steroid receptors. It has been shown that the progestin needs to be given for at least ten, and probably 12 days each month to maximally reduce the estrogen-induced risk of endometrial hyperplasia.[17, 21–27]

However, the addition of a progestin to the hormone replacement regimen has certain disadvantages. In addition to the frequent induction of withdrawal uterine bleeding and certain progestin-induced systemic side effects, such as weight gain, the addition of a progestin could theoretically nullify several of the advantages of estrogen replacement, such as the prevention of atrophic vaginitis, atrophic urethritis, and, most important, myocardial infarction.

Postmenopausally, the decline of ovarian function is associated with a striking increase in low-density lipoprotein (LDL) concentrations and a decline in high-density lipoprotein (HDL)-to-LDL ratio.[28] Administration of exogenous estrogens can reverse this trend[28-31] and may explain why estrogen replacement is associated with a lower incidence of death from myocardial infarction and reduced age-adjusted mortality.[4, 71] The addition of a progestin may reverse the beneficial effect of estrogen on lipoproteins. However, much of the evidence seems to suggest that the type of progestin as well as the dosage is crucial in determining the effect on blood lipid levels. The beneficial effect of replacement therapy with estradiol valerate (2 mg) on HDL cholesterol levels was reduced to a level 20% below that observed prior to treatment with estrogen alone after addition of cyclic norgestrel (0.5 mg/day) or norethindrone acetate (10 mg/day).[28] In contrast, addition of cyclic medroxyprogesterone acetate (10 mg/day), a nonandrogenic progestin, had no such effect.[28, 32] Another study also confirmed that medroxyprogesterone acetate, when used with cyclic conjugated estrogens had no effect on lipoprotein distribution even after 18 months.[33]

A recent study from Ottosson et al.[34] also confirms the previous observations that addition of levo-norgestrel (250 µg/daily) to the last ten days of each treatment cycle (three weeks of daily 2 mg estradiol valerate) will significantly decrease total HDL cholesterol and subfraction HDL_2, the most important lipoprotein subfraction that is believed to be protective in regards to coronary artery disease, to 18% and 28% (respectively) below pretreatment values. However, they also report a less marked but significant decrease in HDL-cholesterol (8%) and HDL_2 (17%), when 10 mg/day medroxyprogesterone acetate is added. If, instead, a newly available preparation of orally active micronized progesterone were used at the end of the treatment cycle, there was no apparent influence on HDL cholesterol or on its subfractions. The authors postulate that this natural hormone may become an attractive alternative to synthetic progestogens.

Additionally, some studies have suggested that lower doses of the 19-nortestosterone derivatives may have a less adverse effect on lipoproteins. Treatment for one year with a cyclic combination pill containing varying levels of estradiol and estriol, with 1 mg norethisterone acetate added for the last 12 days, each month, resulted in no significant changes in lipoproteins.[35] However, in another study,[36] there was a reduction in all serum lipids, triglycerides, cholesterol, and phospholipids after three and 12 months of treatment with continuous estrogen/norethisterone acetate (1 mg) combination. The ratio of LDL cholesterol to HDL cholesterol was unaltered. It is unclear what significance this may have in terms of athrogenicity.

Since the 19-nortestosterone derivatives, norethisterone acetate and levo-norgestrel, appear to lower HDL cholesterol to a greater extent than 17-acetoxy progesterone derivatives, such as medroxyprogesterone acetate,[28] use of the latter type of progestin may be preferable, since the beneficial alterations on lipoprotein levels produced by the estrogen will not be reversed as greatly.

USE OF "NATURAL" ESTROGENS

The choice of estrogen also plays a role in metabolic changes.[37] Although synthetic and "natural" estrogens seem to affect lipoproteins in a similar way when administered orally,[72] their effect on serum triglycerides is different. The synthetic compounds, ethinyl estradiol and mestranol, tend to increase triglycerides level, while the "natural" compounds, estrone sulfate, estradiol valerate, and conjugated equine estrogens (CEE), have no such effect.[29, 38-41] Because the effect of this elevation of triglycerides has not been associated with an increased risk of coronary heart disease, it would appear that either type of estrogen can be used in terms of lipoprotein effect.

Nevertheless, the synthetic estrogens, whether administered orally or vaginally, appear to have a greater effect on liver globulins than the natural estrogens.[37, 42, 43] Since elevation of certain of these globulins, such as factors VII and X, increase the risk of thrombus, while elevation of another, angiotensinogen, may increase blood pressure, it is important that this hepatic effect be as minimal as possible. Using an increase in globulins as a measure of dose response, it has been shown that ethinyl estradiol is about 100 times as potent as CEE, and CEE is about twice as potent as estrone sulfate, another natural estrogen.[37]

CONTRAINDICATIONS: RELATIVE AND ABSOLUTE

After the menopause, most of the circulating estrogen is derived from the extraglandular conversion of androstenedione to estrone. This conversion takes place in the fatty tissue. Therefore, obese women are less likely to be estrogen deficient[44] and are much less likely to benefit from hormone replacement therapy. Because the potential problems of hormone replacement therapy are magnified in certain patients, the postmenopausal patient should be carefully evaluated prior to starting therapy. However, current regimens for estrogen replacement therapy mimic the estrogen milieu of the early follicular phase of a natural cycle and are associated with minimal risk.

Table 23–1 lists the conditions that are either an absolute or relative contraindication for estrogen therapy. Hormone replacement therapy should be withheld in patients with a past history of breast or uterine cancer, active liver disease, and the presence of thrombophlebitis. Progestin-only therapy may be a good alternative in many of these patients.

TABLE 23–1.

Contraindications for Estrogen Therapy

Absolute Contraindications
Previously diagnosed or suspected breast or uterine cancer
Acute liver disease
Active thrombophlebitis or thromboembolic disorders
Relative Contraindications
Chronic hepatic dysfunction
Obesity
Preexisting uterine leiomyoma
A history of thromboembolism or thrombophlebitis
Endometriosis

AVAILABLE PREPARATIONS

Tables 23–2 and 23–3 list currently available estrogens and progestins by their generic and trade names and list the doses available.

ROUTES OF ADMINISTRATION

Oral Administration.—Because of the ease and uniformity of administration, most estrogen replacement therapy regimens rely on the oral route. However, due to the internal hepatic circulation, orally-administered estradiol is mainly metabolized to estrone and its conjugates.[45] After ingestion of oral estrogens, there is a small increase in plasma estradiol but major increases in estrone. An orally-administered dose of 2 mg micronized estradiol will increase circulating estradiol (E_2) three hours after ingestion by 40 pg/ml and increase estrone (E_1) by 250 pg/ml.[46, 47] The change in plasma levels one

TABLE 23–2.

Oral Estrogens Available

GENERIC NAME	BRAND NAME	DOSES AVAILABLE (MG)
Oral		
Conjugated equine estrogens	Premarin, Estrocon	0.3, 0.625, 0.9, 1.25, and 2.5
Piperazine estrone sulfate, Estropipate (ES)	Ogen, Hormonin	0.3, 0.625, 1.25, 2.5, and 5
Esterified estrogens	Estratab, Evex, Menest, Amnestrogen	0.3, 0.625, 1.25, and 2.5
Estradiol valerate	Progynova	1 and 2
Estriol hemisuccinate	Hormonion	1 and 2
Micronized estradiol	Estrace	1 and 2
Estriol		1 and 2
Synthetic		
Diethystilbestrol	Generic	0.1, 0.25, 0.5, 1, 5
Ethinyl estradiol	Estinyl, Feminone	0.02, 0.05, 0.5
Quinestrol	Estrovis	0.1
Mestranol		
Injectable		
Estradiol benzoate	Generic	0.5 mg/ml
Polyestradiol phosphate	Estradurin	40 mg/2 ml
Conjugated equine estrogen	Intravenous Premarin	25 mg/ml
Estrone	Generic	1, 2, 5 mg/ml
Estradiol valerate	Generic	10, 20, 40 mg/ml
	Delestrogen, Estate, Gynogen, Menaval	10, 20, 40 mg/ml
Estradiol cypionate	Generic	5 mg/ml
	Depo-Estradiol	1, 5 mg/ml
	E-Ionate, E-Cypionate	5 mg/ml
Ethinal estradiol	Generic	1 gm powder
Topical–Vaginal		
Estropipate	Ogen	1.5 mg/gm
Conjugated equine estrogen	Premarin	0.625 mg/gm
Dinestrol	DV	0.01% in 90 gm
Diethystilbestrol	Generic	0.1, 0.5 mg (suppositories)
Topical-transdermal	Oestrogel[72]	3 mg
17-β Estradiol	Estraderm (skin patch)[55]	.05 mg/day, .1 mg/day (release rate)

hour after an oral dose of CEE of 1.25 mg is 110 pg/ml of E_1 and between 33 and 58 pg/ml of E_2.[47, 48]

Intramuscular Injection.—Administration of estrogens parenterally avoids the hepatic first-pass effect; thus, smaller dosages can achieve similar levels to higher oral doses, with a higher E_2/E_1 ratio. The drawbacks, however, include initial high peak values, variability in disappearance rates, and discomfort in administration. The injections have to be given at least once a month, since no longer-acting formulations are available.

Vaginal Application.—Parenteral administration of estrogen by vaginal application also bypasses the enterohepatic circulation, resulting in larger increases in plasma E_2 as compared to E_1. Vaginal application of 1 mg of micronized 17-β estradiol cream produces an increase in E_2 of 800 pg/ml and 150 pg/ml of E_1 in three hours (see Fig 12–1).[49] Vaginal cream, however, is often considered difficult to administer, and the variable absorption patterns result in a great variety of bioavailability of the estrogen. Development of vaginal rings for estrogen administration offers some promise.[50, 51]

Subcutaneous Pellets.—Steady concentrations of between 30 and 100 pg/ml of estradiol can be obtained by use of the subcutaneous pellets or capsules containing 25 mg cystal-line 17-β E_2 (Fig 23–1).[52-54] The implants are difficult to remove and have a variable life span. The possible hazards of prolonged action, the inconvenience of adding progestin therapy, and the difficulty in determining the length of action, are disadvantages for their use.

Transdermal Cream.—Percutaneous application of estradiol results in prolonged levels of estradiol without the pronounced increases seen with oral administration. A recently developed transdermal therapeutic system, consisting of a 4-cm disc containing E_2, can produce steady mean concentrations of estradiol and estrone of about 72 pg/ml and 37

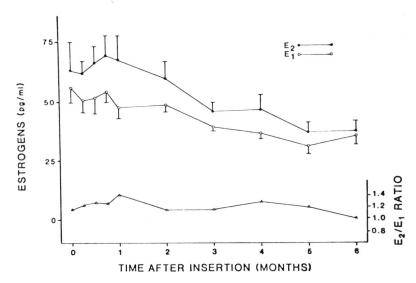

FIG 23–1.
Mean (± SE) serum estradiol (E_2) and estrone (E_1) levels and E_2/E_1 ratios in 22 women after oophorectomy and insertion of one 25 mg E_2 pellet. (From Lobo RA, March CM, Goebelsmann U, et al: Subdermal estradiol pellets following hysterectomy and oophorectomy. *Am J Obstet Gynecol* 1980; 138:714. Used by permission.)

pg/ml, respectively, with limited effects on hepatic function (Fig 23–2).[55] These discs are attached to the skin by adhesives and need to be replaced every three days.

TREATMENT REGIMENS

Progestin Only

Progestins have been shown to have a beneficial effect on calcium metabolism[56, 57] as well as relief of vasomotor symptoms[56-63] when used as a single treatment regimen in postmenopausal patients. The use of progestin therapy is especially appealing for those individuals for whom estrogen therapy is contraindicated, such as patients who have had carcinoma of the breast or endometrium[63] and in those patients who experience intolerable side effects such as mastodynia, fibrocystic breast disease, breakthrough bleeding, or nausea even on low-dose estrogen therapy.

Depomedroxyprogesterone acetate (DMPA) appears to be a suitable substitute for estrogen in the treatment of climacteric symptoms.[56] Lobo et al.[56, 57] demonstrated that 150 mg DMPA once every three months was as effective as an oral, daily dose of 0.625 mg of conjugated equine estrogens in reducing the urinary calcium/creatinine and hy-

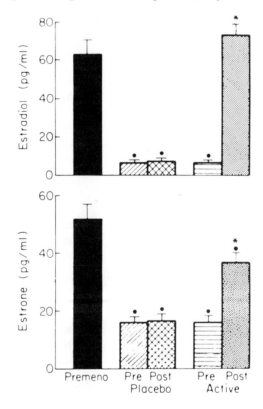

FIG 23–2.
Mean (± SEM) estradiol and estrone serum levels (pg/ml) in premenopausal control subjects and before and at the end of treatment of postmenopausal subjects with placebo or estradiol-containing (active) systems. *Asterisk* denotes significant difference from baseline. *Solid circle* denotes significant difference from premenopausal control subjects. (From Laufer LR, de Fazio JL, Lu JKH, et al: Estrogen replacement therapy by transdermal estradiol administration. *Am J Obstet Gynecol* 1983; 146:533. Used by permission.)

droxyproline/creatinine ratios as well as hot flush episodes. In both treatment groups these ratios were similar to the ratios in premenopausal women. These ratios are felt to be markers of bone resorption and would suggest that this dose may be protective against osteoporosis.

Doses of 50, 100, and 150 mg of DMPA have been shown by other investigators to be equally effective in relieving hot flushes.[62] However, the clearance rate of this method of application is variable, and the steroid can be measured in the blood up to seven months after a single injection. This form of administration also can result in irregular spotting in those patients with an intact uterus. Oral medroxyprogesterone (MPA) has a much more rapid clearance rate and offers an advantage for ease in controlling plasma levels, but is more expensive.

Albrecht et al.[61] in a placebo-controlled, double-blind study, treated six postmenopausal women with 20 mg per day orally of MPA and noted a 92% decrease in vasomotor flushes and reduction in frequency and amplitude of luteinizing hormone (LH) pulses. In another double-blind study,[65] oral MPA, 20 mg daily, was also found to be significantly more effective than placebo in relieving hot flushes.

Other progestins have also been reported to be effective in decreasing vasomotor episodes. Judd et al.[60] demonstrated a dose-response pattern after the oral administration of 0, 20, 40, and 80 mg megestrol acetate (MA) daily for four weeks at each dose level. The oral administration of 10 mg MPA is equivalent to 80 mg MA in reducing the calcium/creatinine ratio, whereas 20 mg MPA/day reduces the calcium/creatinine ratio to the premenopausal range.[63]

Norethisterone has been used as a single progestational agent. Paterson[59] treated 23 menopausal women with daily norethisterone (5 mg) or placebo for a three-month interval. He found that hot flushes were significantly reduced and that serum cholesterol and triglycerides were also significantly lower with the progestin.

As mentioned above, the use of progestins can reverse some of the positive metabolic effects of estrogen therapy, especially those on lipid metabolism. Use of the 17-acetoxy progesterone derivatives, such as medroxyprogesterone acetate, may be preferable to use of the 19-nortestosterone derivatives, norethisterone or megestrol acetate, since they have the least effect on lipid levels. However, recent studies indicate that use of natural oral progesterone in the form of micronized progesterone (200 mg daily) had no effect on HDL-cholesterol or its subfractions.[34] Natural progesterones may become an attractive alternative to the synthetic progestins now available. Table 23–3 lists recommended treatment regimens.

Cyclic

Because unopposed estrogen use has been associated with an increase in endometrial cancer, the most common type of hormone replacement therapy currently in the U.S. is cyclic treatment, consisting of 21–25 days of an oral estrogen with the concurrent administration of a progestin during the last 10–14 days of estrogen treatment. Although it is unclear what optimal dose and duration of progestin treatment is needed to reverse the biochemical and histologic changes in the endometrium associated with postmenopausal estrogen replacement therapy, long duration of progestin treatment is clearly emerging as an important factor.

Paterson[26] suggests that more than ten days each month of progestin therapy is necessary to reverse histologic changes associated with both low-dose or high-dose estrogen. He found an incidence of hyperplasia of 3% in patients taking ten days of proges-

TABLE 23–3.

Progestins Available

GENERIC NAME	BRAND NAME	AVAILABLE DOSAGE (MG)
Oral		
Medroxyprogesterone acetate	Provera	2.5, 5, 10
	Curretabs, Amen	
Megestrol acetate	Megace, Pallace	20, 40
Norethindrone	Norlutin, Nor-	0.35, 5
(Norethisterone)	Q.D., Micronor	
Micronized progesterone	Utrogestin[34]	100
Norethinedrone acetate	Norlutate, Aygestin	5
Norgestrel	Ovrette	.075
Injectable		
Medroxyprogesterone acetate	Depo-Provera	100, 400 mg/ml
	Prodrox	250 mg/ml
Hydroxy Progesterone	Delalutin	125 mg/ml
caproate	Generic	125 mg/ml
Progesterone	Generic	25, 50, 100 mg/ml

togen (norgestrel 0.5 mg) but no hyperplasia when norethisterone was given for more than ten days.

Whitehead suggests that progestin therapy be extended to 12–13 days each month. He bases his conclusion on the biochemical changes induced by progestogen therapy on an estrogen-primed endometrium, such as suppression of DNA synthesis and increase in estradiol dehydrogenase activity.[13, 27] He presents data that the current treatment regimens using 10 mg norethindrone (NET) and 0.5 mg dl norgestrel, can be substantially reduced to at least 1 mg NET or 150 µg dl norgestrel, without loss of the their protective effect. However, he states the minimal effective dose is yet to be determined.[25]

Gibbons et al.[23, 24] confirmed that low-dose progestin therapy may be equally as effective as higher-dose therapy in mediating biochemical and morphological events in the endometrium. They concluded that 5 mg MPA for 11 days per month was as effective as 10 mg in opposing changes stimulated by CEE (0.3, 0.625, and 1.25 mg) in the endometrium in all treatment groups, and 2.5 mg MPA opposed the changes produced by 0.3 and 0.625 mg CEE (Fig 23–3).

There are several studies showing a beneficial effect of low-dose estrogen-progestin treatment in climacteric women. Ylostalo et al.[66] studied 31 perimenopausal women with climacteric symptoms and irregular menstrual patterns. Each patient received estrogen-progestin treatment for six months, according to the following scheme: sodium estrone sulfate (1.5 mg daily) alone for 11 days and then combined with norethisterone acetate (5 mg daily) in group A, and with megestrol acetate (5 mg daily) in group B for the following ten days. There was a drug-free interval of seven days between treatment periods. There was a significantly decreased incidence of climacteric symptoms in both treatment groups. Half of the patients experienced the recurrence of slight climacteric symptoms during the medication-free period. Withdrawal bleeding uniformly occurred during the drug-free periods between treatment cycles and no breakthrough bleeding occurred. Endometrial aspiration cell samples taken after the sixth cycle of treatment revealed no premalignant or hyperplastic changes.

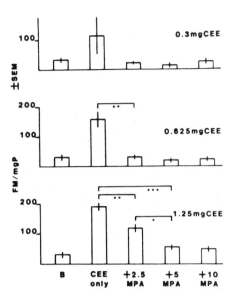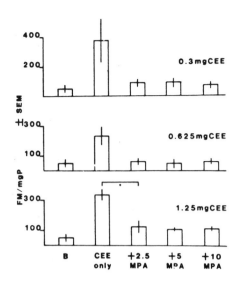

FIG 23–3.
The concentrations of cytosolic *(left) and nuclear (right)* estrogen receptor in the three groups of postmenopausal women receiving no therapy (B), estrogen only (CEE), and estrogen plus various dosages of medroxyprogesterone acetate (MPA). *Left:* * = p <0.025, ** = p <0.01, *** = p <0.001; *Right:* * = p <0.001. (From Gibbons WE, et al: *Am J Obstet Gynecol* 1986; 154:456. Used by permission.)

Christensen et al.[67] randomized 100 volunteers in early menopause to one of three different doses (high, medium, or low) of natural estrogens (micronized 17-β estradiol [E_2] and estriol [E_3]), sequentially combined with norethisterone acetate (1 mg) for 10 of the 28 treatment days or to a placebo group. The high dose contained 4 mg E_2, plus 2 mg E_3; the medium dose contained 2 mg E_2 plus 1 mg E_3; and the low dose contained 1 mg E_2 plus 0.5 mg E_3. Relief of climacteric symptoms (hot flushes) were dose-related, being 70%, 56%, and 33% in the high-, medium-, and low-estrogen groups, respectively, and unchanged in the placebo group. Seventy-eight percent of those patients receiving the high dose had regular withdrawal vaginal bleeding, which was reduced to 64% and 40% in the medium- and low-dose estrogen groups. Bone mass, as measured by photon absorptiometry, was increased in the high and medium groups, was unchanged in the low group, and declined in the placebo group. There was a reduction in serum cholesterol which was dose-related in the three treatment groups, reaching a maximum of 10% in the high-dose group and falling to a low of 3% in the low-dose group. Blood pressure, body weight, and serum triglyceride levels remained unchanged in all groups (Table 23–4).[67] Jensen and Christensen[69] treated 162 postmenopausal women with these same dosage regimens for 42 months. The data also revealed a highly significant ($P < 0.001$) dose-response reduction in climacteric symptoms as compared to the placebo group. There was complete relief of hot flushes with the two highest doses of estradiol and a highly significant ($P < 0.001$) dose-dependent return of symptoms after withdrawal of hormone treatment (Fig 23–4).

TABLE 23–4.

Clinical Data and Pretreatment Values in 87 Postmenopausal Women Divided into Four Treatment Groups*

TREATMENT	AGE (YR) MEAN	AGE (YR) RANGE	MENOPAUSAL AGE (MO) MEAN	MENOPAUSAL AGE (MO) RANGE	KUPPERMAN INDEX (SCORE) MEAN	KUPPERMAN INDEX (SCORE) RANGE	HEIGHT (CM) (MEAN ± 1 SD)	SERUM FSH (U/L) (MEAN ± 1 SD)	SERUM CHOLESTEROL (MMOL/L) (MEAN ± 1 SD)	BONE MASS (UNITS) (MEAN ± 1 SD)
High dose (n = 19)	50.6	45–53	40.1	29–59	5.6	0–18	162.2 ± 4.4	84.2 ± 23.4	5.9 ± 1.0	38.2 ± 5.3
Medium dose (n = 22)	52.7	49–55	44.6	30–61	8.4	0–25	161.2 ± 4.8	82.0 ± 31.4	6.2 ± 1.3	39.0 ± 7.8
Low dose (n = 23)	52.3	47–55	42.3	28–58	8.2	0–30	160.7 ± 6.7	84.3 ± 32.8	5.8 ± 1.2	36.4 ± 6.2
Placebo (n = 23)	50.4	46–55	44.1	29–62	7.2	0–25	162.9 ± 6.9	85.6 ± 34.2	5.6 ± 1.0	36.1 ± 6.0

*From *Am J Obstet Gynecol* 1982; 144:873. Used by permission.

A novel combination of conjugated equine estrogens, 1.5 mg given daily for 21 days, followed by two days of no treatment, followed by five daily doses of 5 mg MPA was tested by Cullberg et al.[68] in 34 postmenopausal women with climacteric complaints. Ten women experienced no bleeding episodes at all following treatment. In the other 24, the instances of bleeding episodes decreased gradually, and after 36 months of treatment, 15 of the 22 women remaining on treatment had no bleeding at all. Endometrial biopsies after six months and 36 months of treatment showed inactive or weakly secretory endometrium in 46 out of 50 endometrial samples. However, in two cases, mild proliferation developed with signs of progestin effect only in small areas, and in two other patients endometrial hyperplasia was found. The authors suggest that these findings emphasize the importance of having at least ten days per month of progestin therapy. Four women complained of dysmenorrhea during the days of bleeding, three women experienced breast tenderness, and two women reported migraine-like headaches during the MPA treatment period. There was a rapid decrease in the number of hot flushes and sweats, and there were no vasomotor symptoms present after six and 36 months of treatment.

Currently in the U.S. the most popular cyclic method is CEE, 0.625 mg for days 1–25 of the month, with 10 mg MPA added the last 10–12 days. Based on recent data, the progestin should be given at least 12–13 days each month.[24, 25] Since about half the patients experience withdrawal bleeding with this regimen, the dose of MPA can be reduced to 5 mg without changing the biochemical parameters in the endometrium. This dose should decrease the incidence of withdrawal bleeding and progestin-associated side effects.

A recommended cyclic treatment regimen is listed in Table 23–5.

Continuous Therapy

A newer approach to estrogen replacement therapy has been the oral regimen of continuous daily treatment with both an estrogen and progestin. This method was developed in order to avoid the withdrawal bleeding experienced by many women on

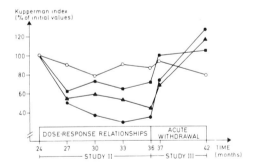

FIG 23–4.
Effect of withdrawal of different doses of estrogen on climacteric symptoms (Kupperman index) in 87 postmenopausal women. The Kupperman index considers 11 symptoms of the menopause including hot flushes, paraethesias, insomnia, and nervousness. These are scored from 0 (none) to 3 (severe) and combined with a multiplication factor of up to 4 (for hot flushes). ● = high dose, 4 mg E_2; ▲ = medium dose, 2 mg E_2; ■ = low dose, 1 mg E_2; ○ = placebo. (From Paterson M, et al: *Br J Obstet Gynaecol* 1980; 87:552. Used by permission.)

cyclic therapy and to reduce the progestogenic side effects seen with higher dose progestin therapy. A recent study[20] using continuous CEE (0.625 or 1.25 mg daily) and low-dose progestin (norethisterone, 0.35 or 1.05 mg daily) observed that amenorrhea was achieved immediately in 65% of the patients on the lower dose estrogen. In those patients experiencing bleeding, the progestin dose was gradually increased by one norethisterone tablet (0.35 mg). Forty-one percent of women in the higher-estrogen group were initially amenorrheic, and all became amenorrheic by increasing the dose of norethisterone to 2.1 mg after one year. After one year, 95.1% of the patients were amenorrheic, and all women remained amenorrheic after that throughout the follow-up of 2.5 years. Half of the patients received an endometrial biopsy after six months of treatment and, regardless of dose, all specimens revealed atrophic or hypoplastic histology. Six patients stopped the treatment because of excessive bloating and breast tenderness, but most patients had no symptoms attributed to the progestin after the first three months. Thirty-three out of 95 patients (mainly those on the 1.25 mg CEE dose) stopped treatment, mainly because of bleeding problems. All patients noticed the same incidence of relief of their climacteric symptoms as after cyclic therapy.

In a similar study evaluating continuous treatment with a combined estrogen-progestin therapy[36, 70] (2 mg E_2, 1 mg E_3, and 1 mg norethisterone acetate), 23 out of 26 women were completely free from vasomotor disturbances after three months of treatment. Evaluation of the endometrial specimens after 6–12 months of treatment revealed that the mucosa was mainly inactive or atrophic. Breakthrough bleeding was reported frequently during the first three months, but was more common in the perimenopausal patients. Of the 11 perimenopausal women in the study, only one had no bleeding, while 11 out of 15 postmenopausal women experienced no bleeding. Side effects included mastalgia in four women, increased irritability in nine, intermittent headaches in six, and a major increase in uterine fibroid growth was noted in two women after one year of treatment.

When comparing the lipid values after three and 12 months of this regimen, these authors report a tendency to approach pretreatment values over time. Although a drop in all lipid values was noted after three months of treatment, there was a reduction of both very low-density lipoprotein (VLDL) triglycerides and HDL cholesterol, thought to be due to the progestogen component. The ratio of LDL cholesterol/HDL cholesterol remained unaltered over a 12-month treatment period. The significance of these changes in terms of atherogenicity is unclear. Since MPA has less adverse effects on lipids, a continuous regimen of 0.625 mg CEE and either 2.5 or 5 mg MPA should produce

TABLE 23–5.

Treatment Regimens

NATURAL ESTROGENS (MG)	PROGESTINS (MG)
Conjugated estrogens (Premarin) 0.625, 1.25	Medroxyprogesterone acetate 5, 10 (Provera)
Estropipate (Ogen) 0.625, 1.25	Norethindrone Norethindrone acetate 2.5, 5, 10
Micronized estradiol (Estrace) 1, 2	Norlutate 1, 5, 10
Estradiol Valerate 1, 2	Norgestrel .5
CYCLIC	
Estrogen days 1–25 + Progestin days 14–25	

endometrial atrophy and a low incidence of bleeding. It is not necessary to have withdrawal bleeding to prevent hyperplasia.

Several recommended treatment regimens for continuous hormone replacement therapy are shown in Table 23–6. Weekday-only progestin-plus-estrogen is used as an alternative to daily treatment. It does lower the total hormone ingested, allows for treatment-free days, and is well received by most patients.

THERAPY FOR WOMEN WITHOUT A UTERUS

The principal beneficial effect of addition of progestin is prevention of endometrial cancer. A similar protective effect of progestins against development of breast cancer has not been clearly demonstrated. Thus, because all synthetic progestins have an adverse affect on lipoproteins and they could increase the risk of heart attack, it is currently recommended that progestins not be given to women who have had a hysterectomy and are receiving estrogen replacement.

MONITORING ESTROGEN REPLACEMENT THERAPY

A complete physical exam with medical history and family history should be performed prior to initiation of therapy. Special attention should be given to blood pressure, breast, abdominal, and pelvic exams, and pap smear. A sampling of endometrium for histology is necessary if there is any prior abnormal bleeding but is unnecessary otherwise prior to treatment. The patient should be fully informed about the risks and benefits of exogenous estrogen therapy, and a written informed consent should be obtained. A baseline mammogram should be performed prior to treatment to avoid giving estrogen to a patient with preexisting subclinical cancer of the breast.

After initiation of therapy, blood pressure should be monitored at three-month and yearly intervals. A pap smear and a breast and pelvic exam should also be repeated at six-month to yearly intervals. After therapy is started, an endometrial biopsy is recommended if any breakthrough bleeding occurs, but it is not necessary if the patient is receiving cyclic estrogen-progestin therapy, and withdrawal bleeding occurs only during the drug-free interval or if no bleeding occurs. Patients on estrogen alone should have endometrial sampling every year by some screening technique. Adequate amounts of calcium for a total of 1.5 gm per day should be ingested in the diet or by supplementation. Women should also be encouraged to continue or start exercise programs daily after the menopause. Walking 2 miles per day is recommended. Repeat mammograms at yearly intervals should be performed on all women in this age group, since the incidence of breast cancer increases with age.

POTENTIAL PROBLEMS AND SOLUTIONS

Estrogen Side Effects.—Nausea, headache, breakthrough bleeding, breast tenderness, and depression may be due to the estrogen component. A drop in the estrogen dose may

TABLE 23–6.

Continuous Treatment Regimen

ES or CEE 0.625 mg + 2.5 or 5 mg MPA[24] daily or weekdays only
CEE 0.625 or 1.25 mg + NET 0.35 to 2.1 mg daily
E_2 2 mg + E_3 1 mg + NET acetate 1 mg daily

be helpful in these patients. If the patient experiences breast tenderness, continuous estrogen progestin therapy should be given.

Progestogen Side Effects.—Some patients may complain of abdominal bloating, headaches, mastalgia, or nervousness. These symptoms are probably related to the dose and duration of the progestin. When these occur, a lower dose of the progestin should be considered, with possible consideration of the low daily continuous protocol of estrogen and progestin.

Withdrawal and Breakthrough Bleeding.—Withdrawal bleeding may be seen in many of the patients using cyclic estrogen and progestin therapy. Data suggest that there is not one single dose of estrogen and progestogen that will control bleeding in all women, but that the ratio of the two hormones needs to be adjusted. Continuous therapy may also be used in an attempt to prevent withdrawal bleeding.

REFERENCES

1. Campbell S, Whitehead MI: Oestrogen therapy and the menopausal syndrome, in Greenblatt RB, Studd JWW (eds): *Clinics in Obstetrics and Gynaecology.* Philadelphia, WB Saunders Co, 1977, pp 31–47.
2. Judd HL, Cleary RE, Creasman WT, et al: Estrogen replacement therapy. *Obstet Gynecol* 1981; 58:267.
3. Erlik Y, Tataryn TV, Meldrum DR, et al: Association of waking episodes with menopausal hot flushes. *JAMA* 1981; 245:1241.
4. Ross RL, Paganini-Hill A, Mack TM, et al: Menopausal estrogen and protection from ischaemic heart disease death. *Lancet* 1981; 1:858.
5. Alffram PA: An epidemiologic study of cervical and trochanteric fractures of the femur in an urban population. *Acta Orthop Scand [Suppl]* 1964; 65:9.
6. Iskrant AP: The etiology of fractured hips in females. *Am J Public Health* 1968; 58:485.
7. Lindsay R, Hart DM, Clark DM: The minimal effective dose of estrogen for prevention of postmenopausal bone loss. *Obstet Gynecol* 1984; 63:759.
8. Henneman PH, Wallach S: A review of the prolonged use of estrogens and androgens in postmenopausal and senile osteoporosis. *Arch Intern Med* 1957; 100:715.
9. Nachtigall LE, Nachtigall RH, Nachtigall RD, et al: Estrogen replacement therapy. 1: A 10-year prospective study in the relationship to osteoporosis. *Obstet Gynecol* 1979; 53:277.
10. Hutchinson TA, Polansky SM, Feinstein AR: Postmenopausal oestrogens protect against fractures of hip and distal radius: A case-control study. *Lancet* 1979; 2:705.
11. Weiss NS, Ure CL, Ballard JH, et al: Decreased risk of fractures of hip and lower forearm with postmenopausal use of estrogen. *N Engl J Med* 1980; 303:1195.
12. Cramer DW, Knapp RC: Review of epidemiologic studies of endometrial cancer and exogenous estrogen. *Obstet Gynecol* 1979; 54:521.
13. Whitehead MI, Townsend PT, Pryse-Davies J, et al: Effects of estrogens and progestins on the biochemistry and morphology of the postmenopausal endometrium. *N Engl J Med* 1981; 305:1599.
14. Mack TM, Pike ML, Henderson BE, et al: Estrogen and endometrial cancer in a retirement community. *N Engl J Med* 1976; 294:1262.
15. McDonald TW, Annegers JF, O'Fallon W, et al: Exogenous estrogens and endometrial carcinoma: Case-control and incidence study. *Am J Obstet Gynecol* 1977; 127:572.
16. Gray LA Sr, Christophenson W, Hoover RN: Estrogens and endometrial carcinoma. *Obstet Gynecol* 1977; 49:385.
17. Studd JWW, Thom MH, Paterson MEL, et al: The prevention and treatment of endometrial pathology in postmenopausal women receiving exogenous estrogens, in Paselto N, Paoletti R, Ambrus JL (eds): *Menopause and Postmenopause.* Lancaster, England, MTP Press Ltd, 1980, pp 127–139.
18. Path FRC, Ryder TA, King RJB: Effects of estrogens and progestins on the biochemistry and morphology of the postmenopausal endometrium. *N Engl J Med* 1985; 305:1599.
19. Thom MH, White PJ, Williams RM, et al: Prevention and treatment of endometrial disease in climacteric women receiving oestrogen therapy. *Lancet* 2:1979; 455.

20. Magos AL, Brincat M, Studd JWW, et al: Amenorrhea and endometrial atrophy with continuous oral estrogen and progestin therapy in postmenopausal women. *Obstet Gynecol* 1985; 65:496.
21. Gambrell RD Jr: Clinical use of progestins in the menopausal patient, dosage and duration. *J Reprod Med* 1982; 27(S):531.
22. Gambrell RD Jr: The menopause: Benefits and risks of estrogen-progestogen replacement therapy. *Fertil Steril* 1982; 37:457.
23. Gibbons WE, Lobo RA, Moyer DV, et al: A comparison of biochemical and morphological events medicated by estrogen + progestin in the endometrium of postmenopausal women, abstract. 30th Annual Medical Society of Gynecological Investigation, Washington DC, March 17–20, 1983, p 167.
24. Gibbons WE, Lobo RA, Moyer DV, et al: A comparison of biochemical and morphological events mediated by estrogen and progestin on the endometrium of postmenopausal women. *Am J Obstet Gynecol* 1986; 154:456.
25. Whitehead MI, Townsend PT, Pryse-Davies J, et al: Effect of various types and dosages of progestogens on the postmenopausal endometrium. *J Reprod Med* 1982; 27(S):539.
26. Paterson M, Wade-Evans T, Struder DW, et al: Endometrial disease after treatment with oestrogens and progestogens in the climacteric. *Br Med J* 1980; 280:822.
27. Whitehead MI, Siddle NC, Townsend PT, et al: The use of progestins and progesterone in the treatment of the climacteric and postmenopausal symptoms, in Bardin CW, Edwin, Milgram, et al (eds): *Progesterone and Progestins*. New York, Raven Press, 1983, p. 287.
28. Hirvonen E, Malkonen M, Manninen V: Effects of different progestogens on lipoproteins during postmenopausal replacement therapy. *N Engl J Med* 1981; 304:560.
29. Paterson M, et al: The effect of various regimens of hormone therapy on serum cholesterol and triglyceride concentrations in postmenopausal women. *Br J Obstet Gynaecol* 1980; 87:552.
30. Blumenfeld Z, Aviram M, Brook G, et al: Changes in lipoproteins and subfraction following oophorectomy and oestrogen replacement in perimenopausal women. *Maturitas* 1983; 5:77.
31. Gustafson A, Svanborg A: Gonadal steroid effects on plasma lipoproteins and individual phospholipids. *J Clin Endocrinol Metab* 1972; 35:103.
32. Silfverstolpe G, Gustafson A, Samsioe G, et al: Lipid metabolic studies in oophorectomized women: Effect on serum lipids and lipoprotein of three synthetic progestogens. *Maturitas* 1982; 4:103.
33. Notelovitz M, Gudat JC, Ware MD, et al: Oestrogen-Progestin therapy and the lipid balance of postmenopausal women. *Maturitas* 1982; 4:301.
34. Ottosson UB, Johansson BG, Von Schoultz B: Subfractions of high-density lipoprotein cholesterol during estrogen replacement therapy: A comparison between progestogens and natural progesterone. *Am J Obstet Gynecol* 1985; 151:746.
35. Fletcher CD, Farish E, Hart DM, et al: Effect on lipoproteins of Trisequens®, a combined hormone preparation. *Maturitas* 1984; 6:279.
36. Mattsson LA, Cullberg G, Sansioe G: A continuous estrogen-progestogen regimen for climacteric complaints. *Acta Obstet Gynecol Scand* 1984; 63:673.
37. Mashchak A, Lobo RA, Donzono-Takano R, et al: Comparison of pharmacodynamic properties of various estrogen formulations. *Am J Obstet Gynecol* 1982; 144:511.
38. Bolton CH, et al: Comparison of the effects of ethinyl estradiol and conjugated equine oestrogens in oophorectomized women. *Clin Endocrinol* 1975; 4:131.
39. Wallentin L, Larson-Cohn U: Metabolic and hormonal effects of postmenopausal oestrogen replacement treatment. *Acta Endocrinol* 1977; 86:597.
40. Gow S, MacGillwray I: Metabolic, hormonal and vascular changes after synthetic oestrogen therapy in oophorectomized women. *Br Med J* 1971; 2:73.
41. Larson-Cohn U, Wallentin L: Metabolic and hormonal effects of postmenopausal oestrogen replacement treatment. *Acta Endocrinol* 1972; 86:583.
42. Lobo RA, Brenner P, Mishell DR: Metabolic parameters and steroid levels in postmenopausal women receiving lower doses of natural estrogen replacement. *Obstet Gynecol* 1983; 62:94.
43. Notelovitz M, Greig HBW: Natural estrogen and antithrombin III activity in postmenopausal women. *J Reprod Medicine* 1976; 16:87.
44. Lucisano A, Acampora MG, Russo N, et al: Ovarian and peripheral plasma levels of progestogens, androgens, and oestrogens in postmenopausal women. *Maturitas* 1984; 6:45.

45. Bolt HM: Metabolism of estrogen—Natural and synthetic. *Pharmacol Ther* 1979; 4:155.

46. Dada OA, Laumas V, Landgred BM, et al: Effect of graded oral doses of oestradiol on circulating hormonal levels. *Acta Endocrinol* 1978; 88:754.

47. Nichols K, Schenkel L, Benson H: 17β estradiol for postmenopausal estrogen replacement therapy. *Obstet Gynecol Surv* 1984; 39:230.

48. Whittaker PG, Morgan MRA, Dean PDG, et al: Serum equilin, oestrone, and oestradiol levels in postmenopausal women receiving conjugated equine oestrogen (Premarin). *Lancet* 1980; 1:14.

49. Rigg LA, Milanes B, Villaneuva B, et al: Efficacy of intravaginal and intranasal administration of micronized estradiol 17β. *J Clin Endocrinol Metab* 1977; 45:1261.

50. Stumpf PG, Maruca J, Santen RJ, et al: Development of a vaginal ring for achieving physiologic levels of 17β estradiol in hypoestrogenic women. *J Clin Endocrinol Metab* 1982; 54:298.

51. Englund DE, Victor A, Johansson EDB: Pharmacokinetic and pharmacodynamic effects of vaginal oestradiol administration from silastic rings in postmenopausal women. *Maturitas* 1981; 3:125.

52. Staland B: Treatment of menopausal oestrogen deficiency symptoms in hysterectomized women by means of 17β-oestradiol pellet. *Acta Obstet Gynecol Scand* 1978; 57:281.

53. Lobo RA, March CM, Goebelsmann U, et al: Subdermal estradiol pellets following hysterectomy and oophorectomy. *Am J Obstet Gynecol* 1980; 138:714.

54. Thom MH, Collins WP, Studd JWW: Hormonal profiles in postmenopausal women after therapy with subcutaneous implants. *Br J Obstet Gynecol* 1981; 88:416.

55. Laufer LR, de Fazio JL, Lu JKH, et al: Estrogen replacement therapy by transdermal estradiol administration. *Am J Obstet Gynecol* 1983; 146:533.

56. Lobo RA, McCormick W, Singer F, et al: Depo-medroxyprogesterone for the treatment of postmenopausal women. *Obstet Gynecol* 1984; 63:1.

57. Lobo RA, Roy S, Shoupe D: Estrogen and progestin effects on urinary calcium and calciotropic hormones in surgically-induced postmenopausal women. *Horm Metabol Res* 1985; 17:370.

58. Mandel FP, Davidson BS, Erlik Y, et al: Effects of progestins on bone metabolism in postmenopausal women. *J Reprod Med* 1982; 47:511.

59. Paterson M: A randomized double-blind cross-over trial into the effect of norethisterone on climacteric symptoms and biochemical profiles. *Br J Obstet Gynecol* 1982; 89:464.

60. Meldrum DR, Erlik Y, Davidson OJ, et al: Effect of megestrol acetate (MA) on flushing and bone metabolism in postmenopausal women, abstract #87. 28th Annual Meeting of the Society of Gynecological Investigation, St Louis, 1981.

61. Albrecht BH, Schrift I, Tulchinsky D, et al: Objective evidence that placebo and oral medroxyprogesterone therapy diminish menopausal vasomotor flushes. *Am J Obstet Gynecol* 1981; 139:631.

62. Morrison JC, Martin DC, Blair RA, et al: The use of medroxyprogesterone acetate for relief of climacteric symptoms. *Am J Obstet Gynecol* 1980; 138:99.

63. Erlik Y, Meldrum DR, Lagasse LD, et al: Effect of megestrol acetate on flushing and bone metabolism in postmenopausal women. *Maturitas* 1981; 3:167.

64. Bullock JL, Massey EM, Gambrell RD: Use of medroxyprogesterone acetate to prevent menopausal symptoms. *Obstet Gynecol* 1985; 46:165.

65. Schiff I, Tulchinsky D, Cramer D, et al: Oral medroxyprogesterone in the treatment of postmenopausal women. *JAMA* 1980; 244:1443.

66. Ylostalo P, Kauppila A, Kivinen S, et al: Endocrine and metabolic effects of low-dose estrogen-progestin treatment in climacteric women. *Obstet Gynecol* 1983; 62:682.

67. Christensen MS, Hagen C, et al: Dose-response evaluation of cyclic estrogen/gestagen in postmenopausal women: Placebo controlled trial of its gynecologic and metabolic actions. *Am J Obstet Gynecol* 1982; 144:873.

68. Cullberg G, Knutsson F, Mattson LA: A new combination of conjugated equine oestrogens and medroxyprogesterone for treatment of climacteric complaints. *Maturitas* 1984; 61:55.

69. Jensen J, Christensen C: Dose-response and withdrawal effects on climacteric symptoms after hormonal replacement therapy: A placebo-controlled therapeutic trial. *Maturitas* 1983; 5:125.

70. Mattsson LA, Culberg G, Samsioe G: Evaluation of a continuous oestrogen—progestogen regimen for climacteric complaints. *Maturitas* 1982; 4:95.

71. Stampfer MJ, Willett WC, Colditz GA, et al: A prospective study of postmenopausal estrogen therapy and coronary heart disease. *N Engl J Med* 1985; 313:1044.
72. DeLignieres B, Basdevant A, Thomas G, et al: Biological effect of estradiol-17β in postmenopausal women: Oral versus percutaneous administration. *J Clin Endocrinol Metab* 1986; 536.

Index

Orgasmic, 133
  capacity after estradiol and testosterone
      implant, 229
  frequency, 226
    after ethinyl estradiol, 227
ORG OD14, 175
Oriabasius, 30
Ortloff of Bavaria, 31
Osteoblasts, 79–80
Osteoclasts, 79–80
Osteopenia, 165
Osteoporosis, 12–14, 188
  (*See also* Bone, loss)
  established, treatment, 180
  fractures in (*see* Fractures, osteoporotic)
  high risk individuals, identification, 87–88
  prevention, 165–186
    calcitonin in, 171, 179
    calcium in, 171, 175–177
    estrogen in, 170–173
    estrogen with progestins in, 171,
      173–175
    exercise in, 171, 179–180
    fluoride in, 171, 178–179
    parathyroid hormone in, 171, 179
    progestin in, 175
    progestin in, with estrogen, 171,
      173–175
    steroids in, anabolic, 171, 175
    thiazides in, 171, 179
    vitamin D in, 171, 178
  risk factors, 173
    established, 12
    possible, 12
  skin in, 105
  treatment
    coherence, 180, 181
    effects on lipids and lipoproteins, 202
Ovaries, 25
  cancer (*see* Cancer, ovarian)
  cyclic behavior, 25
  failure, 25
  function, 24
  involutionary changes in, 26
  tumor frequency, endometrioid and clear-
    cell, 289
Oxandrolone: effects on lipids and
    lipoproteins, 202
Oxazepam: in hot flushes, 148

P

Pancreatitis: estrogen-induced, 240
Parathyroid hormone, 167
  bone turnover and, 80
  in osteoporosis prevention, 171, 179
Parity: and age at menopause, 34

Partner
  marriage, 128
  sex, 130
Passion, 133
Patient-doctor relationship, 232
Pelvic
  relaxation, 72–73
  surgery, 131
Peptides: and bone turnover, 80
Perimenopausal
  complaints, 226
  period, oral contraceptives and breast
    cancer, 268–269
  women, treatment of, 129
Perimenopause: WHO definition, 11
Peripheral temperature (*see* Temperature,
    peripheral)
Personal intimacy: orientation toward, 133
Personality variables: and response to hormone
    therapy, 230–231
pH: vaginal, 67, 68
Pharmacologic agents
  beneficial effects, 139–234
    genitourinary, 151–164
    in hot flushes, 141–150
    on lipids, 187–208
    on lipoproteins, 187–208
    psychologic, 225–234
    sexual, 225–234
  commonly used, 188–189
  in hypertension, effects on lipids and
    lipoproteins, 202–203
  in osteoporosis, effects on lipids and
    lipoproteins, 202
  usage, magnitude and patterns of, 188–189
Pharmacology
  of estrogens, 301–315
  of progestogens, 317–334
  of treatment, 299–351
Phosphorus intake: and bone loss, 85
Photon absorptiometry: dual- and single-beam,
    for bone mass measurement, 12–13,
    87–88, 170
Photoplethysmograph, 104
Physical effects: of progestogens, 330
Physiology: of menopause, 21–138
Pill (*see* Oral contraceptives)
Piperazine estrone sulphate, 226
Pituitary
  adenoma resection, skin resistance,
    peripheral temperature and
    gonadotropin after, 60
  anterior, 25
    response, aging human, 26
  gonadotropins, 25
Pliny the Elder, 30
Polygamous chimpanzee, 23